Healthcare Disparities in Otolaryngology

T0200393

Edited by

Sarah N. Bowe

Department of Otolaryngology—Head and Neck Surgery, San Antonio Uniformed Services Health Education Consortium, JBSA-Fort Sam Houston, TX, United States

Erynne A. Faucett

Department of Otolaryngology—Head and Neck Surgery, University of California-Davis, Sacramento, CA, United States

ELSEVIER

Publisher: Sarah E. Barth
Acquisitions Editor: Jessica L. McCool
Editorial Project Manager: Tracy L. Tufaga
Project Manager: Swapna Srinivasan
Cover Designer: Miles Hitchen

3251 Riverport Lane
St. Louis, Missouri 63043

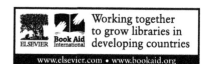

Healthcare Disparities in Otolaryngology

To my wife, Joyce: the backbone of our family. Your unconditional support and patience has given me the drive to continue to pursue my journey in medicine and advocacy.

To my girls, Zola and Jozelyn: born during a time of extreme social unrest and ongoing racial and socioeconomic divide, magnified by a global pandemic—you both continue to inspire me to be better, do better, and learn more.

I love you,

Erynne.

This book is dedicated to my family, whose love and support has been the foundation of my success. To my parents, Don and Lynne, your endless encouragement has made this book possible. To my amazing husband, Bill, and incredible children, Madelyn, Evan, and Charlotte, who have been a constant source of inspiration and strength, I could not have done this without you. With love, Sarah.

Contents

CHAPTER 4   The integration of sex and gender considerations in otolaryngology..41

Sarah N. Bowe and Erynne A. Faucett

Contributors

Patrick Adamcyzk
University of Connecticut School of Medicine, Farmington, CT, United States

Oneida A. Arosarena
Department of Otolaryngology, Lewis Katz School of Medicine at Temple University, Philadelphia, PA, United States; Center for Urban Bioethics, Lewis Katz School of Medicine at Temple University, Philadelphia, PA, United States

Karthik Balakrishnan
Department of Otolaryngology—Head and Neck Surgery, Stanford University School of Medicine, Stanford, CA, United States; Stanford Medicine Children's Health and Lucile Packard Children's Hospital, Palo Alto, CA, United States

Sana Batool
Center for Surgery and Public Health, Brigham and Women's Hospital, Boston, MA, United States; Department of Otolaryngology—Head and Neck Surgery, Harvard Medical School, and Division of Otolaryngology—Head and Neck Surgery, Brigham and Women's Hospital, Dana-Farber Cancer Institute, Boston, MA, United States

Regan W. Bergmark
Center for Surgery and Public Health, Brigham and Women's Hospital, Boston, MA, United States; Department of Otolaryngology—Head and Neck Surgery, Harvard Medical School, and Division of Otolaryngology—Head and Neck Surgery, Brigham and Women's Hospital, Dana-Farber Cancer Institute, Boston, MA, United States

Isaac A. Bernstein
Department of Otolaryngology—Head and Neck Surgery, Stanford University School of Medicine, Stanford, CA, United States

Nikolas Block-Wheeler
Department of Head and Neck Surgery, Kaiser Permanente, East Bay, Oakland, CA, United States

Sarah N. Bowe
Department of Otolaryngology—Head and Neck Surgery, San Antonio Uniformed Services Health Education Consortium, JBSA-Ft. Sam Houston, TX, United States

Matthew L. Bush
Department of Otolaryngology—Head and Neck Surgery, University of Kentucky, Lexington, KY, United States; UK College of Medicine Endowed Chair in Rural Health Policy, Department of Otolaryngology—Head and Neck Surgery, University of Kentucky, Lexington, KY, United States

Scott Randolph Chaiet
Division of Otolaryngology—Head and Neck Surgery, University of Wisconsin
School of Medicine and Public Health, Madison, WI, United States

Michael Collins
University of Connecticut School of Medicine, Farmington, CT, United States

Amanda G. Davis
Department of Otolaryngology—Head and Neck Surgery, University of Kentucky,
Lexington, KY, United States

Sunshine Dwojak-Archambeau
Northwest Permanente Medicine, Portland, OR, United States

Erynne A. Faucett
Department of Otolaryngology—Head and Neck Surgery, University of California-
Davis, Sacramento, CA, United States

Samuel A. Floren
Division of Otolaryngology—Head and Neck Surgery, University of Wisconsin
School of Medicine and Public Health, Madison, WI, United States

Michael Ghiam
Department of Otolaryngology—Head and Neck Surgery, Columbia University
Irving Medical Center, New York-Presbyterian Hospital, New York, NY, United
States

David A. Gudis
Department of Otolaryngology—Head and Neck Surgery, Columbia University
Irving Medical Center, New York-Presbyterian Hospital, New York, NY, United
States

Karen Hawley
Pediatric Otolaryngology, Division of Otolaryngology—Head and Neck Surgery,
Department of Surgery, University of New Mexico, Albuquerque, NM, United
States

Javier J.M. Howard
Department of Otolaryngology—Head and Neck Surgery, School of Medicine,
Stanford University, Stanford, CA, United States

Stacey L. Ishman
Division of Pulmonary and Sleep Medicine, Cincinnati Children's Hospital
Medical Center, Cincinnati, OH, United States; Division of HealthVine, Cincinnati
Children's Hospital Medical Center, Cincinnati, OH, United States; Department of
Otolaryngology—Head and Neck Surgery, College of Medicine, University of
Cincinnati, Cincinnati, OH, United States

Ashok A. Jagasia
Department of Otorhinolaryngology—Head and Neck Surgery, Rush University
Medical Center, Rochester, MN, United States

Ketan Jain-Poster
Department of Head and Neck Surgery, Kaiser Permanente, East Bay, Oakland, CA, United States

Victor O. Jegede
Lewis Katz School of Medicine at Temple University, Philadelphia, PA, United States

Kelly A. Malcolm
Cochlear Center for Hearing & Public Health, Johns Hopkins Bloomberg School of Public Health, Baltimore, MD, United States

Uchechukwu C. Megwalu
Department of Otolaryngology—Head and Neck Surgery, Stanford University School of Medicine, Stanford, CA, United States

Carrie L. Nieman
Cochlear Center for Hearing & Public Health, Johns Hopkins Bloomberg School of Public Health, Baltimore, MD, United States; Department of Otolaryngology—Head and Neck Surgery, Johns Hopkins School of Medicine, Baltimore, MD, United States

Kourosh Parham
Department of Surgery, Division of Otolaryngology, Head and Neck Surgery, University of Connecticut School of Medicine, Farmington, CT, United States

Anaïs Rameau
Sean Parker Institute for Voice, Weill Cornell Medicine, New York, NY, United States

Marissa Schuh
Department of Otolaryngology—Head and Neck Surgery, University of Kentucky, Lexington, KY, United States

Amber Maria Sheth
Department of Surgery, University of Wisconsin School of Medicine and Public Health, Madison, WI, United States

Matthew J. Urban
Department of Otorhinolaryngology—Head and Neck Surgery, Rush University Medical Center, Rochester, MN, United States

Grace M. Wandell
Department of Otolaryngology—Head and Neck Surgery, University of Washington School of Medicine, Seattle, WA, United States

Noriko Yoshikawa
Department of Head and Neck Surgery, Kaiser Permanente, East Bay, Oakland, CA, United States

Acknowledgments

We would like to thank Jess McCool and Elsevier for giving us the opportunity to work on this meaningful and timely project. We are grateful for the guidance and insight of our Editorial Project Manager, Tracy Tufaga, and Senior Project Manager, Swapna Srinivasan, for helping us turn our ideas into a finished product. Finally, we would like to extend our sincere appreciation for all the authors who contributed to this book. Their collective wisdom and insights have made this work much richer and more diverse than we could have ever imagined.

Disclosure

The views expressed herein are those of the author(s) and do not necessarily reflect the official policy or position of the Defense Health Agency, the Brooke Army Medical Center, the Department of Defense, nor any agencies under the U.S. Government.

Introduction to healthcare disparities in otolaryngology

1

Erynne A. Faucett[1], Sarah N. Bowe[2]

[1]*Department of Otolaryngology—Head and Neck Surgery, University of California-Davis, Sacramento, CA, United States;* [2]*Department of Otolaryngology—Head and Neck Surgery, San Antonio Uniformed Services Health Education Consortium, JBSA-Ft. Sam Houston, TX, United States*

Of all the forms of inequality, injustice in healthcare is the most shocking and inhumane.

- Dr. Martin Luther King Jr.

The Medical Committee for Human Rights (MCHR) was organized in New York in the spring of 1964 as a support group for civil rights workers in Mississippi.[1] Overall, more than 100 healthcare professionals, mostly doctors but also nurses, psychologists, and social workers, spent at least a week in Mississippi during what would later be known as "Freedom Summer."[1] The most successful medical volunteers pitched in to help in a variety of ways, as illustrated by Dr. Lee Hoffman in his personal account of his activities in Clarksdale: "Attended a civil rights worker who was beaten over the head .... Played football with local high school boys .... Visited several sick local people, with nurse .... Was arrested for being out after curfew .... Put a lock on a Freedom House .... Attended funeral at request of family of a terminal patient I had seen earlier."[1] After their summer experiences, the participating healthcare professionals made the MCHR a permanent organization with headquarters in New York and chapters in major cities across the country. Over the course of two years in the South, the MCHR made a significant contribution to ending hospital segregation. Members annually picketed the national American Medical Association, which until the late 1960s permitted its affiliate state organizations to deny membership, and subsequently hospital privileges, to Black physicians.[2] The members also operated a free clinic in Mileston, which became the inspiration for MCHR's most enduring and noteworthy contribution to medicine, the comprehensive community health center (CHC).

Dr. Jack Geiger, a young professor at the Harvard School of Public Health, had persuaded a wealthy benefactor to fund the Mileston clinic, but he realized that approach was not sustainable.[1] In December 1964, a memorable meeting took place, where Dr. Geiger began to share his experiences working in apartheid South Africa with Dr. Sidney and Emily Kark. The Karks had developed a healthcare delivery model called community-oriented primary care.[1] Using this model as their

Healthcare Disparities in Otolaryngology. https://doi.org/10.1016/B978-0-443-10714-6.00016-X

1

foundation, the MCHR members created a comprehensive plan, including health services, nutrition programs, preventive medicine, and even environmental interventions. Dr. Geiger took this plan back to Boston and was able to persuade the new federal poverty agency, the Office of Economic Opportunity, to fund two CHCs, the Columbia Point Health Center in Boston, MA and the Delta Health Center in Mound Bayou, MS.[1] As of 2021, there are 1400 CHCs, operating at more than 14,000 locations, and providing care for more than 30 million underserved patients.[3]

It was at the annual MCHR convention in 1966 that Dr. Martin Luther King Jr. voiced the quote noted at the beginning of this chapter.[1] During the 1960s, MCHR activists opposed the Vietnam War, opened free clinics in inner cities, pressured medical schools to enroll more Black students, and supported a woman's right to choose. Having lost most many of its supporters throughout the 1970s to competing groups, the MCHR finally dissolved in 1980, but it had established a long-lasting legacy of CHCs.[4]

In 1971, the National Association of Community Health Centers (NACHC) was founded and has served as the leading national advocacy organization in support of CHCs.[5] In the Spring of 2021, the NACHC board redeveloped its strategic plan, which included six key priorities or pillars. The six pillars start with *equity* and all others relate back to this theme. More explicitly, the first pillar is as follows: "Pillar 1: Center everything we do in a renewed commitment to equity and social justice."[5] Thus, the need to counteract the inequality and injustice that were noted by Dr. Martin Luther King Jr. in 1966 still persists.

Health disparities research has a critical role in advancing equity.[6] Kilbourne and colleagues described three phases of health disparities research: detection, understanding, and reduction/elimination. Most research in otolaryngology-head and neck surgery (OHNS) has focused on detecting disparities, which involves identifying sociodemographic factors, defining health outcomes, and measuring disparities in outcomes among the sociodemographically defined population groups.[6] While detection is an important initial step, it doesn't provide insight into the underlying causes of those disparities, nor does it suggest a path for mitigating disparities and achieving healthy equity.

Over the course of the coronavirus pandemic, studies consistently revealed that COVID-19 disproportionately affected racial and ethnic minority groups.[7] In response to these findings, stakeholders from the OHNS community stated the following, "health care providers perpetuate these disparities when they are unaware of, fail to respond to, or lack the skill to understand the circumstances of at-risk patients."[8] Unfortunately, there are numerous indications that trainees and practicing surgeons are ill-equipped to meet this challenge. In the most recent report from the Accreditation Council for Graduate Medical Education's *Clinical Learning Environment Review*, which included data from June 2017 to February 2020, <5% of participating institutions had a systematic approach to address healthcare disparities among at-risk patients receiving care within their organization.[9] In a survey administered between July 2013 and March 2014 to general surgeon members of the American College of Surgeons, only 38% of respondents reported institutional efforts to address disparities.[10] Thus, there is an evident need to accelerate the incorporation of education focused on healthcare disparities, not only for trainees, who represent the future workforce, but also for those already in practice.

We are motivated to provide you with this series of reflective chapters on crucial topics related to healthcare disparities. Our authors represent a diverse group of leading OHNS experts who have assembled the most up-to-date recommendations for detecting, understanding, and mitigating healthcare disparities in the field. The book begins with specialty-wide perspectives, addressing the impact of healthcare system organization, race and ethnicity, sex and gender, LGBTQ + identity, age, rurality and urbanicity, and health literacy on disparities. The latter part of the book focuses on subspecialty-specific evidence, examining laryngology, rhinology, otology, head and neck oncology, sleep medicine, and facial plastic surgery. We hope that you enjoy this book and that its content spurs you to join us in taking action to move our specialty forward and provide truly equitable patient-centered care.

References

1. Dittmer J. The medical committee for human rights. *AMA J Ethics*. 2014;16(9):745−748. https://doi.org/10.1001/virtualmentor.2014.16.9.mhst1-1409.
2. Baker RB, Washington HA, Olakanmi O, et al. African American physicians and organized medicine, 1846−1968: origins of a racial divide. *JAMA*. 2008;300(3):306. https://doi.org/10.1001/jama.300.3.306.
3. National Association of Community Health Centers. America's Health Centers: 2022 Snapshot. NACHC. Accessed March 25, 2023. https://www.nachc.org/research-and-data/americas-health-centers-2022-snapshot/.
4. Encyclopedia Britanica. Medical Committee for Human Rights. Published November 30, 2015. Accessed March 26, 2023. https://www.britannica.com/topic/Medical-Committee-for-Human-Rights.
5. National Association of Community Health Centers. About NACHC. NACHC. Accessed March 25, 2023. https://www.nachc.org/about/about-nachc/.
6. Megwalu UC, Raol NP, Bergmark R, Osazuwa-Peters N, Brenner MJ. Evidence-based medicine in otolaryngology, part xiii: health disparities research and advancing health equity. *Otolaryngol Neck Surg*. 2022;166(6):1249−1261. https://doi.org/10.1177/01945998221087138.
7. Bowe SN, Megwalu UC, Bergmark RW, Balakrishnan K. Moving beyond detection: charting a path to eliminate health care disparities in otolaryngology. *Otolaryngol Neck Surg*. 2022;166(6):1013−1021. https://doi.org/10.1177/01945998221094460.
8. Prince ADP, Green AR, Brown DJ, et al. The clarion call of the covid-19 pandemic: how medical education can mitigate racial and ethnic disparities. *Acad Med*. 2021;96(11):1518−1523. https://doi.org/10.1097/ACM.0000000000004139.
9. Koh N, Wagner R, Kuhn C, Co J, Weiss K, CLER Program. *CLER National Report of Findings 2021*. Accreditation Council for Graduate Medical Education; 2021. https://doi.org/10.35425/ACGME.0008.
10. Britton BV, Nagarajan N, Zogg CK, et al. US surgeons' perceptions of racial/ethnic disparities in health care: a cross-sectional study. *JAMA Surg*. 2016;151(6):582. https://doi.org/10.1001/jamasurg.2015.4901.

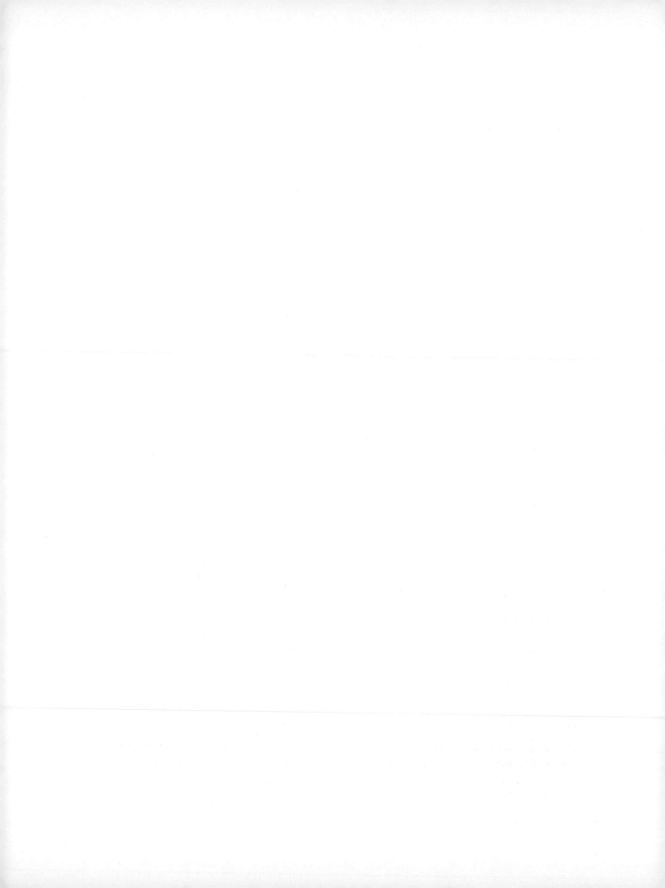

Influence of healthcare system organization on healthcare disparities in otolaryngology

2

Sana Batool[1,2], Regan W. Bergmark[1,2]

[1]*Center for Surgery and Public Health, Brigham and Women's Hospital, Boston, MA, United States;* [2]*Department of Otolaryngology—Head and Neck Surgery, Harvard Medical School, and Division of Otolaryngology—Head and Neck Surgery, Brigham and Women's Hospital, Dana-Farber Cancer Institute, Boston, MA, United States*

Introduction

Numerous studies have demonstrated healthcare disparities across all specialties in medicine in the development of disease, early detection and quality of treatment, and outcomes.[1] Within otolaryngology, non-Hispanic Black males have a higher incidence of more aggressive non-oropharyngeal tumors and distant-stage tumors,[2] and are less likely to receive surgery for oral cavity squamous cell carcinoma compared to non-Hispanic White males.[3] In cancer care, research has shown delayed diagnoses and significantly higher incidence and prevalence of various cancers, with higher morbidity and mortality in patients of minority racial and ethnic background due to poor access to health care.[1] Similar results have been observed for cardiovascular diseases, with racial inequities in treatment following coronary revascularization that have led to higher mortality rates in African American patients.[4] The structure of our healthcare system contributes to these inequities. This chapter focuses on the existing healthcare disparities in otolaryngology, highlights the influence of the United States (US) healthcare system's structure on these disparities, and briefly discusses broad strategies to address the key determinants of these inequities in otolaryngology.

Healthcare system and healthcare disparities

Healthcare disparities are the consequences of many different factors such as social and racial inequities, which make it challenging to isolate a single source of healthcare disparities. One of the major factors is the healthcare system itself which is the focus of this chapter. It is important to note that although the US healthcare system is often entirely blamed for its poor population health such as lower life expectancy

Healthcare Disparities in Otolaryngology. https://doi.org/10.1016/B978-0-443-10714-6.00010-9

compared to other developed countries like Japan, Australia, and Canada,[5] there are many other factors such as personal behaviors and public health that affect an individual's health, which are outside the scope of this chapter.

Definition of health disparity versus healthcare disparity

Health disparity and healthcare disparity are closely related terms but differ in definitions. The National Institutes of Health (NIH) defines "health disparities" as "differences in the incidence, prevalence, mortality, and burden of diseases and other adverse health conditions that exist among specific population groups in the United States."[6] The Institute of Medicine defines "healthcare disparities" as "differences in treatment provided to members of different groups that are not justified by the underlying health conditions or treatment preferences of patients."[1] Within otolaryngology, an example of health disparity is that Black patients have 10% greater risk of mortality within 90 days after treatment of head and neck squamous cell carcinoma compared with White patients,[7] while an example of healthcare disparity is that Black patients are 13% less likely to undergo surgery for oral cavity squamous cell carcinoma compared with White patients.[3] For the purposes of this chapter, we will focus on healthcare disparities as they relate to the structure and organization of the US healthcare system that limits access to high-quality care to certain populations and presents a great challenge to our society (Fig. 2.1).

US healthcare system

The US has the world's most expensive healthcare system,[8] yet it fails to deliver high-quality care to all. It is the structure and organization of this system that has led to unequal access to medical services resulting in healthcare disparities. The US does not have a single nationwide system of health insurance like many countries. Health services are provided by private and public hospitals as well as solo and group practices paid for by a complex mixture of private insurances, individual payments, and public payers that include the federal, state, and local governments. Health insurance in the US, discussed in detail below, is provided by employers for most people and their dependents under 65 years old.

Government programs such as Medicare are for people 65 years old or older or with extremely specific health conditions (e.g., renal failure), while Medicaid is a primarily state-run program for individuals in or near poverty. In 2020, employment-based insurance covered 54.4% of the US population, while 18.4% was covered by Medicare and 17.8% was covered by Medicaid.[9] This leads to some people having multiple health insurances, while others are left completely uninsured.

American physicians have the choice to practice at a private or public practice or hospital anywhere in the country. Physicians are, therefore, often concentrated in urban and suburban areas, while remote rural areas are left with insufficient providers and resource-poor hospitals and practices, resulting in unequal access to care. The US healthcare system is often touted for its state-of-the-art medical technology,

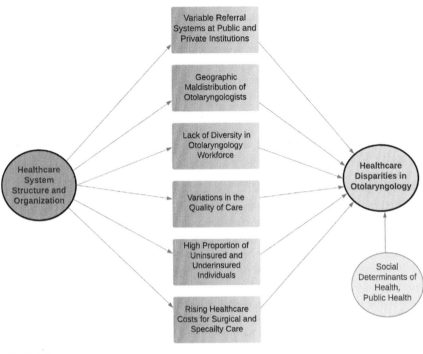

Healthcare System and Disparities in Otolaryngology

FIGURE 2.1

Influence of healthcare system on healthcare disparities in otolaryngology.

highly skilled providers, consumer flexibility to choose their providers, and rigorous biomedical research to advance the medical science. However, it has significant issues such as lack of universal healthcare coverage, geographic maldistribution of hospitals, clinics and providers, and differences in the quality and access to care, all of which have led to healthcare disparities in the US.[10]

Other healthcare systems

There are many different healthcare systems around the world that differ in structure and organization. Unlike the US that spent 16.8% of its GDP on health care in 2019, Canada and the United Kingdom spent only 10.8% and 10.2%, respectively,[8] and have a single payer system that provides universal healthcare coverage for its citizens paid by the government. Germany spent 11.7% of its GDP on healthcare and has a mixed public-private insurance system where citizens are free to choose between public insurance or pay a higher premium for private insurance. Switzerland has a mandatory public health insurance system funded from general tax revenues; however, it has high levels of cost-sharing. France has a universal public insurance system and spent 11.1% of its GDP on health care in 2019.[8] France has low out-of-pocket expenses compared to other European countries as the public insurance covers 70%−80% of costs.[11]

In contrast, Singapore uses a unique system that involves public insurance and mandatory national health savings account, both of which pay for healthcare services. Australia has a universal public health insurance that is funded by citizens' taxes. Many South American countries like Argentina, Brazil, and Colombia also have universal and publicly funded health insurance[10]; however, there is a lack of medical resources in small villages and isolated cities. The US is one of the few developed countries that does not offer a universal publicly funded health insurance to its citizens, which restricts access to care for certain populations.

Healthcare and public health

The integration of health care and public health is crucial in understanding and reducing health and healthcare disparities on a national and global level. While health care refers to addressing illnesses and diseases in individuals, public health encompasses the health of an entire community that includes issues like access to safe drinking water, immunization programs, gun violence, motor vehicle accidents, smoking cessation programs, and housing. It is important to assess public health to develop and implement public policies that promote healthy behaviors and change social, economic, and environmental conditions to improve the health of all people. There is a disconnect between the healthcare system and public health in the US that has hindered the effectiveness of efforts in addressing healthcare disparities.[12] Public health interventions and broader public policy may have a large impact on life expectancy and risk of illnesses but are beyond the scope of this chapter.

Goals of a healthcare system

Healthcare systems around the world have contributed to better health outcomes and increased life expectancy with varying degrees of success,[13] which highlights the importance of the structure of a healthcare system. An ideal health system aims at providing the best possible health outcomes with equal access to affordable, high-quality care to every individual regardless of their age, gender, race, ethnicity, healthcare availability, level of education, socioeconomic status (SES), or geographic distance.[14] Many frameworks and metrics have been developed to assess the quality of a healthcare system, but none has been used consistently on a national or global level.[15,16]

Metrics to measure access to quality surgical care

The Lancet Commission on Global Surgery (LCoGS) released a report in 2015 that highlighted the healthcare disparities in surgical care in low-income and

Table 2.1 Metrics for measuring access to high-quality surgical care proposed by the Lancet Commission on Global Surgery (LCoGS)[17] and their proposed goals by 2030.

Metric	Definition per LCoGS	Proposed goals by 2030 per LCoGS
Access to timely care	"Proportion of population that can access a medical facility with surgical care services within 2 hours"	"Minimum of 80% coverage of essential surgical services per country"
Workforce density	"Number of surgical, anesthetic, and obstetric physicians per 100,000 population"	"100% of countries with at least 20 surgical, anesthetic, and obstetric physicians per 100,000 population"
Case volume	"Number of surgical procedures done per 100,000 population annually"	"100% of countries tracking surgical volume with a minimum 5000 procedures per 100,000 population"
Perioperative mortality	"Percentage of all-cause death before discharge for patients undergoing surgical procedure"	"100% of countries tracking perioperative mortality"
Protection against expenditure	"Proportion of households protected against impoverishing and catastrophic expenditure from direct out-of-pocket payments for surgical care"	"100% protection against impoverishment and catastrophic expenditure from out-of-pocket payments for surgical and anesthesia care"

middle-income countries (LMICs) and proposed a set of core indicators to assess access to affordable, quality surgical care.[17] These core indicators as well as proposed goals for surgical care are summarized in Table 2.1 and include timely access to surgical care, capacity and quality of surgical care, mortality rates, and affordability. These metrics are proposed to be used on a global level to assess access to high-quality surgical care in LMICs but have been applied to high-income countries as well.[18] The concept can be applied on a national level to gauge access to otolaryngologic care for patients.[19]

Disparities and access to care in otolaryngology

Like other fields of medicine, otolaryngology has been noted to have differences in survival, disease recurrence, and overall mortality based on various factors such as race, ethnicity, SES, and insurance status, particularly among head and neck cancer (HNC) patients. A study of 16,771 cancer patients showed that patients with HNC were more likely to be poor, unemployed, publicly insured, less educated, and from a minority race and ethnicity compared to other cancers.[20] HNC patients from minority racial and ethnic groups also tend to present at a later stage compared to nonminority groups, suggesting lack of access to care for patients from minority racial and ethnic groups.[21] Studies have shown that when SES factors such as income, education, insurance, etc., and behavioral factors such as smoking are controlled, no racial and ethnic disparities exist among HNC patients.[21,22] In this section, we discuss the healthcare disparities in otolaryngology that exist due to the structure and organization of the US healthcare system.

Disparities throughout the continuum of care: voltage drop model

Inadequate access to high quality care contributes to disparities in health outcomes. The term "access" has been defined by various organizations and committees. The Institute of Medicine committee defines access as "the timely use of personal health services to achieve the best possible health outcomes."[23] The Institute of Healthcare Improvement defines access as the right patient having the right initial access point, undergoing the right workup and treatment with the right care team in the right setting at the right time.[24] Both definitions cover the entire continuum of care that begins with the initial presentation of a patient with a medical problem and ends with their posttreatment care. This has been described as a conceptual framework using the "voltage drop" model first used by Eisenberg and Power to describe the many steps between potential access to insurance in the US and access to high quality care.[25]

The "voltage drop" framework has been applied to surgical care,[26] which describes that access to care begins with an initial contact with the healthcare system that could be a primary care physician (PCP), emergency department (ED) physician, or a specialist who may recognize the patient's medical problem. The patient's social network, such as a family member or friend, may also encourage the patient to seek care or recommend a particular provider for care. Geographic proximity, insurance status, out-of-pocket costs, and frequent doctor visits may all affect when and where patients present for care. For surgical care, there are then multiple steps to connect with a surgeon, undergo a workup, and potentially undergo surgical intervention and recovery. Presenting at the right time, being connected to the right surgeon at the right place and the right time, undergoing the right procedure and having the right follow up all contribute to the patient's outcome. This framework can also be applied to otolaryngologic care to understand factors known as "resistance points" that affect a patient's continuum of care and influence disparities in access to otolaryngologic care as shown in Fig. 2.2. Some of these factors include access to referring providers, referral patterns, otolaryngology workforce characteristics, geographic location of hospitals and medical practices, insurance coverage, and social determinants of health (SDH) discussed separately in this chapter.

Referral pathways

Surgical care begins with the recognition of the surgical problem either by the patient, community health workers, PCP, ED physician, or family or friends in the

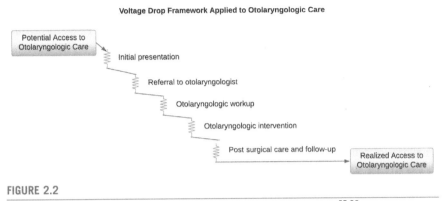

FIGURE 2.2

Conceptual "voltage drop" framework applied to otolaryngologic care.[25,26]

community. Once the problem is identified, the patient is referred to a surgeon for further care. This process of care for a patient occurs in a complex health system in the US. Primary care, urgent care centers, ambulatory surgery centers, and smaller hospitals may provide easier access to care due to their proximity to patients' homes. However, patients needing more complicated surgical care need referral to larger hospitals that might not be close to patients' homes, especially in remote rural areas. This complex health system environment results in a complex referral system that varies from state to state due to different kinds of connections between institutions. As a result of these variations, patients may get lost in the referral process or even experience discontinuity of care without an appropriate follow-up,[27] which may affect certain groups more than others. Patients from historically vulnerable and oppressed groups are more likely to experience delays in care and lower quality care as they travel through their care network.[26]

Otolaryngology is the third most common specialty for referrals by PCPs.[28] Emergency rooms also see many patients with otolaryngologic complaints. In 2011, otolaryngologic conditions such as otitis media, eustachian tube disorders, and vertigo accounted for more than two million ED visits,[29,30] most of which were referred to an otolaryngology clinic for further management. Therefore, the referral system plays a significant role in healthcare disparities in otolaryngology, as delays in referrals lead to delayed care in HNC patients[31] and increased psychosocial and financial burden of disease,[32] which not only exacerbate these disparities but also add to the healthcare costs. A 2015 study showed that delayed referral to otolaryngology for voice complaints led to increased healthcare costs.[33] Another study, in 2020, demonstrated differences in otolaryngology referral mechanisms at a private versus public hospital, both affiliated with the University of Southern California.[34] This study showed that although the time between otolaryngology referrals and first clinic visits was shorter at the public hospital, the referred patients from the tertiary care center received surgical care sooner after their first clinic visit than patients from public hospital. This may be due to differences in the operating room capacity between the two hospitals, better communication between referring providers and specialists at the tertiary care center, or appropriate prior workup of the patients at the tertiary care center that make them eligible for prompt surgical care compared to those at public hospitals who might need further workup by otolaryngologists.

As mentioned above, the first metric "timely access to care" proposed by the LCoGS was defined as "the proportion of population that lived within two hours of a surgical facility for caesarean delivery, laparotomy, and treatment of open fracture."[17] Besides the geographic proximity, this metric is also dependent on the timeliness of referrals to surgeons. PCPs in metropolitan areas or those with ready access to medical resources and tertiary care centers tend to refer their patients for specialty care more frequently.[35] Patients without timely referral to specialists may suffer delayed diagnoses and worse health outcomes. There is a paucity of studies on the referral pathways to otolaryngologists, and more research is needed. Timely referrals may affect access to care; improvements in this system may help remediate existing healthcare disparities.

Otolaryngology workforce characteristics

To improve access to otolaryngologic care in the US, assessment of the existing otolaryngology workforce is crucial. This requires a thorough understanding of the effect of changes in this workforce on access to otolaryngologic care. The geographic distribution, diversity, and subspecialization of this workforce influences access to affordable, high-value otolaryngologic care.

Geographic distribution of otolaryngology workforce

Geography often affects access to care. Despite a higher number of specialized physicians in the US compared to other countries, there is still a disparity in access to specialty care due to the concentration of specialty clinics in urban areas.[36] Two studies found that the percentage of otolaryngologists in urban counties exceeded the percentage of the US population living in urban counties.[37,38] Individuals living in remote, resource-poor areas have to travel farther to get specialty care, which is why rural population finds it difficult to obtain primary and specialty care.[39,40]

Several studies have noted the uneven distribution of otolaryngologists in the US. Otolaryngologists are concentrated in more urban areas. One study found that two thirds of US counties did not have a practicing otolaryngologist.[41] Another study showed that rural counties had fewer otolaryngologists per population, while the high-income urban areas had a higher density of otolaryngologists.[42] In 2016, the US Department of Health and Human Services predicted a deficit of 1620 otolaryngologists by 2025.[43] This shortage will disproportionately affect rural counties. Increasing the number of residency positions has not resulted in improvement in the geographic distribution of residency training sites,[44] leaving the rural areas vulnerable. This disparity in the geographic distribution of otolaryngology residents exists in certain metropolitan areas as well. The average number of otolaryngology residents per 100,000 people across all metropolitan areas in the US is 2.70, but the Phoenix−Mesa−Chandler area in Arizona has the lowest number of residents per 100,0000 people at 0.2.[45] Therefore, we need to develop strategies to streamline referral pathways in rural counties and coordinate and expedite referrals to otolaryngology. Another strategy would be to train PCPs with basic otolaryngology training as well as to develop outreach programs. Although rural outreach systems via visiting consultant clinics were successful in increasing the proportion of rural population within 30-minute drive of an otolaryngologist by 33% in Iowa, the additional travel costs make these clinics unsustainable.[46] The use of a hub-and-spoke model has been successful in enhancing medical care with improved referral services for specialty care in rural communities.[47] This model proposes the development of a main hub or hospital that receives resources for the most intensive medical and surgical services and is complemented by satellite spokes or clinics that offer limited but accessible care to communities.

Diversity of otolaryngology workforce
Several studies have demonstrated the positive effect of a diverse healthcare workforce on the quality of care to patients.[1,48] Racial and ethnic concordance between providers and patients lead to improved communication,[48] increased patient satisfaction,[48] and greater healthcare utilization that minimize delays in care.[49] Physicians from minority racial and ethnic groups are more likely to provide care to patients in medically underserved areas as well as serve low-income, Medicaid, and uninsured patients.[50,51] Therefore, in order to increase access to care and reduce healthcare disparities, it is critical for the otolaryngology workforce to mirror the diversity of the society it serves.[52]

The otolaryngology workforce does not currently reflect the diversity of the US population with respect to race, ethnicity, or gender. In 2016, otolaryngology had the lowest representation of residents and faculty who self-identified as African American compared to all other surgical specialties. People who identify as African American comprise 12.6% of the US population but make up only 2.1% of otolaryngology residents and 2.4% of otolaryngology faculty.[53] Similarly, people of Hispanic ethnicity are underrepresented at all levels in otolaryngology compared to the general US population, with only 5.5% of otolaryngology residents self-identifying as Hispanic versus 17% of the US population.[53] The annual growth rate for individuals identifying as African American and Native American among otolaryngology residents is not statistically significant. Similarly, the growth rate of people of Hispanic ethnicity in the field of otolaryngology is below the growth rate of the US population.[41] The University of Michigan described the small number of Black and Latinx surgeons in otolaryngology by a "leaky pipeline" that helps visualize opportunities to improve diversity at each level.[54]

Women are also still a minority in the field of otolaryngology, accounting for only 17.1% of practicing otolaryngologists in the US in 2020.[41] Although the number of women in otolaryngology residency positions is increasing steadily, with 36.3% positions occupied by women in 2020 compared to 8.1% in 2000, otolaryngology still lags behind other surgical specialties when it comes to diversifying the workforce.[41] It is pertinent to implement strategies nationwide to create a diverse otolaryngologic workforce for the US population that would contribute to the reduction of healthcare disparities.[52,55]

Subspecialization of otolaryngology workforce

Subspecialization also affects the otolaryngology workforce in several ways and may influence access to care. Fellowship-trained otolaryngologists may provide highly subspecialized care but may be more limited in the range of services they choose to provide. The otolaryngology subspecialty may determine their practice location and scope, which may affect the distribution of the workforce and subsequently limit access to otolaryngologic care for certain populations. For instance, 98% of US fellowship-trained head and neck surgeons practice in urban locations and over 70% of them practice at academic institutions.[41] Similarly, 54% of pediatric otolaryngologists practice at academic institutions.[56] The number of fellowship positions has been increasing, with the most drastic increase in rhinology fellowships recently from three positions in 1996 to 29 positions in 2017.[41] This increase in subspecialization in otolaryngology affects access to otolaryngologic care for certain populations, particularly in rural areas with a lower number of local otolaryngologists providing the full spectrum of care to these populations.[57]

Quality of care

Variation in the quality of care is an important mechanism for healthcare disparities based on race and ethnicity, SES, and insurance status. Quality of care is often measured by volume of surgical cases, accreditation of hospitals, and quality metrics scores for medical and surgical conditions.[27] Uninsured patients are at a higher risk of receiving substandard medical care than insured patients.[58] Similarly, racial and ethnic minorities are more likely to receive care at low-quality hospitals than their White counterparts.[27] Although African American patients tend to live closer to high-quality hospitals than White patients, they are less likely to have their surgeries there.[59]

A cross-sectional study found that Medicaid and self-pay insurance status were strongly associated with ED presentation for acute rhinosinusitis among adult and pediatric patient population.[60] In a 2020 study, Ruthberg et al. found that African American patients are 1.5 times more likely to visit the ED for otolaryngologic conditions than White patients.[61] Otolaryngologic care received at the ED may not be as high-quality as at an otolaryngologist's clinic because ED visits have longer wait times without robust patient follow-up and ED providers may not be as thorough in evaluating patients due to patient acuity and time pressures. Furthermore, ED visits often indicate a lack of access to PCPs and specialty clinics. Kangovi et al. proposed that African American or Hispanic patients may prefer hospitals over outpatient care due to easier access and affordability,[62] but this may result in low-quality care received by racial and ethnic minority groups.

The quality of care significantly affects patient outcomes in otolaryngology. Treatment of thyroid cancer at high-quality hospitals is associated with improved survival, where quality was defined by thyroid case volumes, accreditation status, and adherence to American Thyroid Association guidelines.[63] Another study showed that oral cancer patients have improved survival when they receive treatment at high-quality hospitals. However, individuals who identify as Black and Hispanic with oral cancer are less likely to be treated at high-quality hospitals.[64] Therefore, the quality of otolaryngologic care is another compounding factor that influences healthcare disparities.

Insurance status and healthcare cost

The US healthcare system is the world's most expensive healthcare system,[8] yet it lacks universal health insurance or a centralized healthcare organization that makes it challenging to provide equitable access to high-quality, affordable care. The US healthcare system has undergone multiple health reforms over the past few decades to try to address access, cost, and quality of care. The most recent major reform is the Affordable Care Act (ACA) implemented in March 2010, which aimed at increasing access by expanding health insurance coverage, improving quality of care, and reducing costs through bundled payments.[65] Access to care and cost of care are both interconnected and significantly affect healthcare disparities. Unequal access to care due to lack of insurance coverage not only leads to rising costs to the patients but also burdens the healthcare system financially which further worsens healthcare disparities.

Affordable Care Act in the US
The implementation of the ACA expanded Medicaid and decreased the number of uninsured Americans from 50 million to 27 million. This increased cancer screenings among the American population, which improved the timing of patient presentation with acute surgical diseases.[66] It decreased the spending for hospitals and physician group practices by $278.5 million and $255 million, respectively, through bundled payment programs. While the ACA has its own shortcomings, it has significantly improved access to care and reduced healthcare disparities in the US.

Cost to the patients
Impact of no insurance or underinsurance on access to care: Although the ACA decreased the number of uninsured Americans by 20 million, there are still many Americans who remain uninsured and unable to afford medical care.[67] In 2019, 28.9 million nonelderly individuals were uninsured in the US. Among these uninsured individuals, 82.6% belonged to families with incomes below 400% of the federal poverty level (FPL). Individuals who identified as Hispanic, Black, American Indian/Alaska Native, and Native Hawaiians and Other Pacific Islander all had higher uninsured rates than White people.[67] High healthcare costs and lack of insurance coverage most significantly impact low-income individuals from minority

racial and ethnic groups who delay seeking medical care or completely forego their care. For instance, uninsured and Medicaid patients were more likely to present with unresectable oropharyngeal cancer and have worse disease-specific survival than patients with other insurance types.[68] The association between Black race and unresectable disease is eliminated after adjusting for insurance status,[68] highlighting that insurance status is one of the drivers of racial and ethnic healthcare disparities. After Medicaid expansion through the ACA, there was a decrease in the number of uninsured people and an increase in early stage HNC patients from low-SES counties,[69] showing that expanded insurance coverage aids in earlier presentation of HNC.

Financial burden of healthcare services on patients: Lack of health insurance coverage does not only lead to delayed care and consequently poor health for the uninsured and underinsured, but it also creates financial burden, putting patients at risk of impoverishment due to high out-of-pocket costs. Out-of-pocket costs include deductibles, coinsurance, and copayments for insurance-covered services as well as the cost of services that are not covered.[70] When uninsured individuals seek medical care, they incur higher out-of-pocket costs. For instance, uninsured diabetes patients have an annual out-of-pocket expense of $1446 on average.[71] The insured individuals are also affected by high costs of healthcare services. Hospitals request higher reimbursements for insured patients to compensate for the care of uninsured patients, referred to as cost-sharing, which results in higher deductibles and co-payments leading to higher out-of-pocket payments. One study found that at the 90th percentile of out-of-pocket spending, individuals with high-deductible and low-deductible plans spent $1072 and $338 more compared to no-deductible plans, respectively,[72] which highlights cost-related access barriers even for the insured patients.

This financial burden is particularly relevant to HNC. One study found that compared to other cancers, HNC patients are more often of a minority race and poorer, lacking private insurance with total median medical expenses greater by $2171 compared to non-HNC patients.[20] Insurance coverage does not necessarily protect against out-of-pocket costs, particularly for HNC patients who are low-income with out-of-pocket expenses constituting a larger percentage of income for these patients compared to non-HNC patients.[20] This study also noted that medical expenses are particularly high within the first year of HNC diagnosis, most likely due to the costly treatments, and need for long-term health services such as tracheostomy care, dental care, speech therapy, etc. Studies have also looked at the catastrophic expenditure incurred as a result of accessing care which is defined as an expenditure over 40% of nonfood household expenditure and includes nonmedical costs such as transportation and lodging that may not be accounted for in out-of-pocket costs.[73] Approximately 150 million individuals face catastrophic expenditure while accessing healthcare services globally, 22% of whom are accessing surgical care.[73] These catastrophic expenditures further add to the financial burden of HNC patients.

Cost to the healthcare system

The high cost of health care in the US affects all stakeholders, including patients, providers, payers, and the rest of the healthcare system. One study found that the most common pediatric surgical diagnoses had an increase of 37% in the average hospital charges, but the average cost of those diagnoses increased only by 11% from 2006 to 2012.[74] The total hospital charges for surgical diagnoses increased more than twofold between 2000 and 2012.[75] Consequently, private insurances reduce premium costs by increasing deductibles and co-payments as well as restricting patients' choice of providers and hospitals, which may exclude bigger academic and cancer referral centers.[76] The low-income or middle-class Americans who are unable to afford higher co-payments may delay or forego medical care, which ultimately results in downstream health problems and higher medical costs.[66] When Medicare added new co-payments for patients, outpatient visits decreased but hospital admissions increased, raising the total healthcare costs.[77] Wealthy Americans also may turn to "concierge" medicine services, which offer longer visits with providers and access to a wide range of specialists, and may be associated with increased use of diagnostic studies, driving the cost of health care even higher.[78]

Mergers and acquisitions

One of the consequences of rising healthcare costs is hospital mergers and acquisitions that has been changing the healthcare landscape across the US. This occurs when a larger hospital absorbs local smaller hospitals and physician practices and merge them into a bigger unified system to control costs and manage care for most of a region's population. A positive impact of this is the elimination of financial burden on smaller hospitals and practices, but it gives monopolistic pricing power to larger hospital systems. An example is the Mass General Brigham System that has merged the Brigham and Women's Hospital and Massachusetts General Hospital along with many other smaller hospitals in Massachusetts into one system. Rural hospitals have been a common acquisition for bigger hospitals, which could be beneficial as this results in improved access to expanded medical services and advanced technologies to rural populations.[79] Proponents of hospital mergers and acquisitions claim that this leads to greater efficiency of care with reduced costs and better patient outcomes. However, one study looked at 246 hospitals that merged or were acquired between 2009 and 2013 and reported that these mergers and acquisitions did not improve quality of care or reduce costs.[80]

Social determinants of health

Healthcare disparities in the incidence, progression, and outcome of diseases based on SES have been studied and documented for many years, which have resulted in the coining of term "Social determinants of health (SDH)" that refer to the race, ethnicity, gender, education level, household income, etc., of an individual. Poverty predisposes individuals to poorer emotional and physical health due to poorer health habits and lower access to medical care.[81] Individuals from racial and ethnic minority groups tend to receive lower quality of care than nonminority individuals even when controlled for other SES factors such as income level and insurance status.[1] SDH play a major role in timely access to high-quality care and has been discussed in more detail in Chapter 3 "The Contribution of Racial and Ethnic Biases to Disparate Health Outcomes in Otolaryngology."

Effects of COVID-19 pandemic on healthcare disparities

When the COVID-19 pandemic hit the US in early 2020, it highlighted numerous long-standing healthcare disparities among racial and ethnic minority groups. New York City saw the most striking differences in infection rates as well as morbidity and mortality due to COVID-19 between racial and ethnic minority and nonminority communities. Deaths from COVID-19 infection occurred at rates of 19.8 and 22.8 per 100,000 people for individuals who identify as Black and Hispanic, respectively, compared to 10.2 for those who identify as White.[82] Similarly in Louisiana, 39.7% of COVID-19 patients needed hospitalization of whom 76.9% were Black patients.[83] Magesh et al. reported that decreased access to care was positively correlated with COVID-19 infections among Hispanic and African American populations,[84] which also translated to higher rates of deaths for these racial and ethnic groups.

The COVID-19 pandemic affected many medical specialties, but the surgical specialties including otolaryngology were particularly influenced. Most elective and semielective surgeries as well as outpatient practices were stopped in the early months of pandemic. Otolaryngology was one of the specialties with the highest reduction in surgical volume and outpatient visits in the US.[85] For instance, Massachusetts noted a 63% decrease in otolaryngology office visits and a greater decrease in OR procedures compared to in-office procedures.[86] Another study showed that there was an increase in the number of advanced orbital emergencies due to underlying otolaryngologic diseases such as acute sinusitis during the pandemic.[87] A recent report by Harvard School of Public Health noted that one in four rural households had a member who could not access medical care during the pandemic,[88] demonstrating that the pandemic further limited access to care for rural America. This decline in otolaryngologic care likely delayed the diagnoses of many otolaryngologic conditions including HNCs, particularly for those who already had decreased access to care and were at risk of delayed presentation of their pathology.[82] This includes uninsured or underinsured individuals with low SES, those from racial and ethnic minority groups, those living in rural remote areas as well as those with limited English proficiency and limited access to internet and electronic devices needed for telemedicine appointments. However, there is currently little data on the effects of COVID-19 pandemic on these individuals in otolaryngology.

Interventions to reduce healthcare disparities in otolaryngology

The National Academy of Medicine issued the report "Unequal Treatment: Confronting Racial and Ethnic Disparities in Healthcare" in 2002, bringing national attention to this issue. This was followed by numerous studies that highlighted healthcare disparities within otolaryngology and served as a call to action for otolaryngologists to mitigate these disparities. However, the Accreditation Council for Graduate Medical Education reported that less than 5% of participating institutions had a systematic approach to address healthcare disparities within their organizations between 2017 and 2020.[89] It is time that we move beyond the "detection phase" and identify solutions as well as implement strategies to reduce and eventually eliminate healthcare disparities.[27] Table 2.2 highlights a few systemic and individual level strategies to address healthcare disparities in otolaryngology.

Table 2.2 Interventions to mitigate healthcare disparities in otolaryngology.

Components of otolaryngologic care	Recommended interventions	Examples
Referral pathways	Improve the referral system	Streamline the referral system by developing referral guidelines to be used on a national level so that hospitals serving minority patients have an adequate referral procedure in place to coordinate and expedite proper otolaryngologic care to patients on a timely basis.
Otolaryngology workforce	Increase availability of otolaryngologic care services	Expand otolaryngologic care to remote rural areas, so those communities are not solely dependent on outreach clinics that may delay their care. This could be accomplished by adapting the hub-and-spoke model of care.
	Diversify the otolaryngology workforce	Increase exposure of underrepresented in medicine (UIM) students to otolaryngology during medical school and expand institutional efforts in residency recruitment.
	Increase awareness among otolaryngologists	Encourage open discussions about literature on health disparities among otolaryngologists, so each provider could make efforts on an individual level to address implicit bias and mitigate these disparities.

Continued

Table 2.2 Interventions to mitigate healthcare disparities in otolaryngology.—*cont'd*

Components of otolaryngologic care	Recommended interventions	Examples
Quality of otolaryngologic care	Better support for low-quality hospitals	Invest in developmental support programs for low-quality hospitals to improve access to high-quality care for minority communities.
		Provide greater financial support through medicaid and other programs to minority-serving and safety-net hospitals.
	Improve system-wide communication	Promote communication across the entire care delivery process from community to tertiary care centers, for example, via system-wide connectivity.
Costs of otolaryngologic care	Reduce cost to patients	Expand medicaid and other government health insurance programs to improve insurance coverage of specialty services and decrease co-payments.
	Reduce cost to the system	Decrease administrative costs; increase transparency of hospital charges to insurance companies and patients; and increase access to primary and preventive care.
Research and education	Evaluate otolaryngologic clinical outcomes for diverse patients	Develop robust institutional monitoring systems to increase transparency and accountability related to healthcare disparities in otolaryngology.
	Make patient education a priority	Implement culturally appropriate patient education programs to increase their knowledge of when and how to best access care for otolaryngologic diseases as well as participate actively in their treatment plans.

References

1. Smedley BD, Stith AY, Nelson AR, eds. *Unequal Treatment: Confronting Racial and Ethnic Disparities in Health Care*. National Academies Press (US); 2003. https://doi.org/10.17226/12875.
2. Peterson CE, Khosla S, Chen LF, et al. Racial differences in head and neck squamous cell carcinomas among non-Hispanic black and white males identified through the National

Cancer Database (1998−2012). *J Cancer Res Clin Oncol*. 2016;142(8):1715−1726. https://doi.org/10.1007/s00432-016-2182-8.

3. Lewis CM, Ajmani GS, Kyrillos A, et al. Racial disparities in the choice of definitive treatment for squamous cell carcinoma of the oral cavity. *Head Neck*. 2018;40(11): 2372−2382. https://doi.org/10.1002/hed.25341.

4. Peterson ED, Shaw LK, DeLong ER, Pryor DB, Califf RM, Mark DB. Racial variation in the use of coronary-revascularization procedures. Are the differences real? Do they matter? *N Engl J Med*. 1997;336(7):480−486. https://doi.org/10.1056/NEJM199702133360706.

5. Preston SH, Ho J. *Low Life Expectancy in the United States: Is the Health Care System at Fault?* National Academies Press (US); 2010. https://www.ncbi.nlm.nih.gov/books/ NBK62584/. Accessed September 27, 2022.

6. Braveman PA, Kumanyika S, Fielding J, et al. Health disparities and health equity: the issue is justice. *Am J Publ Health*. 2011;101(Suppl 1):S149−S155. https://doi.org/ 10.2105/AJPH.2010.300062.

7. Gaubatz ME, Bukatko AR, Simpson MC, et al. Racial and socioeconomic disparities associated with 90-day mortality among patients with head and neck cancer in the United States. *Oral Oncol*. 2019;89:95−101. https://doi.org/10.1016/j.oraloncology.2018.12.023.

8. Health - OECD Data. Accessed September 7, 2022. https://data.oecd.org/health.htm.

9. Bureau UC. Health Insurance Coverage in the United States: 2020. Census.gov. Published September 14, 2021. Accessed September 19, 2022. https://www.census.gov/ library/publications/2021/demo/p60-274.html.

10. Healthcare Systems Around the World. Accessed September 7, 2022. https://www.news-medical.net/health/Healthcare-Systems-Around-the-World.aspx.

11. Carroll AE, Frakt A. The best health care system in the world: which one would you pick? *N Y Times*; September 18, 2017. https://www.nytimes.com/interactive/2017/09/ 18/upshot/best-health-care-system-country-bracket.html.

12. Lurie N, Fremont A. Building bridges between health care and public health: a critical piece of the health reform infrastructure. *JAMA J Am Med Assoc*. 2009;302(1):84−86. https://doi.org/10.1001/jama.2009.959.

13. Organization World Health. *The World Health Report : 2000 : Health Systems : Improving Performance*. 2000.

14. Optimal Access. ACS. Accessed September 7, 2022. https://www.facs.org/about-acs/ statements/optimal-access/.

15. Burstin H, Leatherman S, Goldmann D. The evolution of healthcare quality measurement in the United States. *J Intern Med*. 2016;279(2):154−159. https://doi.org/ 10.1111/joim.12471.

16. Wakefield MK. The quality chasm series: implications for nursing. In: Hughes RG, ed. *Patient Safety and Quality: An Evidence-Based Handbook for Nurses. Advances in Patient Safety*. Agency for Healthcare Research and Quality (US); 2008. http://www.ncbi. nlm.nih.gov/books/NBK2677/. Accessed September 20, 2022.

17. Meara JG, Leather AJM, Hagander L, et al. Global Surgery 2030: evidence and solutions for achieving health, welfare, and economic development. *Lancet*. 2015;386(9993): 569−624. https://doi.org/10.1016/S0140-6736(15)60160-X.

18. Truche P, Semco RS, Hansen NF, et al. Association between surgery, anesthesia and obstetric (SAO) workforce and emergent surgical and obstetric mortality among United States hospital referral regions. *Ann Surg*. February 17, 2022. https://doi.org/10.1097/ SLA.0000000000005421.

19. Shrime MG, Dare A, Alkire BC, Meara JG. A global country-level comparison of the financial burden of surgery. *Br J Surg*. 2016;103(11):1453−1461. https://doi.org/10.1002/bjs.10249.

20. Massa ST, Osazuwa-Peters N, Adjei Boakye E, Walker RJ, Ward GM. Comparison of the financial burden of survivors of head and neck cancer with other cancer survivors. *JAMA Otolaryngol Head Neck Surg*. 2019;145(3):239−249. https://doi.org/10.1001/jamaoto.2018.3982.

21. Ragin CC, Langevin SM, Marzouk M, Grandis J, Taioli E. Determinants of head and neck cancer survival by race. *Head Neck*. 2011;33(8):1092−1098. https://doi.org/10.1002/hed.21584.

22. Du XL, Liu CC. Racial/Ethnic disparities in socioeconomic status, diagnosis, treatment and survival among medicare-insured men and women with head and neck cancer. *J Health Care Poor Underserved*. 2010;21(3):913−930. https://doi.org/10.1353/hpu.0.0331.

23. Institute of medicine (US) committee on monitoring access to personal health care services. In: Millman M, ed. *Access to Health Care in America*. National Academies Press (US); 1993. http://www.ncbi.nlm.nih.gov/books/NBK235882/. Accessed September 7, 2022.

24. Rutherford PA, Provost LP, Kotagal UR, Luther K, Anderson A. Achieving hospital-wide patient flow | IHI - Institute for Healthcare Improvement. Accessed September 7, 2022. https://www.ihi.org:443/resources/Pages/IHIWhitePapers/Achieving-Hospital-wide-Patient-Flow.aspx.

25. Eisenberg JM, Power EJ. Transforming insurance coverage into quality health care: voltage drops from potential to delivered quality. *JAMA*. 2000;284(16):2100−2107. https://doi.org/10.1001/jama.284.16.2100.

26. Bergmark RW, Burks CA, Schnipper JL, Weissman JS. Understanding and investigating access to surgical care. *Ann Surg*. 2022;275(3):492−495. https://doi.org/10.1097/SLA.0000000000005212.

27. Bowe SN, Megwalu UC, Bergmark RW, Balakrishnan K. Moving beyond detection: charting a path to eliminate health care disparities in otolaryngology. *Otolaryngol Head Neck Surg Off J Am Acad Otolaryngol-Head Neck Surg*. 2022;166(6):1013−1021. https://doi.org/10.1177/01945998221094460.

28. Forrest CB, Nutting PA, Starfield B, von Schrader S. Family physicians' referral decisions: results from the ASPN referral study. *J Fam Pract*. 2002;51(3):215−222.

29. Saber Tehrani AS, Coughlan D, Hsieh YH, et al. Rising annual costs of dizziness presentations to U.S. emergency departments. *Acad Emerg Med Off J Soc Acad Emerg Med*. 2013;20(7):689−696. https://doi.org/10.1111/acem.12168.

30. Kozin ED, Sethi RKV, Remenschneider AK, et al. Epidemiology of otologic diagnoses in United States emergency departments. *Laryngoscope*. 2015;125(8):1926−1933. https://doi.org/10.1002/lary.25197.

31. Rapoport Y, Kreitler S, Chaitchik S, Algor R, Weissler K. Psychosocial problems in head-and-neck cancer patients and their change with time since diagnosis. *Ann Oncol Off J Eur Soc Med Oncol*. 1993;4(1):69−73. https://doi.org/10.1093/oxfordjournals.annonc.a058365.

32. Avoidable costs in U.S. Healthcare. http://offers.premierinc.com/rs/381-NBB-525/images/Avoidable_Costs_in%20_US_Healthcare-IHII_AvoidableCosts_2013%5B1%5D.pdf.

33. Cohen SM, Kim J, Roy N, Courey M. Delayed otolaryngology referral for voice disorders increases health care costs. *Am J Med.* 2015;128(4). https://doi.org/10.1016/j.amjmed.2014.10.040, 426.e11-426.e18.
34. Bertelsen C, Choi JS, Jackanich A, Ge M, Sun GH, Chambers T. Comparison of referral pathways in otolaryngology at a public versus private academic center. *Ann Otol Rhinol Laryngol.* 2020;129(4):369−375. https://doi.org/10.1177/0003489419887990.
35. Sobal J, Muncie HL, Valente CM, Levine DM, DeForge BR. Self-reported referral patterns in practices of family/general practitioners, internists, and obstetricians/gynecologists. *J Community Health.* 1988;13(3):171−183. https://doi.org/10.1007/BF01324242.
36. Cyr ME, Etchin AG, Guthrie BJ, Benneyan JC. Access to specialty healthcare in urban versus rural US populations: a systematic literature review. *BMC Health Serv Res.* 2019; 19(1):974. https://doi.org/10.1186/s12913-019-4815-5.
37. Liu DH, Ge M, Smith SS, Park C, Ference EH. Geographic distribution of otolaryngology advance practice providers and physicians. *Otolaryngol Head Neck Surg Off J Am Acad Otolaryngol Head Neck Surg.* 2022;167(1):48−55. https://doi.org/10.1177/01945998211040408.
38. Vickery TW, Weterings R, Cabrera-Muffly C. Geographic distribution of otolaryngologists in the United States. *Ear Nose Throat J.* 2016;95(6):218−223.
39. Casey MM, Thiede Call K, Klingner JM. Are rural residents less likely to obtain recommended preventive healthcare services? *Am J Prev Med.* 2001;21(3):182−188. https://doi.org/10.1016/s0749-3797(01)00349-x.
40. Aboagye JK, Kaiser HE, Hayanga AJ. Rural-urban differences in access to specialist providers of colorectal cancer care in the United States: a physician workforce issue. *JAMA Surg.* 2014;149(6):537−543. https://doi.org/10.1001/jamasurg.2013.5062.
41. Cass LM, Smith JB. The current state of the otolaryngology workforce. *Otolaryngol Clin.* 2020;53(5):915−926. https://doi.org/10.1016/j.otc.2020.05.016.
42. Gadkaree SK, McCarty JC, Siu J, et al. Variation in the geographic distribution of the otolaryngology workforce: a national geospatial analysis. *Otolaryngol Head Neck Surg Off J Am Acad Otolaryngol Head Neck Surg.* 2020;162(5):649−657. https://doi.org/10.1177/0194599820908860.
43. US department of health and human services, health resources and services administration, national center for health workforce analysis. National and regional projections of supply and demand for surgical specialty practitioners: 2013−2025. Published online December 2016:15.
44. *Locations and Types of Graduate Training Were Largely Unchanged, and Federal Efforts May Not Be Sufficient to Meet Needs, Report GAO-17-411*; May 2017. https://www.gao.gov/assets/690/684946.pdf.
45. Smith DH, Case HF, Quereshy HA, et al. Geographic distribution of otolaryngology training programs and potential opportunities for strategic program growth. *Laryngoscope.* August 23, 2022. https://doi.org/10.1002/lary.30361.
46. Gruca TS, Nam I, Tracy R. Reaching rural patients through otolaryngology visiting consultant clinics. *Otolaryngol Head Neck Surg Off J Am Acad Otolaryngol Head Neck Surg.* 2014;151(6):895−898. https://doi.org/10.1177/0194599814553398.
47. Elrod JK, Fortenberry JL. The hub-and-spoke organization design revisited: a lifeline for rural hospitals. *BMC Health Serv Res.* 2017;17(Suppl 4):795. https://doi.org/10.1186/s12913-017-2755-5.

48. Cooper-Patrick L, Gallo JJ, Gonzales JJ, et al. Race, gender, and partnership in the patient-physician relationship. *JAMA*. 1999;282(6):583−589. https://doi.org/10.1001/jama.282.6.583.

49. LaVeist TA, Nuru-Jeter A, Jones KE. The association of doctor-patient race concordance with health services utilization. *J Publ Health Pol*. 2003;24(3−4):312−323.

50. Komaromy M, Grumbach K, Drake M, et al. The role of black and Hispanic physicians in providing health care for underserved populations. *N Engl J Med*. 1996;334(20): 1305−1310. https://doi.org/10.1056/NEJM199605163342006.

51. Rabinowitz HK, Diamond JJ, Veloski JJ, Gayle JA. The impact of multiple predictors on generalist physicians' care of underserved populations. *Am J Publ Health*. 2000;90(8): 1225−1228. https://doi.org/10.2105/ajph.90.8.1225.

52. Burks CA, Russell TI, Goss D, et al. Strategies to increase racial and ethnic diversity in the surgical workforce: a state of the art review. *Otolaryngol Head Neck Surg Off J Am Acad Otolaryngol Head Neck Surg*. 2022;166(6):1182−1191. https://doi.org/10.1177/01945998221094461.

53. Ukatu CC, Welby Berra L, Wu Q, Franzese C. The state of diversity based on race, ethnicity, and sex in otolaryngology in 2016. *Laryngoscope*. 2020;130(12): E795−E800. https://doi.org/10.1002/lary.28447.

54. Truesdale CM, Baugh RF, Brenner MJ, et al. Prioritizing diversity in otolaryngology-head and neck surgery: starting a conversation. *Otolaryngol Head Neck Surg Off J Am Acad Otolaryngol Head Neck Surg*. 2021;164(2):229−233. https://doi.org/10.1177/0194599820960722.

55. Meyer TK, Bergmark R, Zatz M, Sardesai MG, Litvack JR, Starks Acosta A. Barriers pushed aside: insights on career and family success from women leaders in academic otolaryngology. *Otolaryngol Head Neck Surg Off J Am Acad Otolaryngol Head Neck Surg*. 2019;161(2):257−264. https://doi.org/10.1177/0194599819841608.

56. Espinel A, Poley M, Zalzal GH, Chan K, Preciado D. Trends in U.S. Pediatric otolaryngology fellowship training. *JAMA Otolaryngol Head Neck Surg*. 2015;141(10):919−922. https://doi.org/10.1001/jamaoto.2015.1570.

57. Winters R, Pou A, Friedlander P. A "medical mission" at home: the needs of rural America in terms of otolaryngology care. *J Rural Health Off J Am Rural Health Assoc Natl Rural Health Care Assoc*. 2011;27(3):297−301. https://doi.org/10.1111/j.1748-0361.2010.00343.x.

58. Burstin HR, Lipsitz SR, Brennan TA. Socioeconomic status and risk for substandard medical care. *JAMA*. 1992;268(17):2383−2387.

59. Dimick J, Ruhter J, Sarrazin MV, Birkmeyer JD. Black patients more likely than whites to undergo surgery at low-quality hospitals in segregated regions. *Health Aff Proj Hope*. 2013;32(6):1046−1053. https://doi.org/10.1377/hlthaff.2011.1365.

60. Bergmark RW, Ishman SL, Phillips KM, Cunningham MJ, Sedaghat AR. Emergency department use for acute rhinosinusitis: insurance dependent for children and adults. *Laryngoscope*. 2018;128(2):299−303. https://doi.org/10.1002/lary.26671.

61. Ruthberg JS, Khan HA, Knusel KD, Rabah NM, Otteson TD. Health disparities in the access and cost of health care for otolaryngologic conditions. *Otolaryngol Head Neck Surg Off J Am Acad Otolaryngol Head Neck Surg*. 2020;162(4):479−488. https://doi.org/10.1177/0194599820904369.

62. Kangovi S, Barg FK, Carter T, Long JA, Shannon R, Grande D. Understanding why patients of low socioeconomic status prefer hospitals over ambulatory care. *Health Aff Proj Hope*. 2013;32(7):1196−1203. https://doi.org/10.1377/hlthaff.2012.0825.

63. Megwalu UC, Ma Y, Hernandez-Boussard T, Divi V, Gomez SL. The impact of hospital quality on thyroid cancer survival. *Otolaryngol Head Neck Surg Off J Am Acad Otolaryngol Head Neck Surg.* 2020;162(3):269–276. https://doi.org/10.1177/0194599819900760.

64. Megwalu UC, Ma Y. Racial/ethnic disparities in use of high-quality hospitals among oral cancer patients in California. *Laryngoscope.* 2022;132(4):793–800. https://doi.org/10.1002/lary.29830.

65. Neiman PU, Tsai TC, Bergmark RW, Ibrahim A, Nathan H, Scott JW. The affordable care act at 10 Years: evaluating the evidence and navigating an uncertain future. *J Surg Res.* 2021;263:102–109. https://doi.org/10.1016/j.jss.2020.12.056.

66. Dickman SL, Himmelstein DU, Woolhandler S. Inequality and the health-care system in the USA. *Lancet Lond Engl.* 2017;389(10077):1431–1441. https://doi.org/10.1016/S0140-6736(17)30398-7.

67. Tolbert J. *Nov 06 ADP, 2020. Key Facts about the Uninsured Population. KFF*; November 6, 2020. https://www.kff.org/uninsured/issue-brief/key-facts-about-the-uninsured-population/. Accessed September 20, 2022.

68. Shukla N, Ma Y, Megwalu UC. The role of insurance status as a mediator of racial disparities in oropharyngeal cancer outcomes. *Head Neck.* 2021;43(10):3116–3124. https://doi.org/10.1002/hed.26807.

69. Osazuwa-Peters N, Barnes JM, Megwalu U, et al. State Medicaid expansion status, insurance coverage and stage at diagnosis in head and neck cancer patients. *Oral Oncol.* 2020;110:104870. https://doi.org/10.1016/j.oraloncology.2020.104870.

70. Out-of-Pocket Costs—Glossary. HealthCare.gov. Accessed September 21, 2022. https://www.healthcare.gov/glossary/out-of-pocket-costs.

71. Garfield RL, Damico A. Medicaid expansion under health reform may increase service use and improve access for low-income adults with diabetes. *Health Aff Proj Hope.* 2012;31(1):159–167. https://doi.org/10.1377/hlthaff.2011.0903.

72. Segel JE, Kullgren JT. Health insurance deductibles and their associations with out-of-pocket spending and affordability barriers among US adults with chronic conditions. *JAMA Intern Med.* 2017;177(3):433–436. https://doi.org/10.1001/jamainternmed.2016.8419.

73. Shrime MG, Dare AJ, Alkire BC, O'Neill K, Meara JG. Catastrophic expenditure to pay for surgery: a global estimate. *Lancet Global Health.* 2015;3(0 2):S38–S44. https://doi.org/10.1016/S2214-109X(15)70085-9.

74. Marvin K, Ambrosio A, Brigger M. The increasing cost of pediatric otolaryngology care. *Int J Pediatr Otorhinolaryngol.* 2019;123:175–180. https://doi.org/10.1016/j.ijporl.2019.05.011.

75. Harsha WJ, Perkins JA, Lewis CW, Manning SC. Head and neck endocrine surgery in children: 1997 and 2000. *Arch Otolaryngol Head Neck Surg.* 2005;131(7):564–570. https://doi.org/10.1001/archotol.131.7.564.

76. Schleicher SM, Mullangi S, Feeley TW. Effects of narrow networks on access to high-quality cancer care. *JAMA Oncol.* 2016;2(4):427–428. https://doi.org/10.1001/jamaoncol.2015.6125.

77. Schoen C, Osborn R, Squires D, Doty MM. Access, affordability, and insurance complexity are often worse in the United States compared to ten other countries. *Health Aff Proj Hope.* 2013;32(12):2205–2215. https://doi.org/10.1377/hlthaff.2013.0879.

78. Pines JM, Meisel ZF. Concierge medicine vs. Patient-centered medical homes: can better access to care help reduce health care costs? | TIME.com. TIME. https://healthland.time.

com/2012/01/23/does-better-access-to-health-care-really-help-lower-costs/; January 23, 2012. Accessed September 21, 2022.

79. Noles MJ, Reiter KL, Boortz-Marx J, Pink G. Rural hospital mergers and acquisitions: which hospitals are being acquired and how are they performing afterward? *J Healthc Manag Am Coll Healthc Exec*. 2015;60(6):395–407.

80. Stark R. Hospital mergers don't improve quality of care. https://www.washingtonpolicy.org/publications/detail/hospital-mergers-dont-improve-quality-of-care; January 2, 2020. Accessed September 7, 2022.

81. Mendes E. In U.S., health disparities across incomes are wide-ranging. Gallup.com. https://news.gallup.com/poll/143696/Health-Disparities-Across-Incomes-Wide-Ranging.aspx; October 18, 2010. Accessed September 7, 2022.

82. Burks CA, Ortega G, Bergmark RW. COVID-19, disparities, and opportunities for equity in otolaryngology-unequal America. *JAMA Otolaryngol Head Neck Surg*. 2020;146(11): 995–996. https://doi.org/10.1001/jamaoto.2020.2874.

83. Price-Haywood EG, Burton J, Fort D, Seoane L. Hospitalization and mortality among black patients and white patients with covid-19. *N Engl J Med*. 2020;382(26): 2534–2543. https://doi.org/10.1056/NEJMsa2011686.

84. Magesh S, John D, Li WT, et al. Disparities in COVID-19 outcomes by race, ethnicity, and socioeconomic status: a systematic-review and meta-analysis. *JAMA Netw Open*. 2021;4(11):e2134147. https://doi.org/10.1001/jamanetworkopen.2021.34147.

85. Losenegger T, Urban MJ, Jagasia AJ. Challenges in the delivery of rural otolaryngology care during the COVID-19 pandemic. *Otolaryngol Head Neck Surg Off J Am Acad Otolaryngol Head Neck Surg*. 2021;165(1):5–6. https://doi.org/10.1177/0194599821 995146.

86. Patel VM, Kominsky E, Tham T, et al. The impact of the COVID-19 pandemic on otolaryngologic emergency department visits at two major NYC hospital systems. *Am J Otolaryngol*. 2021;42(5):103123. https://doi.org/10.1016/j.amjoto.2021.103123.

87. Fastenberg JH, Bottalico D, Kennedy WA, Sheikh A, Setzen M, Rodgers R. The impact of the pandemic on otolaryngology patients with negative COVID-19 status: commentary and insights from orbital emergencies. *Otolaryngol Head Neck Surg Off J Am Acad Otolaryngol Head Neck Surg*. 2020;163(3):444–446. https://doi.org/10.1177/0194599820931082.

88. *The Impact of Coronavirus on Households in Rural America*; October 2020. https://cdn1.sph.harvard.edu/wp-content/uploads/sites/94/2020/10/Rural-Report_100520-FINAL.pdf.

89. Koh N, Wagner R, Newton R, Kuhn C. *CLER National Report of Findings 2021*. 2021.

The contribution of racial and ethnic biases to disparities across the care cycle and to outcomes in otolaryngology

Karthik Balakrishnan[1,2]

[1]*Department of Otolaryngology—Head and Neck Surgery, Stanford University School of Medicine, Stanford, CA, United States;* [2]*Stanford Medicine Children's Health and Lucile Packard Children's Hospital, Palo Alto, CA, United States*

Introduction

The title of this chapter suggests that it focuses on race and ethnicity as specific drivers of disparate health outcomes in otolaryngologic disease. Indeed, many readers will be well aware of the literature supporting the relationship between these components of patient identity and health outcomes. However, from the start of this chapter, it is essential to view the effects of race and ethnicity in the context of the overall lived experience of each patient and the interactions of these aspects of individual patients with the social, economic, legal, geographic, and historic systems in which patients live and seek health care. David Stevenson and colleagues thus describe the driving forces behind health disparities as a combination of the *genome* and the *exposome*[1]; they define the latter as the combined environment in which an individual exists and in which that individual's ancestors existed. The interplay between genome and exposome is immensely complex and only just beginning to be investigated and understood in health care as a whole, much less in otolaryngology. That said, this chapter will attempt to incorporate this approach as much as possible in discussing how race and ethnicity relate to health outcomes.

Another important note is that the chapter will focus on race and ethnicity and does not address other essential aspects of individuals' identity such as gender, education, and socioeconomic status, except in passing. The author encourages readers to study other chapters in this textbook to better understand these topics.

Race and ethnicity

While the terms *race* and *ethnicity* are often used interchangeably or in combination (the author admits to having published studies that commit this error), they have

Healthcare Disparities in Otolaryngology. https://doi.org/10.1016/B978-0-443-10714-6.00009-2

quite different meanings. *Race* refers to artificially constructed categories based on physical characteristics, such as skin color. While these categories have no basis in genetic differences and are based on a combination of social constructs and self-identification, they continue to be used inappropriately as a proxy for genetic groups.[2] As this chapter will discuss, race's contribution to disparate health outcomes is most likely due to associated social factors such as systemic racism and access to optimal care rather than direct effects on health.

In contrast, *ethnicity* refers to shared beliefs and cultural practices.[2] Ethnicity may reflect genuine groups based on self-identification and may be associated with practices and behaviors that indeed affect health outcomes. For example, certain populations in the Kashmir valley of South Asia have elevated rates of cutaneous cancer of the abdominal wall related to chronic use of contact heat sources, so-called "kangri cancer."[3]

Genetics

Despite the now widely accepted conclusion that race is based on socially imposed divisions rather than group genetic differences,[3] researchers continue to examine the contribution of genetic factors to racial disparities in health outcomes. In some cases, this approach can be productive. For example, a recent study identified differences in prevalence of mutations in *TP53* and *JAK3*, and in tumor-infiltrating lymphocyte counts, when comparing Black and non-Latinx White patients, and that methylation of certain promoters correlated with various socioeconomic measures.[4] This study is an admirable effort to understand aspects of the interaction between genome and exposome in order to support the development of individualized treatment for head and neck cancer patients. However, its interpretation comes with some risk: without careful consideration, a reader of that manuscript might conclude that Black patients with head and neck cancer are a genetically distinct group with specific risk factors. The authors, in contrast, suggest that apparent racial differences in head and neck cancer outcomes are in fact the result of interactions between genetic, disease, and social elements, and they clearly explain the limitations to currently available data in clarifying these interactions. This author encourages readers to contrast this approach with the more common, less-nuanced approach of simply dividing patients by race (self-identified or externally assigned) and proceeding with analysis of genetic data using race as a covariate; this latter method inappropriately treats race as a true biological identifier.

Even with careful attention to a nuanced analysis like that done by Guerrero-Preston and colleagues, there is risk. For example, Duello and colleagues point out that any sample of "Black" patients may not generate data generalizable to any other "Black" patient, due to genome- and exposome-level heterogeneity that melds socially imposed and self-selected categories.[2] It may be more useful to focus on the specific genetic markers studied, to consider social factors associated with race as separate covariates, and to consider race specifically with regard to the potential effects of systemic racism on outcomes.

Available data

A further limitation in interpreting studies of race- and ethnicity-related health outcome disparities is the inequality of available data for many groups. Most studies examine Black patients in relation to White patients, or non-White patients collectively compared to White patients. While Black patients deserve a great deal of attention due to the long history of systemic racism that they have experienced, other groups are less well studied. Many authors call out the small numbers of Native American and Alaska Native patients in their data. An illustrative example is a recent study specifically examining head and neck cancer in these particular groups, which included 51,289 patients overall but only 320 Native American and Alaska Native individuals (0.62% of the total study sample). This study used a major state-based health registry.[5] A similar study of head and neck cancer presentation in Native Hawaiian and Other Pacific Islander patients using the national SEER database included 469 individuals in the group of interest, out of 76,473 subjects overall (0.61%).[6] Furthermore, many clinical trials do not recruit subjects in a way that reflects the composition of the US population. The effect is that populations that may experience disadvantage throughout the otolaryngology health care process may not be adequately reflected in published data, making studies of disparate outcomes even more challenging to interpret. A final caveat is that most of the data presented in this chapter are drawn from studies of patients in the United States.

The remainder of this chapter reviews existing data on the relationship between race, ethnicity, and otolaryngology health outcomes. Without referring to the artificial construct of race, and without including studies that interweave race and ethnicity, there would be little data to discuss, and the chapter would be impossible to write. The author therefore humbly asks that readers keep in mind the caveats raised above. These caveats do not negate the genuine health disparities described, but they should raise questions in the reader's mind about the true drivers that lie between race, ethnicity, and outcomes that deserve further attention.

Head and neck cancer, laryngology, and endocrine surgery

Among the subspecialties in otolaryngology, head and neck oncology presents the broadest range of studies on the relationship between race and health outcomes. The associated disparities are present throughout the care cycle, from stage at presentation through treatment outcomes and survival. Given the preponderance of data in this subspecialty, this chapter discusses head and neck cancer care in depth and will cover other subspecialties in otolaryngology more succinctly, with the understanding that similar mechanisms drive treatment and outcome disparities in those areas.

Presentation

The current literature suggests that race and ethnicity are associated with differential cancer stage at presentation. However, the specific patterns of association are inconsistent, suggesting again that race and ethnicity are not optimal ways to divide patients for prognosis. For example, one study suggests that for sinus cancer, age at presentation tends to be younger for non-White individuals, while those who identify as Hispanic may be more likely to present with regional or distant disease[7]; other studies have not shown this association.[8] Similarly, a 2021 study finds that American Indian and Alaska Native patients in California have the highest rates of Stage IV head and neck cancer at presentation compared to other races, while Black patients have a lower five-year survival rate than other races.[5] Contrary to what a reader might expect, the authors also found that White patients had the second-highest risk of Stage IV disease at presentation; the published data do not allow the reader to explain these findings.

Studies of head and neck squamous cell carcinoma as an overall disease entity suggest that various non-White groups may be more likely to present with advanced disease or inoperable cancers, when compared to White patients.[6,9]

These differences in presentation are likely due to multiple complex factors separate from (but related to) race. For example, Native American and Alaska Native populations overall have very high rates of cigarette smoking, but this observation is confounded by associations with younger age, fewer years of education, and lower family income or poverty,[10] all of which individuals within these populations may experience more often due to current and historical systemic racism and disadvantage.

Travel distance appears to be another important predictor of stage at presentation,[11] though the relationship is more complex than just geographic distributions of different racial groups. For example, long travel may indicate treatment at an academic medical center, while nonprivate insurance and lower income may reduce patients' likelihood of traveling for care.[12] Indeed, the relationship is quite layered, with Black and Hispanic patients' being less likely to travel for radiation therapy but more likely to travel for treatment at centers that may have more expertise.[12]

Treatment

As with disease presentation, treatment recommendations and decisions appear to vary by race and ethnicity. For example, Black patients with lower-stage (T1–T3) laryngeal squamous cell carcinoma may be more likely to undergo total laryngectomy than White patients and also more likely to undergo primary radiation therapy for T4 disease.[13] One major contributor to these different treatment patterns is differences in what treatment is recommended to patients of different races. A 2020 study found that non-Hispanic Black patients were less likely to be offered surgery for any head and neck cancer site than non-Hispanic White patients, despite increased rates of surgery in both groups over time.[14] The same study, and others, have found that non-Hispanic Black patients were less likely to accept recommended surgery.[14,15] A higher likelihood of refusing recommended cancer surgery has been observed in Black patients with cancers of various types, but refusal of surgery cannot be understood simply through race-based analysis. For example, pediatric patients with well-differentiated thyroid cancer do not show differences by race in proceeding with recommended surgery.[16] Many factors affect the decision to proceed with surgery, including insurance, marital status (perhaps reflecting available support in the home), site of the cancer, age, sex, and geography.[15,17,18] In addition, an essential result of the exposome of some individuals is decreased trust in medical providers and in the health care system, which may also affect patients' treatment decisions. This lack of trust varies in part by race; Black lung cancer patients, for example, have lower trust in physicians and feel that physicians are less informative, supportive, and partnering (when compared to White patients).[19] Trust and perceived discrimination in turn have significant effects on treatment adherence for a wide variety of diseases.[20] In addition, even efforts to promote shared decision-making and build trust may not include essential components such as family and community input, depending on the patient.[21]

An added component of these differences is likely due to differential access to high-quality care. Multiple factors may decrease a patient's likelihood of receiving cancer care consistent with current guidelines, including race, insurance status, education, and whether the patient is treated at an academic medical center.[22] Similarly, a 2021 study found that Black patients tended to receive lower-quality head and neck cancer care than White patients overall, with these quality differences and hospital characteristics (volume and safety-net role) explaining more than 11% of excess mortality in Black patients[23]; this association of race with care at hospitals of differing quality has been corroborated by other studies.[24]

Survival and other outcomes

As with treatment, many studies have identified differences in head and neck cancer outcomes for various racial and ethnic groups. Multiple studies have identified excess mortality in non-White patients in respect to both disease-specific and overall survival.[23,25]

Again, multiple factors apart from race itself likely drive these differences. Disease-related and hospital factors may explain a large proportion of these outcome disparities.[23] In addition, race interacts with other factors such as sex,[25] marital status,[25] insurance status,[9] etc. Some authors have found that even with adjustment for these factors, Black patients in particular experience excess mortality that cannot be fully explained. In contrast, other authors have suggested that controlling for various aspects of socioeconomic status may completely explain this excess mortality.[26] If there is indeed a component of excess mortality that cannot be explained through these large-scale statistical adjustments, as-yet unstudied components of the exposome may explain it. For example, lack of access to healthy food, safe open spaces, and leisure time may contribute to a lack of physical activity, which in turn has been linked to obesity and increased cancer risk.[27] Adverse childhood experiences may similarly increase the risk of cancer[28]; exposure to these experiences varies by race, possibly because of disparities in family income and family resilience.[29]

Head and neck cancer outcome studies tend to focus on survival, but other outcomes are of course also important to patients and vary by race. For instance, voice outcomes after thyroid surgery appear to be worse in Black patients, who have a higher risk of objective and subjective voice impairment three to six months into the postoperative period.[30] Similarly, as noted earlier, total laryngectomy is more commonly performed in Black patients than White patients. Voice preservation therapy for laryngeal cancer patients was less often used in Black patients with laryngeal cancer when compared to White, Hispanic, and Asian individuals, throughout the period 1991–2008.[31] Patients of non-White race were also more likely to be listed as a "no-show" for voice therapy appointments, whereas the ability to be seen in a multidisciplinary voice clinic decreased no-show rates[32]; readers may hypothesize that factors such as travel distance, employment, and childcare support likely influence these relationships to some degree. Race is not a direct predictor of outcomes after medialization laryngoplasty, but significant medical comorbidity is a predictor,[33] and this may mediate the relationship between race and outcomes.

Finally, end-of-life care for head and neck cancer patients also appears to vary by race, with some groups more or less likely to die at home or in hospice care.[34] Again, other variables such as sex, age, and cancer subsite also influence this outcome. Furthermore, the results of this particular study do not make clear how much of these differences are driven by patient preference versus differences that are imposed on the patient.

Rhinology

Sinonasal malignancies are discussed to some degree in the previous section. This section will focus on sinusitis (specifically chronic rhinosinusitis), given the commonality of this disease. The majority of studies of sinusitis outcomes do not include information on race and ethnicity; those studies that do include data appear to underrepresent non-White patients relative to the US population.[35,36] In the available data, putting aside concerns of generalizability, the incidence of sinusitis appears to vary by race,[35] though the relative contributions of major confounders such as environmental pollutants and smoking remains unclear.

Among patients with sinusitis, presenting symptoms do not appear to vary consistently by race. One study suggested that Black patients with sinusitis were more likely to be unable to work (while the question did not specify whether this was due to the sinusitis, the incremental change in patients unable to work with vs. without sinusitis was greatest among Black patients).[35] The authors performed a smaller analysis of a single cohort of patients who underwent surgery and found that while quality of life varied by race, disease severity by imaging, endoscopy, or olfaction scores did not, suggesting that the disease's effect on patients' ability to work and patient-perceived symptoms is modified by other factors in the patient's life. Although the study did not offer suggestions, readers might consider forces such as environmental stress, comorbidity, etc., as well as issues of delayed care as noted later in this section. However, a separate study suggests that patient-reported disease severity measures are not different by race at presentation.[37]

In respect to presentation, Black patients were more likely to seek evaluation in the emergency department for concerns related to sinusitis.[35] Insurance status may play a role in this; Black and Hispanic patients were more likely than other groups to report delaying care due to concerns about cost and were less likely to have insurance covering emergency department visits,[35] though residential zip code income did not predict patient reported severity at baseline.[37] As with head and neck cancer, patients seeking care at different hospitals have different experiences; those served at public hospitals are less likely to be White and more likely to have longer duration of symptoms and polyposis.[38] As with the conditions previously discussed, the effects of race on outcomes appear to be mediated by a variety of social and economic factors rather than the intrinsic effects of race itself.

At least one study has examined biological aspects of chronic rhinosinusitis by race. The authors found that Black patients had more eosinophils per high-powered field on histopathologic analysis, which might correlate with their finding of higher patient-reported severity scores in this group. However, similar findings were associated with patients with public insurance, and controlling for insurance status eliminated the association with Black race, suggesting again that financial, access, social, or environmental issues may be the true driver of disease severity that apparently varies by race.[39]

In terms of treatment, at least one study suggests that race, insurance, and residential area income do not predict oral antibiotic or steroid use[37]; the same holds true when comparing public versus private hospital patients.[38] However, patients treated at public hospitals were less likely to follow up and had to wait about three weeks longer for surgery on average when compared to those treated at private hospitals.[38] Despite this delay, the two groups had similar rates of revision surgery. However, public hospital patients were more likely to have more severe asthma, again possibly related to environmental factors or access to care rather than race itself. Asian American patients are less likely to undergo endoscopic sinus surgery despite the lack of difference from other groups in subjective and objective baseline severity; this may be related to language barriers rather than insurance status, based on one study.[40] After surgery, Black and Latinx patients are less likely to receive treatment from an allergist, and Black patients tended to have worse patient-reported outcomes despite similar baseline scores.[41]

With regard to pediatric sinus surgery, Black and Hispanic patients have been found to require urgent and emergent operations more frequent than White patients, while Hispanic children have increased rates of postoperative complications.[42]

Adult and pediatric sleep surgery

As with the other conditions discussed in this chapter, outcomes in sleep apnea and sleep-disordered breathing cannot be understood through the lens of race alone. Multiple forces may affect the quality of an individual's sleep, including their work or school schedules, home environment, childcare obligations or availability, comorbidities such as obesity, substance use, other medications, and so on. In addition, sleep surgery studies underrepresent non-White groups (and women), impairing generalizability.[43] That said, at least one systematic review found that lower socioeconomic status predicted higher risk of obstructive sleep apnea for both adult and pediatric patients.[44] Another systematic review that specifically examined the role of ethnic minority identity confirmed the association of lower socioeconomic status with elevated obstructive sleep apnea risk while demonstrating no specific independent relationship between ethnicity and disease severity.[45]

In terms of diagnosis, children of Black or Hispanic identity were less likely to attend referral appointments, perhaps explained by the findings that children from areas of higher social vulnerability were also less likely to attend, as were children with public insurance.[46] Children of non-White race are more likely to undergo preoperative sleep study, while obesity and other comorbidities may mediate this relationship, the association persists in multivariable adjusted analysis.[47] Black children specifically are more likely to undergo both preoperative and postoperative sleep study.[47] However, in children with obstructive sleep apnea, obesity is more common among Black, Hispanic, and Native American patients,[48] suggesting that simply adjusting for obesity may not clarify the role of race. Other studies have demonstrated that children whose mothers have less than a high-school education or who live in more urban areas are more likely to have obstructive sleep apnea and more severe disease[49]; structural inequities are likely contributors to racial differences in parental education or residential geography.

Among children undergoing sleep endoscopy-directed surgery for obstructive sleep apnea, White race was associated with higher likelihood of surgical success, defined as obstructive apnea-hypopnea index less than five events per hour.[50] While obesity predicted a lower success rate, the adjusted model in this study continued to show that Black race was associated with a lower likelihood of surgical success. The authors cite multiple previous studies showing the same relationship and hypothesize that genetic factors may mediate this association, which is unconvincing based on the arguments made earlier in the chapter.

Otology

Among otologic procedures, cochlear implantation has been best studied with regard to outcome disparities. While many studies do not include analysis by race, insurance status is a commonly studied variable. A recent systematic review suggests that socioeconomic status and parental education level are major drivers of cochlear implant outcomes in children.[51] Studied outcomes included sentence complexity and length, vocabulary, global language development, and cognitive measures; it is important to note that findings were not consistent across all studies analyzed. Given the known association between age (or pre- vs. postlingual status) and outcomes, another study examined which patients who met audiometric criteria for implantation did not receive referral for implantation.[52] The authors found that children with married parents and private insurance were more likely to be referred, though the insurance finding dropped out in multivariable analysis. Parental marital status remained a significant predictor regardless of managing otolaryngologist or area income; area income itself was reported as a "marginally significant" predictor based on the statistical cutoffs for this study. Another study of pediatric patients found that publicly insured children were less likely to receive sequential bilateral implants; this group also had a significantly higher complication rate and higher likelihood of missing follow-up visits.[53] Public insurance or no insurance coverage also predicted delayed sound recognition and imitation in pediatric patients.[54] At least one study has identified Black or Hispanic identity as an independent predictor of delayed implantation, even when children have private insurance; publicly insured White children were more likely to be implanted in the first two years of life compared to privately insured Black children.[55] This finding suggests that racial disparities in access to care or treatment decisions may be a factor in differential outcomes.

Meanwhile, another study of adult patients found that non-White race predicted longer time to implantation, while insurance type was not predictive.[56] That study also demonstrated that non-White race was associated with higher pure-tone thresholds, lower speech recognition scores, and lower likelihood of preimplantation hearing aid use. The authors note that race appears to be an independent predictor and cite previous literature indicating that non-White patients with severe hearing loss are less likely to undergo aural rehabilitation.

Facial plastic and reconstructive surgery

Studies of racial disparities in this subspecialty are largely lacking. Readers may make some inferences from the existing literature, which contains many discussions of operative and technical nuance based on race. For example, many studies reference racial differences in skin character. This holds true even for less invasive and temporary procedures such as nonsurgical rhinoplasty; a recent study of this procedure suggests that both anatomy and patient expectations vary with ethnicity.[57] Other authors also suggest the importance of cultural sensitivity and understanding of patient expectations,[58] though the dominant focus of the literature on White skin, despite the cognitive differentiation of racial skin types (whether or not these can truly be divided as such), suggest that more targeted research into different patient groups is needed.

Meanwhile, racial disparities in pediatric facial plastic surgery appear in analyses of cleft palate operations. Black (emergent admissions, increased length of stay, higher hospital charges, fistula, and other complications), Hispanic (higher hospital charges), and Asian/Pacific Islander (accidental puncture and fistula) children showed differential outcomes when compared to White children undergoing cleft palate repair; the authors suggest that non-White patients may undergo surgery at a later age, which may contribute to these outcomes.[59]

Pediatric otolaryngology

Several studies of pediatric conditions have been discussed in other sections of this chapter; this section will briefly address a few additional areas. A recent global analysis of health disparities in pediatric otolaryngology concluded that many common conditions and procedures demonstrate aspects of inequity, including tonsillectomy, ear tubes, and tracheostomy.[60] For example, a recent study of prescribing patterns after pediatric tonsillectomy suggested that Hispanic identity was associated with dispensing of lower quantities of opioids.[61]

Children undergoing tracheostomy also demonstrate differences by race. Black children are more likely to have a tracheostomy placed and are more likely to have associated airway and pulmonary problems such as airway stenosis and bronchopulmonary dysplasia[62]; they also have differential outcomes with longer hospital stay on average.[62,63] Hispanic children are less likely to undergo tracheostomy.[64] In-hospital and overall mortality and 30-day readmission do not appear to vary by race.[63,64] It is unclear why these racial differences exist, whether in relation to quality of care, cultural or social factors affecting parental decision about tracheostomy, issues of trust in health care providers, etc.

Summary

The above data make clear that race and ethnicity are associated with differential experiences and outcomes throughout the care cycle of various otolaryngologic conditions, and almost certainly the care cycle of any conditions not explicitly discussed here. However, to simply state this association grossly oversimplifies the ways in which race and ethnicity contribute to outcomes. While race and ethnicity cannot be defined genetically, they are social constructs or groupings that lead to systematic differences in the lived experiences of individuals in different groups. These experiences drive health outcomes in complex ways through the "exposome," in addition to which individuals may directly receive differential treatment by health care providers and systems due to their race or ethnicity. While the current result is that many individuals experience disadvantage in health outcomes, a deeper understanding of these complexities may eventually lead to more individualized care that accounts for both genome and exposome and creates greater equity in outcomes.[65] Beyond that, awareness of these complexities will ideally drive systemic changes to create not just equity but also justice for all patients receiving care from our specialty.

References

1. Stevenson DK, Wong RJ, Aghaeepour N, et al. Understanding health disparities. *J Perinatol.* 2019;39:354–358.

2. Duello TM, Rivedal S, Wickland C, et al. Race and genetics vs. "race" in genetics: a systematic review of the use of African ancestry in genetic studies. *Evol Med Public Health*. 2021;19:232−245.

3. Wani I. Kangri cancer. *Surgery*. 2010;147:586−588.

4. Guerrero-Preston R, Lawson F, Rodriguez-Torres S, et al. *JAK3* variant, immune signatures, DNA methylation, and social determinants linked to survival racial disparities in head and neck cancer patients. *Cancer Prev Res*. 2019;12:255−270.

5. Warren BR, Grandis JR, Johnson DE, et al. Head and neck cancer among American Indian and Alaska Native populations in California, 2009−2018. *Cancers*. 2021;13:5195.

6. Moon PK, Ma Y, Megwalu UC. Head and neck cancer stage at presentation and survival outcomes among Native Hawaiian and Other Pacific Islander patients compared with Asian and White patients. *JAMA Otolaryngol Head Neck Surg*. 2022;148:636−645.

7. Sharma RK, Schlosser RJ, Beswick DM, et al. Racial and ethnic disparities in paranasal sinus malignancies. *Int Forum Allergy Rhinol*. 2021;11:1557−1569.

8. Low CM, Balakrishnan K, Smith BM, et al. Sinonasal adenocarcinoma: population-based analysis of demographic and socioeconomic disparities. *Head Neck*. 2021;43:2946−2953.

9. Gourin CG, Podolsky RH. Racial disparities in patients with head and neck squamous cell carcinoma. *Laryngoscope*. 2006;116:1093−1106.

10. Odani S, Armour BS, Graffunder CM, et al. Prevalence and disparities in tobacco product use among American Indians/Alaska Natives—United States, 2010−2015. *MMWR Morb Mortal Wkly Rep*. 2017;66:1374−1378.

11. Morse E, Lohia S, Dooley LM. Travel distance is associated with stage at presentation and laryngectomy rates among patients with laryngeal cancer. *J Surg Oncol*. 2021;124:1272−1283.

12. Graboyes EM, Ellis MA, Li H, et al. Racial and ethnic disparities in travel for head and neck cancer treatment and the impact of travel distance on survival. *Cancer*. 2018;124:3181−3191.

13. Shin JY, Truong MT. Racial disparities in laryngeal cancer treatment and outcome: a population-based analysis of 24,069 patients. *Laryngoscope*. 2015;125:1667−1674.

14. Nocon CC, Ajmani GS, Bhayani MK. A contemporary analysis of racial disparities in recommended and received treatment for head and neck cancer. *Cancer*. 2020;126:381−389.

15. Crippen MM, Elias ML, Weisberger JS, et al. Refusal of cancer-directed surgery in head and neck squamous cell carcinoma patients. *Laryngoscope*. 2019;129:1368−1373.

16. Gruszczynski NR, Low CM, Choby G, et al. Effects of social determinants of health on pediatric thyroid cancer outcomes in the United States. *Otolaryngol Head Neck Surg*. 2022;166:1045−1054.

17. Sahovaler A, Gualtieri T, Palma D, et al. Head and neck cancer patients declining curative treatment: a case series and literature review. *Acta Otorhinolaryngol Ital*. 2021;41:18−23.

18. Amini A, Verma V, Li R, et al. Factors predicting for patient refusal of head and neck cancer therapy. *Head Neck*. 2020;42:33−42.

19. Gordon HS, Street Jr RL, Sharf BF, Kelly PA, Souchek J. Racial differences in trust and lung cancer patients' perceptions of physician communication. *J Clin Oncol*. 2006;24:904−909.

20. Cuffee YL, Hargraves JL, Rosal M, et al. Reported racial discrimination, trust in physicians, and medication adherence among inner-city African American with hypertension. *Am J Publ Health*. 2013;103:e55−e62.

21. Mead EL, Doorenbos AZ, Javid SH, et al. Shared decision-making for cancer care among racial and ethnic minorities: a systematic review. *Am J Publ Health*. 2013;103: e15−e29.

22. Graboyes EM, Garrett-Mayer E, Sharma AK, et al. Adherence to National Comprehensive Cancer Network guidelines for time to initiation of postoperative radiation therapy for patients with head and neck cancer. *Cancer*. 2017;123:2651−2660.

23. Jassal JS, Cramer JD. Explaining racial disparities in surgically treated head and neck cancer. *Laryngoscope*. 2021;131:1053−1059.

24. Megwalu UC, Ma Y. Racial/ethnic disparities in use of high-quality hospitals among oral cancer patients in California. *Laryngoscope*. 2022;132:793−800.

25. Taylor DB, Osazuwa-Peters OL, Okafor SI, et al. Differential outcomes among survivors of head and neck cancer belonging to racial and ethnic minority groups. *JAMA Otolaryngol Head Neck Surg*. 2022;148:119−127.

26. Lenze NR, Farquhar D, Sheth S, et al. Socioeconomic status drives racial disparities in HPV-negative head and neck cancer outcomes. *Laryngoscope*. 2021;131:1301−1309.

27. Friedenreich CM, Ryder-Burbidge C, McNeil J. Physical activity, obesity, and sedentary behavior in cancer etiology: epidemiologic evidence and biologic mechanisms. *Mol Oncol*. 2021;15:790−800.

28. Hughes K, Bellis MA, Hardcastle KA, et al. The effect of multiple adverse childhood experiences on health: a systematic review and meta-analysis. *Lancet Public Health*. 2017;2:e356−e366.

29. Goldstein E, Topitzes J, Miller-Cribbs J, et al. Influence of race/ethnicity and income on the link between adverse childhood experiences and child flourishing. *Pediatr Res*. 2021; 89:1861−1869.

30. Vicente DA, Solomon NP, Avital I, et al. Voice outcomes after total thyroidectomy, partial thyroidectomy, or non-neck surgery using a prospective multifactorial assessment. *J Am Coll Surg*. 2014;219:152−163.

31. Hou W-H, Daly ME, Lee NY, et al. Racial disparities in the use of voice preservation therapy for locally advanced laryngeal cancer. *Arch Otolaryngol Head Neck Surg*. 2012;138:644−649.

32. Vamosi BE, Mikhail L, Gustin RL. Predicting no show in voice therapy: avoiding the missed appointment cycle. *J Voice*. 2020;35:604−608.

33. Ekbom DC, Orbelo DM, Sangaralingham LR, et al. Medialization laryngoplasty/arytenoid adduction: US outcomes, discharge status, and utilization trends. *Laryngoscope*. 2019;129:952−960.

34. Stephens SJ, Chino F, Williamson H, et al. Evaluating for disparities in place of death for head and neck cancer patients in the United States utilizing the CDC WONDER database. *Oral Oncol*. 2020;102, 104555.

35. Soler ZM, Mace JC, Litvack JR, et al. Chronic rhinosinusitis, race, and ethnicity. *Am J Rhinol Allergy*. 2012;26:110−116.

36. Spielman DB, Liebowitz A, Kelebeyev S. Race in rhinology clinical trials: a decade of disparity. *Laryngoscope*. 2021;131:1722−1728.

37. Bergmark RW, Hoehle LP, Chyou D, et al. Association of socioeconomic status, race and insurance status with chronic rhinosinusitis patient-reported outcome measures. *Otolaryngol Head Neck Surg*. 2018;158:571−579.

38. Duerson W, Lafer M, Ahmed O. Health care disparities in undergoing endoscopic sinus surgery for chronic rhinosinusitis: differences in disease presentation and access to care. *Ann Otol Rhinol Laryngol.* 2019;128:608−613.

39. Kuhar HN, Ganti A, Eggerstedt M, et al. The impact of race and insurance status on baseline histopathology profile in patients with chronic rhinosinusitis. *Int Forum Allergy Rhinol.* 2019;9:665−673.

40. Orozco FR, Gao J, Hur K. Treatment decision-making among Asian Americans with chronic rhinosinusitis. *Int Forum Allergy Rhinol.* 2022;12:1558−1561.

41. Konsur E, Rigg L, Moore D, et al. Race and ethnicity define disparate clinical outcomes in chronic rhinosinusitis. *Ann Allergy Asthma Immunol.* 2022;129:737−741.

42. Pecha PP, Hamberis A, Patel TA, et al. Racial disparities in pediatric endoscopic sinus surgery. *Laryngoscope.* 2021;131:E1369−E1374.

43. Debbaneh P, Ramirez K, Block-Wheeler N, et al. Representation of race and sex in sleep surgery studies. *Otolaryngol Head Neck Surg.* 2022;166:1204−1210.

44. Sosso FAE, Matos E. Socioeconomic disparities in obstructive sleep apnea: a systematic review of empirical research. *Sleep Breath.* 2021;25:1729−1739.

45. Gulgielmi O, Lanteri P, Garbarino S. Association between socioeconomic status, belonging to an ethnic minority and obstructive sleep apnea: a systematic review of the literature. *Sleep Med.* 2019;57:100−106.

46. Yan F, Pearce JL, Ford ME. Examining associations between neighborhood-level social vulnerability and care for children with sleep-disordered breathing. *Otolaryngol Head Neck Surg.* 2022;166:1118−1126.

47. Qian ZJ, Howard JM, Cohen SM, et al. Use of polysomnography and CPAP in children who received adenotonsillectomy, US 2004 to 2018. *Laryngoscope.* March 14, 2022;133: 184−188.

48. Bachrach K, Danis DO, Cohen MB, et al. The relationship between obstructive sleep apnea and pediatric obesity: a nationwide analysis. *Ann Otol Rhinol Laryngol.* 2022;131: 520−526.

49. Park JW, Hamoda MM, Almeida FR, et al. Socioeconomic inequalities in pediatric obstructive sleep apnea. *J Clin Sleep Med.* 2022;18:637−645.

50. He S, Peddireddy NS, Smith DF, et al. Outcomes of drug-induced sleep endoscopy-directed surgery for pediatric obstructive sleep apnea. *Otolaryngol Head Neck Surg.* 2018;158:559−565.

51. Omar M, Qatanani AM, Douglas NO, et al. Sociodemographic disparities in pediatric cochlear implantation outcomes: a systematic review. *Am J Otolaryngol Head Neck Med Surg.* 2022;43, 103608.

52. Wiley S, Meinzen-Derr J. Access to cochlear implant candidacy evaluations: who is *not* making it to the team evaluations? *Int J Audiol.* 2009;48:74−79.

53. Chang DT, Ko AB, Murray GS, et al. Impact of socioeconomic status on access and outcomes. *Arch Otolaryngol Head Neck Surg.* 2010;136:648−657.

54. Tolan M, Serpas A, McElroy K, et al. Delays in sound recognition and imitation in underinsured children receiving cochlear implantation. *JAMA Otolaryngol Head Neck Surg.* 2017;143:60−64.

55. Liu X, Rosa-Lugo LI, Cosby JL, et al. Racial and insurance inequalities in access to early pediatric cochlear implantation. *Otolaryngol Head Neck Surg.* 2021;164:667−674.

56. Dorhnoffer JR, Holcomb MA, Meyer TA, et al. Factors influencing time to cochlear implantation. *Otol Neurotol.* 2020;41:173−177.

57. Ziade G, Mojallal A, Ho-Asjoe M, et al. Ethnicity and nonsurgical rhinoplasty. *Aesthet Surg J*. 2022:1−7.
58. Lam SM. Preface: considerations in non-Caucasian facial plastic surgery. *Facial Plast Clin N Am*. 2010;18:xiii.
59. Wu RT, Peck CJ, Shultz BN, et al. Racial disparities in cleft palate repair. *Plast Reconstr Surg*. 2019;143:1738−1745.
60. Pattisapu P, Raol NP. Healthcare equity in pediatric otolaryngology. *Otolaryngol Clin*. 2022;55:1287−1299.
61. Qian ZJ, Alyono JC, Jin MC, et al. Opioid prescribing patterns following pediatric tonsillectomy in the United States, 2009−2017. *Laryngoscope*. 2021;131:E1722−E1729.
62. Brown C, Shah GB, Mitchell RB, et al. The incidence of pediatric tracheostomy and its association among Black children. *Otolaryngol Head Neck Surg*. 2021;164:206−211.
63. Friesen TL, Zamora SM, Rahmanian R, et al. Predictors of pediatric tracheostomy outcomes in the United States. *Otolaryngol Head Neck Surg*. 2020;163:591−599.
64. Johnson RF, Brown CM, Beams DR, et al. Racial influences on pediatric tracheostomy outcomes. *Laryngoscope*. 2022;132:1118−1124.
65. Bowe SN, Megwalu UC, Bergmark RW, et al. Moving beyond detection: charting a path to eliminate health care disparities in otolaryngology. *Otolaryngol Head Neck Surg*. 2022;166:1013−1021.

The integration of sex and gender considerations in otolaryngology

4

Sarah N. Bowe[1], Erynne A. Faucett[2]

[1]*Department of Otolaryngology—Head and Neck Surgery, San Antonio Uniformed Services Health Education Consortium, JBSA-Ft. Sam Houston, TX, United States;* [2]*Department of Otolaryngology—Head and Neck Surgery, University of California-Davis, Sacramento, CA, United States*

Historical perspectives

The results of mostly single-sex investigations, in addition to the many studies that have not reported the sex of animals, cells, or tissues used, have contributed to an incomplete evidence base about sex-based influences on biology and health and spurred numerous policy changes. One of the first funding organizations to discuss the appropriate use of women and minority groups in research was the National Institute of Health (NIH) in 1993.[1] A component of the NIH Revitalization Act states that "in the case of any clinical trial in which women or members of minority groups will be included as subjects, the Director of NIH shall ensure that the trial is designed and carried out in a manner sufficient to provide for valid analysis of whether the variables being studied in the trial affect women or members of minority groups, as the case may be, differently than other subjects."[1] Thus, this language clearly illustrated the importance of sex inclusion, reporting, and analysis for clinical studies. Reporting policies by biomedical journals have also evolved over time. In 1978, the International Committee of Medical Journal Editors (ICMJE) produced the first Uniform Requirements for Manuscripts Submitted to Biomedical Journals to standardize manuscript format and preparation across journals.[2] Since that time, the document has been renamed and provides "Recommendations for the Conduct, Reporting, Editing, and Publication of Scholarly Work in Medical Journals." The most recent update, in May 2022, encourages the "correct use of the terms sex (when reporting biological factors) and gender (identity, psychosocial, or cultural factors)," as well as the incorporation of these concepts throughout the methods, results, and discussion sections of an article.[3] In 2016, an editorial in the *Journal of American Medical Association (JAMA)* noted that "more work is needed to standardize the way sex and gender are reported and elucidate the way these characteristics function independently and together to influence health and health care."[4] The authors concluded with the following recommendations for reporting in research articles: (1) use the terms *sex* when reporting biological factors and *gender* when reporting gender

Healthcare Disparities in Otolaryngology. https://doi.org/10.1016/B978-0-443-10714-6.00015-8

identity or psychosocial or cultural factors; (2) disaggregate demographic and all outcome data by sex, gender, or both; (3) report the methods used to obtain information on sex, gender, or both; and (4) note all limitations of these methods. Coincidentally, the Sex and Gender Equity in Research (SAGER) guidelines were released that same year and represented the culmination of a four-year development process commissioned by the European Association of Science Editors.[5] The guidelines, along with their accompanying checklist, are designed to guide authors in preparing their manuscripts, but can also be instrumental during the research design process. Likewise, the guidelines can be utilized by the editorial community to support the review of manuscripts before consideration for publication.

Definitions

Sex and gender are complex constructs that are interrelated, but conceptually distinct. This chapter discusses the role of sex (biological construct) and gender (social construct) in research and reporting. Sex generally refers to a set of biological attributes that are associated with anatomical and physiological features (e.g., chromosomes, external genitalia, gonads, hormones, and secondary sex characteristics).[6] A binary sex categorization (i.e., female or male) is usually designated at birth ('sex assigned at birth'), most often based solely on the visible external genitalia of the newborn. Gender generally refers to a set of social attributes that links gender identity and gender expression, including expectations about behaviors, characteristics, and status that occur in a historical and cultural context and may vary across societies and over time. Like sex, a binary categorization (i.e., female/male or woman/man) is usually emphasized; however, gender attributes are fluid, with more than two-thirds of women and men reporting gender-related characteristics traditionally attributed to the opposite sex.[7] Gender influences how people view themselves and each other, how they behave and interact, and how power is distributed in society. As such, gender is an equally important variable as biological sex, influencing the behavior of patients, clinicians, and communities (Fig. 4.1).

Sex and gender are often used interchangeably but are distinct constructs. While both are frequently portrayed as binary and unchanging, they instead exist on a continuum with additional sex categorizations and gender identities, including intersex/differences in sex development (DSD), transgender, or nonbinary/gender diverse. The growing visibility of the intersex and transgender populations, as well as efforts to improve the measurement of sex and gender across many scientific fields, "has brought to light the limitations of these assumptions and demonstrated the need to reconsider how sex, gender, and the relationship between them are conceptualized."[6] The collection of sex and gender variables occurs routinely in administrative and research data and thus can have far-reaching consequences for sexual and gender minorities in health care. Between 2021 and 2022, 19 NIH entities, in association with the National Academies, collaborated to produce a comprehensive report on "Measuring Sex, Gender Identity, and Sexual Orientation," further supporting this necessary work.

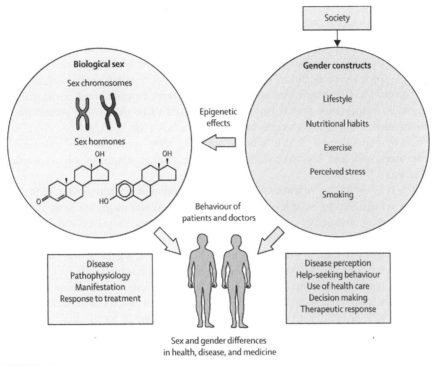

FIGURE 4.1

Interrelation between sex and gender in health, disease, and medicine.

Credit: The Lancet.

Sex and gender in medicine

Having established the importance of sex and gender as modifiers of health and disease, we will begin by summarizing their influences on the most common causes of death in the United States.[7] In 2021, nine of the ten leading causes of death remained the same as in 2020.[8] The top leading cause in 2021 was heart disease, followed by cancer and COVID-19. In most diseases, efforts to separate the effects of sex and gender are incomplete, so throughout the next sections, we will often refer to the differences among women and men. However, in instances in which the comments refer specifically to biological factors, female and male will be used. As knowledge regarding pathophysiology, diagnosis, and treatment of disease is primarily based on men, comments will be focused on how women differ from men. Additionally, we acknowledge that both sex and gender have typically been conceptualized as binary, yet this does not capture the multidimensional nature of these constructs or their underlying complexity for those with intersex traits or those identifying with or expressing gender diversity. However, the available literature has not included this more expansive view on sex and gender; as a result, there will be little reference to categories beyond those of women and men or females and males.

Heart disease

Heart disease is the leading cause of death in the United States, accounting for 20.1% of all deaths in 2021.[8] Ischemic heart disease and heart failure are the major contributors to heart disease mortality. Ischemic heart disease is the most recognized example for integrating the concepts of sex and gender, which shapes distinct disease outcomes. Compared with men, women suffering from ischemic heart disease are older; a difference that is historically believed to be due to the protection of endogenous estrogens, although more recent studies have begun to refute this simplistic explanation.[9,10] Still, women suffering from ischemic heart disease are underdiagnosed and less likely to have a prehospital diagnosis of myocardial infarction.[11,12]

The reasons for this disparity reflect the intersection of sex and gender. First, biological sex differences exist regarding pathogenesis. While males are more likely to be affected by obstructive coronary artery disease of large vessels, coronary microvascular dysfunction leading to chronic myocardial ischemia without obstructive coronary artery disease is more likely in females. Second, a gender bias contributes to the absence of recognition of ischemic heart disease presentation in women. Both men and women with ischemic heart disease who score high on feminine roles and personality traits, on questionnaires designed to ascertain aspects of gender, are at an increased risk of recurrent ischemic disease, independent of female sex.[13]

Women suffering from ischemic heart disease are also less likely to receive evidence-based treatment and when having an acute myocardial infarction, they are less likely to receive reperfusion.[11,12] Women presenting with an acute myocardial infarction treated by male emergency physicians have higher mortality rates than those treated by female physicians.[14] Interestingly, male physicians are more effective at treating women presenting with acute myocardial infarction when they work with more female colleagues and when they have more experience treating female patients. Treatment disparities can also be corrected by improving emergency recognition and management of ST-elevation myocardial infarction in general with the use of standardized protocols and systems.[15]

Cancer

Cancers are the second leading cause of death, accounting for 17.5% of all deaths in 2021.[8] More men develop cancer than women; with few exceptions (e.g., meningioma, thyroid cancer, lung cancer in nonsmokers), nonreproductive cancers exhibit a 2:1 male predominance.[16] In some cases, including oropharyngeal, laryngeal, esophageal, and bladder cancer, the male versus female incidence ratios can be as high as 4:1. Male predominance in those cancers that affect both sexes is evident globally, in all races, and at all ages.[16] This higher cancer risk can be partially explained by gender influences, such as dietary habits or smoking and alcohol consumption; however, this elevated risk still persists even after appropriate adjustment for these risk factors.[17] Moreover, a male bias in incidence and survival also exists before puberty and the adoption of high-risk behaviors.[18]

The fundamental role of sex, in addition to gender, in cancer biology is supported by the nearly universal male predominance in cancer incidence, as well as noted differential outcomes.[7] Sex-specific biology includes broad genetic differences (XX vs. XY chromosomes), escape from X-inactivation in female individuals (which allows the expression of both alleles of X-encoded tumor suppressor genes in female cells), Y chromosome-encoded oncogenes, and chromatin remodeling effects of in-utero testicular testosterone in male cells.[19–21] These differences exert an influence on several of the hallmarks of cancer, including angiogenesis, immunity, growth regulation, and metabolism, which contribute to cancer predisposition and outcomes.[22,23]

Additionally, the treatment of cancer will be improved by incorporating sex- and gender-specific approaches. Previously, little was known about the effect of patients' sex on the efficacy of immune checkpoint inhibitors as cancer treatment.[24] Conforti et al. performed a systematic review and meta-analysis of randomized controlled trials (RCTs) of immune checkpoint inhibitors (ipilimumab, tremelimumab, nivolumab, or pembrolizumab) that reported overall survival according to patients' sex. Immune checkpoint inhibitors were found to improve overall survival for patients with advanced cancers, such as melanoma and nonsmall-cell lung cancer, but the magnitude of benefit was sex-dependent, with a significantly higher overall survival in males compared to females.[24] Future research should focus on improving the effectiveness of immunotherapies in females, potentially exploring different immunotherapeutic approaches between the sexes.

More recently, sex-based differences in adverse events (AEs) in patients receiving immunotherapy, targeted therapy, or chemotherapy have been examined.[25] Females had a 34% increased risk of severe AEs compared with males, including a 49% increased risk among those receiving immunotherapy. Females also experienced an increased risk of severe symptomatic AEs among all treatments, but especially immunotherapy. In addition, females receiving chemotherapy or immunotherapy experienced increased severe hematologic AEs.[25] The greater severity of both symptomatic and hematologic AEs indicates that sex-based differences exist. However, it is also possible that this could reflect variation in the rate and extent of reporting AEs, which would represent a gender-based interpretation on the results. In this study, the disparities noted by sex were found in objectively reported side effects, including lab test results, which would not be influenced by gender. Regardless, particularly large sex differences were observed for patients receiving immunotherapy, suggesting that studying AEs from these agents should be a priority and include efforts to examine the influence of both sex and gender on the findings.

COVID-19

The still-ongoing coronavirus pandemic showcases how profoundly clinical outcomes can be affected by sex and gender. Sex, a biological attribute, and gender, a social construct, may both influence an individual's susceptibility, vulnerability, and exposure to infectious disease.[26] Immune function differs between the sexes; the sex hormones, estrogens and androgens which exist in varying functional levels, respectively, in females and males are cited as the underlying cause for the differential immune response to COVID-19.[27] Evidence shows that estrogen modulates the immune system to protect females from severe inflammation, whereas androgen has been implicated in overactivation of immune cells, cytokine storm, and the resultant severe inflammation, which predisposes males to severe COVID-19. The innate recognition and response to viruses as well as downstream adaptive immune responses during viral infections also differ between females and males. Furthermore, sex differences in the expression and activity of angiotensin-converting enzyme 2, the COVID-19 receptor, has been identified as another potential source of variability in pathogenesis.[28]

Differential disease prevalence between men and women may also be related to cultural roles and gender norms that influence the risk for contracting COVID-19, such as a higher likelihood of employment in essential services (e.g., health care, service industries) for women compared with men.[26] Gender inequality and biases within a society or health care system may also impact who receives a medical test. Tadiri and colleagues sought to investigate whether gender inequality was associated with sex ratios of SARS-CoV-2 positivity and death from COVID-19.[26] The authors found that institutionalized gender inequality, as measured by the United Nations Development Project's Gender Inequality Index, was positively associated with the male:female ratio of reported cases of COVID-19 among counties that reported sex-disaggregated data. While their findings suggest that gender inequality could play a role in epidemiological differences by sex, it is also possible that this reflects differential access to health care and testing resources. Expectantly, the authors conclude that continued investigation of both biological (i.e., sex) and social (i.e., gender) variables and their influence on COVID-19 exposure and vulnerability are necessary.[26]

Unfortunately, despite the implications of sex and gender for COVID-19 diagnosis, treatment, and prognosis, these variables are still rarely accounted for. As vaccination is one of the key responses to the COVID-19 pandemic, it is vital that sex and gender differences be acknowledged, measured, and analyzed in clinical research.[29] Yet, in 75 clinical trials on COVID-19 vaccines, only 24% presented their main outcome data (i.e., vaccine effectiveness and safety profile) disaggregated by sex. Furthermore, only 13% included sex and/or gender as a point in their discussion section.[29] Thus, despite preexisting and increasing calls from funders, research governance bodies, academic journals, and publishers, sex and gender dimensions continue to go overlooked within the very recent body of research on COVID-19 vaccines.

Sex and gender in surgery
General surgery basic and preclinical research

Basic science and translational research serves as the foundation for clinical research, thus there is an imperative to understand sex-based differences in models of disease. Yoon and colleagues performed the first study within any surgical discipline to determine whether a sex bias exists within the basic science and translational literature.[30] All original manuscripts published in the *Annals of Surgery*, *American Journal of Surgery*, *JAMA Surgery*, *Journal of Surgical Research*, and *Surgery* from January 1, 2022 to December 31, 2012 were reviewed. Pertinent variables included the sex of each animal (if specified), the sex of the cells used (if specified), and the presence of sex-based reporting. Sex-based reporting was defined as presenting the results of both females and males separately. The authors also sought to assess sex-based disparities and reporting over time. They examined manuscripts from the *Journal of Surgical Research* during the calendar years 1991, 2001, and 2011 for the previously listed variables.

A total of 618 publications reported the use of animals and/or cells.[30] Of these, 199 (32%) did not specify the sex of the animals or cells. Of those publications that did specify the sex, 333 (80%) studied only males, 71 (17%) only females, and 13 (3%) both sexes. Out of the 618 publications, 531 (86%) included animals. Of these, 117 (22%) did not specify the sex. For those that did specify, 331 (80%) studied only males, 70 (17%) only females, and 11(3%) both sexes. One hundred and eighteen (19%) publications included research using cells. Of these, a larger percentage (90; 75%) failed to specify sex compared to animal studies. Of those publications that did specify sex, 20 (71%) included only males, 6 (21%) only females, and 2 (7%) both sexes.

Out of the 618 studies, only 13 included both females and males.[30] For the animal studies, 8 (62%) matched the number of females and males, and 7 (54%) provided sex-based reporting. For the cell studies, none matched females and males or included sex-base reporting. When evaluating publications over time, the authors noted that animal studies included a greater absolute number of males and number of male-only animal publications in more recent years compared to earlier years.

The authors recognized that sex-conscious research is the responsibility of numerous communities and entities and provide a series of recommendations.[30] First, journals should adjust the author guidelines to require all studies to state the sex of the animal or cell used. They indicated that they communicated with the editors for each of the studied journals and at the time of the publication, two of the journals had implemented the changes and the other three had stated that they would make the changes. Second, they proposed that the Federal Drug Administration should require in the inclusion of both females and males in preclinical and clinical research, along with sex-based reporting of all results. Third, they suggested that the NIH take a stronger stance and require equal representation of females and males in all preclinical funded research. Lastly, the authors implored industry to incorporate better representation and analysis of sex within studies.

General surgery clinical research

As an extension of their previous work, Mansukhanin and colleagues set out to determine if sex bias existed in human surgical clinical research.[31] Adequately controlling for sex as a variable with inclusion, data reporting, and data analysis is critical as data derived from clinical research serve as the foundation for evidence-based medicine. The authors evaluated original manuscripts published from January 1, 2011 through December 31, 2012 in the top five ranked American nonspecialty journals, *Annals of Surgery, American Journal of Surgery, JAMA Surgery, Journal of Surgical Research*, and *Surgery*. The authors evaluated the presence of sex-based data reporting, which included sex-based reporting of data, analysis of data by sex, and inclusion of sex-based results in the discussion section. The degree of sex matching was also calculated. The lesser number of subjects (female or male) was defined as the numerator and the greater number as the denominator. The percent matching was calculated as the ratio of the numerator/denominator multiplied by 100. A 50% matching of female and male subjects would include 25 females and 50 females ($25/50 \times 100 = 50\%$).

Of the 1303 manuscripts that were reviewed, 1078 (83%) stated the sex of the subjects included in the study, while 225 (17%) did not.[31] While there was a consistent pattern among all five journals, a significant difference was identified. The *American Journal of Surgery* had the most with sex not stated (26%) compared to the *Annals of Surgery* that had the least (8%). Of all the studies included, only 38% reported data separately for male and female subjects, only 33% performed statistical analysis on data collected by sex, and only 23% of articles addressed sex-based results in the discussion section. There was notable variability between specialties; colorectal, oncological, endocrine, and thoracic surgery were the highest performers in sex-based data reporting, analysis, and discussion of the data. In contrast, breast, bariatric, and cardiac surgery were the lowest performers. There was also a significant difference in overall distribution of female, male, and unspecified subjects by specialty.

While the implications of these findings are far-reaching, the authors highlight three important points.[31] First, drugs, therapies, and devices may be developed that are effective for only one sex. Second, for therapies or drugs that are reported to have an overall low efficacy when the data are aggregated, it may be abandoned, but it could have greater efficacy in one sex versus the other. Third, therapies may be developed that have undesirable side effects in one sex compared to the other. Additionally, the authors acknowledge that there was specification regarding the difference between sex and gender, such that their study focused solely on the differences between phenotypic female and male sex. Regardless, performing independent data reporting and analysis can yield discoveries that are valuable to all individuals.

Orthopedic surgery basic and preclinical research

With an awareness that sex bias in basic and preclinical research was identified in general surgery, Bryant et al. decided to examine the orthopedic literature.[32] A review of all basic science and translational research articles published from January 1, 2014 to December 31, 2014 was undertaken in the following journals: *The Journal of Bone and Joint Surgery, Clinical Orthopaedics and Relations Research, The Bone and Joint Journal*, and *Journal of Orthopaedic Research*. Variables included the following: number of female and male specimens (for animal and cadaver studies); sex of animals, cells, or cadavers (female only, male only, or both female and male); and presence of sex-based reporting of data (defined as reporting of results by sex). To assess for changes in sex-specific reporting over time, articles in the *Journal of Orthopaedic Research* were evaluated in 1994, 2004, and 2014.

Two hundred and fifty articles met inclusion criteria with 122 (49%) animal studies, 71 (28%) cell studies, and 57 (23%) human cadaver studies.[32] In 88 (35%) articles, there was no reporting of the sex of animals, cells, or cadavers. Of the 162 articles that did report sex, 40 (25%) used only females, 69 (43%) used only males, and 53 (33%) used both sexes; of those using both sexes, only 7 (13%) performed sex-based reporting of their data.

The authors reported the sex of the animal in 99/122 (81%) of the studies.[32] Thirty-two (32%) used only females, 60 (61%) used only males, and 7 (7%) both sexes. In the seven studies that used both sexes, only one (14%) performed sex-based analysis. Of the 71 cell studies, 44 (62%) did not provide details on sex. Of the 27 (38%) that did, 15 (56%) used both sexes, 6 (22%) only females, and 6 (22%) only males. Of those utilizing both sexes, 2/15 (13%) provided sex-based reporting. Regarding the cadaver studies, 21/57 (37%) did not specify the sex of the specimen. Of the 36 studies that did, 31 (86%) utilized both sexes, 2 (6%) only females, and 3 (8%) only males. Sex-based reporting was performed for 4/31 (13%) of the cadaver studies.

When looking at sex-specific result reporting, 4/7 (57%) articles analyzed the impact of sex on outcome measures, with all four finding sex-specific differences.[32] In the other three articles, details were provided on specimen sex; however, there was no additional analysis about the impact on outcome measures. When the *Journal of Orthopaedic Research* publications were evaluated over time, 104 total articles reported the sex of the specimen used, 25 (24%) used both sexes, 31 (30%) females only, and 48 (46%) males only. There was a significant increase in articles specifying sex, and no other significant findings were present.

Given the known influence of sex on outcomes, the authors suggest that reporting of sex in orthopedic research should be mandatory.[32] They recommended that research on animals, cells, or cadavers be performed on both sexes and simultaneously encouraged journals to mandate such study. At a minimum, if only one sex is used, the authors stated that researchers should have to justify the use of only a single-sex model.

Orthopedic surgery clinical research

Recognizing that significant differences have been identified in the prevalence of orthopedic conditions and treatment outcomes between females and males within individuals studies, Hettrich et al. aimed to evaluate whether this had changed over time or was different based on journal type (i.e., general orthopedics vs. subspecialty).[33] Two general orthopedic journals were selected, *Journal of Bone and Joint Surgery (American Volume)* and *Clinical Orthopedics and Related Research*, as well as three subspecialty journals, *Journal of Shoulder and Elbow Surgery, Spine*, and *American Journal of Sports Medicine*. Issues published during even-numbered months of 2000, 2005, and 2010 were critically assessed for the presence of sex-specific analyses. To be marked as having a sex-specific analysis, an article had to include sex in a multifactorial statistical model.

Overall, the proportion of sex-specific analyses increased between 2000 and 2005 (19% and 27%, respectively), but did not subsequently increase in 2010 (30%).[33] Specialty journals had significantly higher reporting rates than general orthopedic journals in 2000 (28% compared to 12%, respectively), but not in 2005 (33%−23%, respectively) or 2010 (33%−28%, respectively). While there was some improvement over time, 70% of the included clinical studies did not perform sex-specific analysis. Understanding how females and males may have different presentations for the same diagnosis or may have different treatment responses based on sex can ultimately improve patient care and outcomes.

The foundational work of Yoon and colleagues has also been used as a model for evaluating sex bias in hand surgery.[34] Four major hand and upper extremity publications, *Journal of Hand Surgery (American Volume), Hand, Journal of Hand Surgery (European Volume)*, and *Plastic and Reconstructive Surgery*, were reviewed from January 1, 2014 to December 31, 2015. Compared with the findings of Mansukhani et al., most hand surgery studies stated the sex of participants, 90%, compared to 83% in general surgery.[31,34] Of all the studies included, only 23% performed statistical analysis on data collected by sex in hand surgery, compared to 33% in general surgery. In contrast, 32% of hand surgery articles addressed sex-based results in the discussion session, compared to 23% in general surgery.[31,34]

Overall, the different journals had similar distributions of studies where sex was stated, sex-based analysis was performed, and sex-based differences were discussed.[34] While there was an overall higher percentage of female participants compared to male participants within the included studies, most studies included more male participants. There was also variation noted among the journals; *Plastic and Reconstructive Surgery* and *Journal of Hand Surgery (European Volume)* were weighted toward male-predominant studies, while *Hand* and *Journal of Hand Surgery (American Volume)* were more equitably distributed.[34]

Like the general surgery literature, Kalliainen and colleagues noted a paucity of evidence regarding sex-based analysis and discussion. As a result, they urged the hand surgery community to address this knowledge gap in future research endeavors.

Sex and gender in otolaryngology

Despite known sex-based differences in diseases of the head and neck, such as thyroid disease and head and neck cancer, limited data exist regarding sex bias in the broader otolaryngology literature. Stephenson and colleagues sought to determine if sex bias exists within general otolaryngology basic science and translational research.[35] Published original articles with animal subjects, human subject cells, or commercial cell lines in all 2016 and 2017 issues of *The Laryngoscope*, *Otolaryngology-Head and Neck Surgery*, and *JAMA Otolaryngology-Head and Neck Surgery* were reviewed. Variables included reporting of cell or animal sex, breakdown of subjects by sex, sex-based statistical analysis, and presence of any statistically significant sex differences.

Of the 144 basic/translational research articles, sex was not reported in 48% (69/144).[35] Of the 75 studies that reported sex, 22 (29%) included both sexes, and 11 (15%) analyzed data by sex. One hundred and five articles used animal subjects, of which 54 (52%) did not report the sex of the subjects. Of the 50 studies that reported sex, animals of single sex were used in 48 (96%) studies and only 3 (6%) analyzed data by sex. Fifty-four studies used commercial cell lines or human/animal subject cells; 26 (48%) reported sex. Data analysis by sex was included in 8 (15%) articles. The authors noted that despite efforts from the NIH to address the sex bias present across all medical and surgical fields, otolaryngology research continues to exhibit results that are just as poor, if not worse, than other surgical literature.

Farzal et al. expanded their evaluation of sex bias within the otolaryngology literature to include original clinical studies.[36] The authors reviewed all articles in 2016 in *The Laryngoscope*, *Otolaryngology-Head and Neck Surgery*, and *JAMA Otolaryngology-Head and Neck Surgery*. Pertinent data included the number/sex of subjects, >50% sex matching (SM $_{\geq 50}$), and sex-based statistical analysis. To analyze whether studies met a minimum standard for sex matching, the SM$_{\geq 50}$ criteria (which indicates that at least half as many participants of the lesser-represented sex compared to the majority sex were included), previously described by Mansukhani and colleagues, were utilized.[31] A total of 1209 articles were included, with the most common being head and neck (n = 196, 71%) and otology (n = 110, 18%).[36] A total of 544/600 studies (91%) reported participant sex, whereas 56 studies (9%) did not. Sex-based statistical analysis was performed in 280/600 studies (47%). Neither sex-reporting rates nor sex-based analysis rates were different between the three journals.

Among otolaryngology subspecialties, the head and neck surgery literature most frequently performed sex-based statistical analysis (54%), followed by pediatric otolaryngology (52%) and rhinology (48%).[36] SM $_{\geq 50}$ was the highest in pediatric otolaryngology (87%) and otology (82%) and the lowest in head and neck surgery (41%) and sleep medicine (30%). The disciplines least frequently performing statistical analysis by sex included facial plastics, laryngology, and sleep medicine (33% each).

Overall, sex-matching rates were higher in certain disciplines compared to others; however, some discrepancies may be appropriate depending on the underlying nature of the study.[36] For instance, in head and neck surgery, some diseases have a sex predisposition, such as a higher prevalence of oral cavity and oropharyngeal cancers in men and thyroid disorders/cancer in women. This may influence the ability to engage in sex-matching if a study is retrospective in nature and patients are evaluated over a certain timeframe. However, such findings support the intention to perform sex-matching of individuals in prospective studies to better analyze outcomes by sex.

Farzal and colleagues performed subset analysis on 30 RCTs.[36] Two studies (7%) did not state participant sex. Nineteen RCTs (68%) met SM $_{\geq 50}$, whereas twelve (40%) performed sex-based analysis. This rate of statistical analysis by sex was less than that found in the overall clinical otolaryngology literature. With RCTs serving as the basis for new treatment recommendations or departures from existing treatment algorithms, the authors implored the otolaryngology community to achieve higher standards of sex inclusion, reporting, and analysis, particularly in RCTs, which by their nature provide the ability to control this starting at the design phase.

Sex and gender in the otolaryngology subspecialties
Otology

Regarding the auditory system, males show longer delays in auditory brainstem responses and distortion product otoacoustic emissions than females, a phenomenon typically attributed to the slightly longer length of the male cochlea.[37] The presence of these differences has implications for the function of the auditory system and its susceptibility to noise-induced hearing loss (NIHL). The question of sex-specific effects is best studied in animals, where noise exposure can be precisely controlled. Lauer and Schrode sought to establish a baseline in basic and preclinical studies of NIHL for the five-year period prior to the implementation of the mandate to include sex as a biological variable in NIH-funded research.[37]

Publications indexed in PubMed were reviewed from January 1, 2011 to December 31, 2015.[37] The search term "noise induced hearing loss" yielded 1209 articles. After inclusion and exclusion criteria were applied, the authors were left with 210 studies. Variables included the total number of subjects, sex of subjects (female, male, both, not specified), total number of female and male subjects, data reported separately by sex, effects of ovarian hormones or cycles, and sex-specific data reported when both sexes were tested. The sex of the animals used was stated in 154 studies (73%), whereas 56 studies (27%) did not report sex.[37] The total number of studies reporting use of only male participants followed a similar pattern to the total number of NIHL studies overall. The percentage of male-only studies increased from 2011 (37%) to 2015 (56%). The total number and percentage of studies reporting the use of both sexes dropped in half from 2011 (20%) to 2015 (10%). Only two studies (1%) reported sex-specific results.

The data indicate that sex bias in basic and preclinical research worsened in the years prior to the NIH mandate.[37] These findings are consistent with data from the broader biomedical literature. Beery and Zuker examined sex bias in research on mammals in 10 biological fields.[38] Male bias was evident in eight disciplines and most prominent in neuroscience, of which auditory neuroscience can be considered a subfield. Over the course of evaluating six or more decades of literature, the authors found increased male bias in neuroscience and biomedical research over time.

Rhinology

Stephenson and colleagues noted a gap in analyzing the rhinology literature and sought to determine whether sex bias and underreporting existed within rhinology basic science, translational research, and clinical studies.[39] Published original manuscripts in all 2016 issues of *Rhinology, American Journal of Rhinology and Allergy*, and *International Forum of Allergy and Rhinology* were reviewed. Studies were examined for mention of cell, animal, or human sex, sex breakdown, sex matching (SM $_{\geq 50}$), sex-based analysis, and presence of statistically significant sex differences in the results. Between sex and gender, "sex" is reported more frequently than "gender" as a demographic variable in clinical studies. This was the case in 100% of reviewed studies, none of which provided any discussion of the sex versus gender demographics; thus, the authors continued to utilize the term sex throughout their article.

Within the basic science and translational research literature, sex breakdown was provided in 55% (24/44) of human cell/tissue and animal studies.[39] Of the 24 studies that reported subject sex, 2 (8.3%) performed sex-based analysis. Four additional cell studies used commercial cell lines, none of which reported cell sex. Within the clinical research, sex was specified in 93% (188/202) of the included studies and SM $_{\geq 50}$ was noted in 82% (154/188) of those studies.[39] Sex-based statistical analysis was not performed in 97/102 (48%) studies. Out of the 105 (52%) studies that included sex-based analysis, 29 (28%) reported at least one statistically significant difference based on sex. Concerningly, sex underreporting and lack of sex-based data analysis was prevalent in the existing rhinology literature, particularly for basic science research, which serves as the foundation for future animal and clinical studies.

In 2022, spurred by the previous work of Stephenson et al., Ramkumar and colleagues proceeded with a scoping review to evaluate the contemporary literature on sex-based differences in rhinology, with a particular focus on anatomy, physiology, disease burden, treatment outcomes, and impact on quality of life (QoL).[39,40] The authors performed a scoping review according to Preferred Reporting Items for Systematic Review and Meta-Analysis guidelines. A combination of keywords was utilized: "rhinology" with the following, "sex," "gender," "hormones," "sex hormones," "pregnancy," "menopause," and "chronic rhinosinusitis."[40]

A qualitative analysis was performed after classifying articles into three major categories, notably, anatomy, physiology, and rhinologic pathology.[40] Significant differences were identified in nasal, sinus, and skull base anatomy based on biological sex. Baseline physiology of females and males varied, particularly influenced by hormonal changes, which include those of puberty and perimenopause/menopause. In respect to rhinologic pathology, the authors presented sex-based differences relating to chronic rhinosinusitis, rhinitis, olfactory dysfunction, and sinonasal malignancies. The authors stated that there is a paucity of literature and further research is needed to offer evidence-based treatment guidelines based on sex as a biological variable.

Laryngology

Within laryngology, the impact of female hormones on the voice, anatomical variations in the larynx, and differences in the pathophysiology of laryngeal disease have been associated with clinically significant differences in sex-based outcomes.[41] Knowing this, Pasick et al. decided to assess the broader laryngology literature for evidence of sex bias both within research and publishing. The authors reviewed articles from 2019 in seven otolaryngology journals: *JAMA Otolaryngology-Head and Neck Surgery*, *The Laryngoscope*, *Otolaryngology-Head and Neck Surgery*, *Annals of Otology, Rhinology, and Laryngology*, *Journal of Voice*, *Logopedics Phoniatrics Vocology*, and *Folia Phoniatrica et Logopaedica*. Study data were extracted, including the number of subjects, sex of subjects, and whether sex-based analysis was performed. In addition, the presence of sex-matching (SM $_{\geq 50}$) was determined.

A total of 259 patient-centered, original articles met the inclusion criteria; only 14 (5%) did not report sex.[41] Of those reporting sex, 17 (52%) included only female, 10 (4%) only male, and 2 (1%) male-to-female transgender individuals. SM $_{\geq 50}$ was reached in 114/259 (44%) studies. Ninety five (37%) studies performed sex-based analysis. Uniquely, this review identified two studies that included exclusively male-to-female participants. The estimated prevalence of transgender individuals is between 0.5% and 1.3% for birth-assigned males and 0.4% and 1.2% for birth-assigned females.[42] Thus, within the laryngology literature, there is burgeoning recognition and support to study aspects of otolaryngology specific to the transgender population (For further information, consider referring to Chapter 6: Transgender Care in Otolaryngology: An Emerging Field).

Bibliometric data were also assessed and included the sexes of all study authors and the position of study authors.[41] Author sex was determined by a manual internet search. When sex could not be ascertained, a "baby name guesser," which has been used in previous studies, was incorporated into the study. Forty-one percent of first and senior authors were female. Studies with female first and/or senior authors did not differ in rates of SM $_{\geq 50}$ or sex-based analysis compared to studies with male first and senior author. This finding was like that of Xiao and colleagues, who performed a bibliometric analysis of the broader surgical literature.[43] No sex-based differences occurred between female and male authors in sex reporting, sex-based analysis, or discussion of the data.

Sex and gender reporting policies in preeminent biomedical journals

Recently, Bibb and colleagues identified a segment of prominent biomedical journals in order to analyze their sex and gender reporting policies.[44] Cross-sectional analysis of 20 journals with the highest 2020 impact factor for each of the 10 largest US medical specialties was performed. The authors evaluated whether the included journals:

(1) had a sex and/or gender reporting policy; (2) distinguished between or defined sex and gender; (3) required researchers to report their methods for determining sex and/or gender; and (4) required collection of both sex and gender. Guidelines for 190 journals were analyzed, because 10 journals are among the top 20 for two different specialties. Among the 190 journals, 65 (34%) stated a policy for reporting sex and/or gender in their author guidelines; 46 (24%) explicitly distinguished between or defined the terms *gender* and *sex*; 31 (16%) recommended or required researchers to report their methods for determining sex and gender; and 3 (2%) required researchers to report both sex and gender demographics. Among the 10 specialties, obstetrics and gynecology had the largest percentage of journals with a sex and gender reporting policy (13/20; 65%), while ophthalmology had the smallest percentage (5/20; 25%). Overall, the authors found a paucity of policies outlining appropriate collection and reporting of sex and gender variables. While researchers must be held accountable for appropriate design and reporting, the adoption of journal guidelines would encourage greater inclusion, rigor, and reproducibility of future studies.

Sex and gender reporting policies in preeminent otolaryngology journals

Using the study by Bibb et al. as a model, we performed a cross-sectional analysis of the top 20 journals within the otorhinolaryngology subject category using the SCImago Journal and Country Rank.[44] The SCImago Journal and Country Rank was utilized as it is a publicly available portal that includes the journals and country scientific indicators developed from the information contained in the Scopus database.[45,46] The journals were assessed by the chapter authors to determine whether they: (1) had a sex and/or gender reporting policy; (2) distinguished between or defined sex and gender; (3) required researchers to report their methods for determining sex and/or gender; and (4) required collection of both sex and gender. In addition, the journals' publisher was also recorded, because author guidelines may be directed by the supporting publisher.

Among the 20 journals, 6 (30%) stated a policy for reporting sex and/or gender in their author guidelines; 6 (30%) explicitly distinguished between or defined the terms *gender* and *sex*; 5 (25%) recommended or required researchers to report their methods for determining sex and gender; and 0 (0%) required researchers to report both sex and gender demographics (Table 4.1).

Generally, if there was a policy for reporting sex and/or gender, then the policy explicitly distinguished between *gender* and *sex* and recommended or required that researchers reported their methods. There was only one journal, *Ear and Hearing*, that fulfilled the first two criteria, but did not require reporting of the methods. In some cases, there was not a universal publisher policy, because there was variation between journals produced by a given publisher; this was noted with the Springer Nature journals. In other cases, the publisher had a foundational policy that was utilized by all

Table 4.1 Characteristics of sex- and gender-based reporting policies in preeminent otolaryngology journals.

Journal*	Stated sex and/or gender reporting policy	Distinguish between or define sex and gender	Require reporting of methods used to determine sex and/or gender	Require collection of both sex and gender	Publisher
Rhinology	N	N	N	N	International Rhinologic Society
International forum of allergy and Rhinology	N	N	N	N	John Wiley and sons
JAMA	Y	Y	Y	N	American Medical Association
Otolaryngology—Head and Neck Surgery	N	N	N	N	SAGE publications/John Wiley and sons
Otolaryngology—Head and Neck Surgery	Y	Y	Y	N	Springer Nature
Journal of Otolaryngology—Head and Neck Surgery	Y	Y		N	Lippincott Williams and Wilkins
Ear and Hearing	Y	Y	N	N	Elsevier
Journal of cranio-maxillofacial Surgery	Y	Y	Y	N	
Laryngoscope	N	N	N	N	John Wiley and sons
Head and Neck	N	N	N	N	John Wiley and sons
Trends in Hearing	N	N	N	N	SAGE Publications
American journal of speech-Language Pathology	N	N	N	N	American speech-Language-Hearing Association
International journal of Oral and maxillofacial Surgery	Y	Y	Y	N	Elsevier

Journal					Publisher
Otology and neurotology	N	N	N	N	Wolters Kluwer Health
European archives of oto-rhino-Laryngology	N	N	N	N	Springer Nature
Journal of the Association for Research in Otolaryngology	N	N	N	N	Springer Nature
American journal of Rhinology and allergy	N	N	N	N	SAGE Publications
Clinical Otolaryngology	N	N	N	N	John Wiley and sons
Clinical and experimental Otorhinolaryngology	Y	Y	Y	N	Korean Society of Otorhinolaryngology
Orthodontics and craniofacial Research	N	N	N	N	John Wiley and sons
Audiology and neurotology	N	N	N	N	Karger Publishers
Total (Y/20; %)	6/20; 30%	6/20; 30%	5/20; 25%	0/20; 0%	

* Journals are listed in order as the top 20 according to SCImago Journal and Country Rank.

their journals; this was noted with Elsevier. Furthermore, upon reviewing numerous reporting policies, we believe that those provided by Elsevier are the most thorough and highly recommend that researchers and journals reference and/or adopt similar guidelines moving forward. The Elsevier reporting policies are noted below:

Elsevier reporting policies
Reporting sex- and gender-based analyses[47]
Reporting guidance

For research involving or pertaining to humans, animals, or eukaryotic cells, investigators should integrate sex and gender-based analyses (SGBA) into their research design according to funder/sponsor requirements and best practices within a field. Authors should address the sex and/or gender dimensions of their research in their article. In cases where they cannot, they should discuss this as a limitation to their research's generalizability. Importantly, authors should explicitly state what definitions of sex and/or gender they are applying to enhance the precision, rigor, and reproducibility of their research and to avoid ambiguity or conflation of terms and the constructs to which they refer (see Definitions section below). Authors can refer to the SAGER guidelines and the SAGER guidelines checklist. These offer systematic approaches to the use and editorial review of sex and gender information in study design, data analysis, outcome reporting, and research interpretation—however, please note there is no single, universally agreed-upon set of guidelines for defining sex and gender.

Best practice on sex and gender reporting in research[48]

Our guides for authors advise you on the use of inclusive language, discussed further in this *Authors' Update* article on using language to empower. We have introduced a section on reporting sex- and gender-based analyses including the use of the SAGER guidelines which recognize the importance of sex and gender within the research itself, a dimension of analysis that has a critical impact on research quality and outcomes. In addition to the guidance in our guides for authors on definitions and the SAGER guidelines, the resources below offer further insight around sex and gender in research studies:

- Institute of Gender and Health, Canadian Institutes of Health Research (updated April 2020)
- Albert K, Delano M. Sex trouble: sex/gender slippage, sex confusion, and sex obsession in machine learning using electronic health records. *Patterns (N Y)*. 2022;3(8):100534. Published 2022 Aug 12. https://doi.org/10.1016/j.patter.2022.100534
- DiMarco M, Zhao H, Boulicault M, Richardson SS. Why "sex as a biological variable" conflicts with precision medicine initiatives. *Cell Rep Med*. 2022;3(4):100550. https://doi.org/10.1016/j.xcrm.2022.100550

- Kronk CA, Everhart AR, Ashley F, et al. Transgender data collection in the electronic health record: current concepts and issues. *J Am Med Inform Assoc.* 2022;29(2):271−284. https://doi.org/10.1093/jamia/ocab136
- Schiebinger L. Sex, gender, and intersectional puzzles in health and biomedicine research. *Med (N Y).* 2022;3(5):284−287. https://doi.org/10.1016/j.medj.2022.04.003
- German Research Foundation (DFG), (Aug 2021; review checklist)
- Office of Research on Women's Health, National Institutes of Health (updated 2021)
- European Institute for Gender Equality, European Commission (2016)
- American Psychological Association style guide (2020)
- Hunt L, et al. A Framework for sex, gender, and diversity analysis in research. *Science.* 2022;377(6614):1492−1495.
- Stites SD, et al. Measuring sex and gender in U.S. Alzheimer's disease and related dementias (ADRD) research. *Alzheimer's & Dementia.* 2022;17(S3): e055012.

Summary and recommendations

The studies included throughout this chapter illustrate that sex as a biological variable in science and medicine has been increasingly well understood, yet the same cannot be said for gender as a sociocultural variable. Tannenbaum and colleagues declared that in order "to reach the full potential of sex and gender analysis for discovery and innovation, it is important to integrate sex and gender analysis, where relevant, into the design of research from the very beginning."[49] To achieve this, interlocking policies need to be implemented within the three pillars of research: funding agencies, peer-reviewed journals, and educational organizations.

Government-led funding agencies took the lead, starting as early as 1993 with the NIH Revitalization Act, mandating the inclusion of women in NIH clinical trials.[1] However, many investigators did not follow this mandate, and those who did still did not analyze the results by sex.[50] Fortunately, more recent requirements from other funding organizations, such as the Canadian Institutes of Health Research (CIHR), have shown promise. Johnson and colleagues conducted a descriptive statistical analysis to identify trends in application data from three research funding competitions (December 2010, June 2011, and December 2011).[51] The CIHR had introduced a policy in 2010 that required applicants to report how sex and/or gender would be accounted for in the research protocol or justify their exclusion. The authors noted that the proportion of applicants responding affirmatively to the questions on sex and gender increased over time (48% in December 2011 compared to 26% in December 2010). (Further details on "Major Granting Agencies' Policies for Integrating Sex and Gender Analysis into the Design of Research" can be found here: https://static-content.springer.com/esm/art%3A10.1038%2Fs41586-019-165 7-6/MediaObjects/41586_2019_1657_MOESM1_ESM.pdf).[49]

While peer-reviewed journals have increasingly developed editorial policies advocating for sex and gender analysis, there is still a lot of room for growth. Recall that across a broad segment of biomedical journals (n = 190), only 65 (34%) stated a policy for reporting sex and/or gender in their author guidelines.[44] Additionally, among the 20 otolaryngology journals reviewed, only 6 (30%) had a policy for reporting sex and/or gender in their reporting policies. (Further details on "Peer-Reviewed Journals' Author and Reviewer Guidelines for Evaluating Sex and Gender Analysis in Manuscripts" can be found here: https://static-content.springer.com/esm/art%3A10.1038%2Fs41586-019-1657-6/MediaObjects/41586_2019_1657_MOESM1_ESM.pdf).[49]

While funding agencies and journals may have policies in place, researchers and reviewers ultimately need foundational education in sex and gender analysis. For instance, the European Commission, which has had policies in place since 2014, found that fewer than expected funded research proposals incorporated sex and gender analysis and correlated this with an "absence of training on gender issues."[52] Several initiatives have been developed to fill this gap. Gendered Innovations is a global, collaborative project initiated from Stanford University in 2009 and supported by the European Commission and the US National Science Foundation that hosts an educational platform that provides instruction on sex, gender, and intersectional analysis, incorporating a case-study approach (https://genderedinnovations.stanford.edu/index.html).[53] The CIHR has developed a series of online training modules for integrating sex and gender analysis into biomedical research (https://cihr-irsc.gc.ca/e/50836.html).[54] And, even publishers have developed educational content, such as Elsevier's Researcher Academy (https://researcheracademy.elsevier.com/communicating-research/inclusion-diversity-researchers/integrate-sex-gender-intersectional-analysis), to support further learning about sex and gender analysis. These resources, among others, should be incorporated into the training of students, residents, and fellows and offered to those already further along the educational path who have missed the opportunity in more traditional educational environments.[55]

Efforts to bring sex and gender into the mainstream of modern medical education, research, and practice are urgently needed to enhance equity by ensuring that research findings are applicable for all members of society.

References

1. Studies I of M (US) C on E and LIR to the I of W in C Mastroianni AC, Faden R, Federman D. *NIH Revitalization Act of 1993 Public Law 103-43*. National Academies Press (US); 1994. https://www.ncbi.nlm.nih.gov/books/NBK236531/. Accessed March 24, 2023.
2. International Committee of Medical Journal Editors. History of the Recommendations. Accessed March 25, 2023. https://www.icmje.org/recommendations/browse/about-the-recommendations/history-of-the-recommendations.html.

3. International Committee of Medical Journal Editors. Recommendations for the Conduct, Reporting, Editing, and Publication of Scholarly Work in Medical Journals. Accessed March 25, 2023. https://www.icmje.org/icmje-recommendations.pdf.

4. Clayton JA, Tannenbaum C. Reporting sex, gender, or both in clinical research? *JAMA*. 2016;316(18):1863. https://doi.org/10.1001/jama.2016.16405.

5. Heidari S, Babor TF, De Castro P, Tort S, Curno M. Sex and gender equity in research: rationale for the SAGER guidelines and recommended use. *Res Integr Peer Rev*. 2016; 1(1):2. https://doi.org/10.1186/s41073-016-0007-6.

6. *National Academies of Sciences, Engineering, and Medicine. Measuring Sex, Gender Identity, and Sexual Orientation*. National Academies Press; 2022. https://doi.org/ 10.17226/26424.

7. Mauvais-Jarvis F, Bairey Merz N, Barnes PJ, et al. Sex and gender: modifiers of health, disease, and medicine. *Lancet*. 2020;396(10250):565–582. https://doi.org/10.1016/ S0140-6736(20)31561-0.

8. National Center for Health Statistics. *Mortality in the United States*. Centers for Disease Control and Prevention; 2021. https://doi.org/10.15620/cdc:122516.

9. Mehta LS, Beckie TM, DeVon HA, et al. Acute myocardial infarction in women: a scientific statement from the american heart association. *Circulation*. 2016;133(9): 916–947. https://doi.org/10.1161/CIR.0000000000000351.

10. Honigberg MC, Zekavat SM, Aragam K, et al. Association of premature natural and surgical menopause with incident cardiovascular disease. *JAMA*. 2019;322(24):2411. https://doi.org/10.1001/jama.2019.19191.

11. Bugiardini R, Ricci B, Cenko E, et al. Delayed care and mortality among women and men with myocardial infarction. *J Am Heart Assoc*. 2017;6(8):e005968. https:// doi.org/10.1161/JAHA.117.005968.

12. D'Onofrio G, Safdar B, Lichtman JH, et al. Sex differences in reperfusion in young patients with st-segment–elevation myocardial infarction: results from the virgo study. *Circulation*. 2015;131(15):1324–1332. https://doi.org/10.1161/CIRCULATIONAHA.114.012293.

13. Pelletier R, Khan NA, Cox J, et al. Sex versus gender-related characteristics. *J Am Coll Cardiol*. 2016;67(2):127–135. https://doi.org/10.1016/j.jacc.2015.10.067.

14. Greenwood BN, Carnahan S, Huang L. Patient–physician gender concordance and increased mortality among female heart attack patients. *Proc Natl Acad Sci USA*. 2018;115(34):8569–8574. https://doi.org/10.1073/pnas.1800097115.

15. Wei J, Mehta PK, Grey E, et al. Sex-based differences in quality of care and outcomes in a health system using a standardized STEMI protocol. *Am Heart J*. 2017;191:30–36. https://doi.org/10.1016/j.ahj.2017.06.005.

16. Wagner AD, Oertelt-Prigione S, Adjei A, et al. Gender medicine and oncology: report and consensus of an ESMO workshop. *Ann Oncol*. 2019;30(12):1914–1924. https:// doi.org/10.1093/annonc/mdz414.

17. McCartney G, Mahmood L, Leyland AH, Batty GD, Hunt K. Contribution of smoking-related and alcohol-related deaths to the gender gap in mortality: evidence from 30 European countries. *Tobac Control*. 2011;20(2):166–168. https://doi.org/10.1136/tc.2010. 037929.

18. Williams LA, Richardson M, Marcotte EL, Poynter JN, Spector LG. Sex ratio among childhood cancers by single year of age. *Pediatr Blood Cancer*. 2019;66(6):e27620. https://doi.org/10.1002/pbc.27620.

19. Dunford A, Weinstock DM, Savova V, et al. Tumor-suppressor genes that escape from X-inactivation contribute to cancer sex bias. *Nat Genet*. 2017;49(1):10–16. https://doi.org/ 10.1038/ng.3726.

20. Li Y, Zhang DJ, Qiu Y, Kido T, Lau YFC. The Y-located proto-oncogene TSPY exacerbates and its X-homologue TSPX inhibits transactivation functions of androgen receptor and its constitutively active variants. *Hum Mol Genet*. 2017;26(5):901−912. https://doi.org/10.1093/hmg/ddx005.

21. Arnold AP. The organizational−activational hypothesis as the foundation for a unified theory of sexual differentiation of all mammalian tissues. *Horm Behav*. 2009;55(5):570−578. https://doi.org/10.1016/j.yhbeh.2009.03.011.

22. Hanahan D, Weinberg RA. Hallmarks of cancer: the next generation. *Cell*. 2011;144(5):646−674. https://doi.org/10.1016/j.cell.2011.02.013.

23. Rubin JB, Lagas JS, Broestl L, et al. Sex differences in cancer mechanisms. *Biol Sex Differ*. 2020;11(1):17. https://doi.org/10.1186/s13293-020-00291-x.

24. Conforti F, Pala L, Bagnardi V, et al. Cancer immunotherapy efficacy and patients' sex: a systematic review and meta-analysis. *Lancet Oncol*. 2018;19(6):737−746. https://doi.org/10.1016/S1470-2045(18)30261-4.

25. Unger JM, Vaidya R, Albain KS, et al. Sex differences in risk of severe adverse events in patients receiving immunotherapy, targeted therapy, or chemotherapy in cancer clinical trials. *J Clin Oncol*. 2022;40(13):1474−1486. https://doi.org/10.1200/JCO.21.02377.

26. Tadiri CP, Gisinger T, Kautzky-Willer A, et al. The influence of sex and gender domains on COVID-19 cases and mortality. *Can Med Assoc J*. 2020;192(36):E1041−E1045. https://doi.org/10.1503/cmaj.200971.

27. Acheampong DO, Barffour IK, Boye A, Aninagyei E, Ocansey S, Morna MT. Male predisposition to severe COVID-19: review of evidence and potential therapeutic prospects. *Biomed Pharmacother*. 2020;131:110748. https://doi.org/10.1016/j.biopha.2020.110748.

28. Klein SL, Dhakal S, Ursin RL, Deshpande S, Sandberg K, Mauvais-Jarvis F. Biological sex impacts COVID-19 outcomesCoyne CB, ed. *PLoS Pathog*. 2020;16(6):e1008570. https://doi.org/10.1371/journal.ppat.1008570.

29. Heidari S, Palmer-Ross A, Goodman T. A systematic review of the sex and gender reporting in covid-19 clinical trials. *Vaccines*. 2021;9(11):1322. https://doi.org/10.3390/vaccines9111322.

30. Yoon DY, Mansukhani NA, Stubbs VC, Helenowski IB, Woodruff TK, Kibbe MR. Sex bias exists in basic science and translational surgical research. *Surgery*. 2014;156(3):508−516. https://doi.org/10.1016/j.surg.2014.07.001.

31. Mansukhani NA, Yoon DY, Teter KA, et al. Sex bias exists in human surgical clinical research. *JAMA Surg*. 2016;151(11):1022. https://doi.org/10.1001/jamasurg.2016.2032.

32. Bryant J, Yi P, Miller L, Peek K, Lee D. Potential sex bias exists in orthopaedic basic science and translational research. *J Bone Jt Surg*. 2018;100(2):124−130. https://doi.org/10.2106/JBJS.17.00458.

33. Hettrich CM, Hammoud S, LaMont LE, Arendt EA, Hannafin JA. Sex-specific analysis of data in high-impact orthopaedic journals: how are we doing? *Clin Orthop*. 2015;473(12):3700−3704. https://doi.org/10.1007/s11999-015-4457-9.

34. Kalliainen LK, Wisecarver I, Cummings A, Stone J. Sex bias in hand surgery research. *J Hand Surg*. 2018;43(11):1026−1029. https://doi.org/10.1016/j.jhsa.2018.03.026.

35. Stephenson ED, Farzal Z, Kilpatrick LA, Senior BA, Zanation AM. Sex bias in basic science and translational otolaryngology research. *Laryngoscope*. 2019;129(3):613−618. https://doi.org/10.1002/lary.27498.

36. Farzal Z, Stephenson ED, Kilpatrick LA, Senior BA, Zanation AM. Sex bias: is it pervasive in otolaryngology clinical research? *Laryngoscope*. 2019;129(4):858−864. https://doi.org/10.1002/lary.27497.

37. Lauer A, Schrode K. Sex bias in basic and preclinical noise-induced hearing loss research. *Noise Health*. 2017;19(90):207. https://doi.org/10.4103/nah.NAH_12_17.

38. Beery AK, Zucker I. Sex bias in neuroscience and biomedical research. *Neurosci Biobehav Rev*. 2011;35(3):565−572. https://doi.org/10.1016/j.neubiorev.2010.07.002.

39. Stephenson ED, Farzal Z, Zanation AM, Senior BA. Sex bias in rhinology research: sex bias in rhinology research. *Int Forum Allergy Rhinol*. 2018;8(12):1469−1475. https://doi.org/10.1002/alr.22179.

40. Ramkumar SP, Brar T, Marks L, Marino MJ, Lal D. Biological sex as a modulator in rhinologic anatomy, physiology, and pathology: a scoping review. *Int Forum Allergy Rhinol*. 2023;15:alr.23135. https://doi.org/10.1002/alr.23135. Published online February.

41. Pasick LJ, Yeakel H, Sataloff RT. Sex bias in laryngology research and publishing. *J Voice*. 2022;36(3):389−395. https://doi.org/10.1016/j.jvoice.2020.06.021.

42. Winter S, Diamond M, Green J, et al. Transgender people: health at the margins of society. *Lancet*. 2016;388(10042):390−400. https://doi.org/10.1016/S0140-6736(16)00683-8.

43. Xiao N, Mansukhani NA, Mendes de Oliveira DF, Kibbe MR. Association of author gender with sex bias in surgical research. *JAMA Surg*. 2018;153(7):663. https://doi.org/10.1001/jamasurg.2018.0040.

44. Bibb LA, Adkins BD, Booth GS, Shelton KM, Jacobs JW. Analysis of sex and gender reporting policies in preeminent biomedical journals. *JAMA Netw Open*. 2022;5(8):e2230277. https://doi.org/10.1001/jamanetworkopen.2022.30277.

45. Scopus. SJR - About Us. SCImago Journal and Country Rank. Accessed March 19, 2023. https://www.scimagojr.com/aboutus.php.

46. Scopus. Journal Rankings on Otorhinolaryngology. SCImago Journal and Country Rank. Accessed March 19, 2023. https://www.scimagojr.com/journalrank.php?category=2733&year=2021.

47. Elsevier. Guide for authors. Elsevier Connect. Accessed March 19, 2023. https://www.elsevier.com/journals/journal-of-cranio-maxillofacial-surgery/1010-5182/guide-for-authors.

48. Elsevier. EDI. Elsevier Connect. Accessed March 19, 2023. https://www.elsevier.com/authors/policies-and-guidelines/edi.

49. Tannenbaum C, Ellis RP, Eyssel F, Zou J, Schiebinger L. Sex and gender analysis improves science and engineering. *Nature*. 2019;575(7781):137−146. https://doi.org/10.1038/s41586-019-1657-6.

50. Geller SE, Koch AR, Roesch P, Filut A, Hallgren E, Carnes M. The more things change, the more they stay the same: a study to evaluate compliance with inclusion and assessment of women and minorities in randomized controlled trials. *Acad Med*. 2018;93(4):630−635. https://doi.org/10.1097/ACM.0000000000002027.

51. Johnson J, Sharman Z, Vissandjée B, Stewart DE. Does a change in health research funding policy related to the integration of sex and gender have an impact?Wicherts JM, ed. *PLoS One*. 2014;9(6):e99900. https://doi.org/10.1371/journal.pone.0099900.

52. *Directorate-General for Research and Innovation (European Commission)*. Interim Evaluation: Gender Equality as a Crosscutting Issue in Horizon 2020. Publications Office of the European Union; 2017. https://data.europa.eu/doi/10.2777/054612. Accessed March 24, 2023.

53. Stanford University. Gendered Innovations in Science, Health and Medicine, Engineering and Environment. Accessed March 24, 2023. https://genderedinnovations.stanford.edu/index.html.

54. Canadian Institutes of Health Research. *How to Integrate Sex and Gender into Research.* Government of Canada; February 12, 2018. https://cihr-irsc.gc.ca/e/50836.html. Accessed March 24, 2023.

55. Khamisy-Farah R, Bragazzi NL. How to integrate sex and gender medicine into medical and allied health profession undergraduate, graduate, and post-graduate education: insights from a rapid systematic literature review and a thematic meta-synthesis. *J Personalized Med.* 2022;12(4):612. https://doi.org/10.3390/jpm12040612.

Improving LGBTQ healthcare in the otolaryngology community

5

Ketan Jain-Poster, Nikolas Block-Wheeler, Noriko Yoshikawa

Department of Head and Neck Surgery, Kaiser Permanente, East Bay, Oakland, CA, United States

Introduction

Otolaryngologists are uniquely situated to provide care for the lesbian, gay, transgender, bisexual, and queer (LGBTQ) community. One area in particular, feminizing procedures for transgender and gender-nonconforming individuals, has increased dramatically, particularly as more insurance providers join in recognizing these procedures as medically necessary. Yet, regardless of the procedure, all otolaryngology providers should be equipped to provide excellent care to all members of the LGBTQ community, whether for care related to their gender or sexual identity or concerns unrelated.

Significant strides in LGBTQ health care have been made over the years (with occasional backtracking); however, much more are needed. Historically a vulnerable population due to systemic discrimination, LGBTQ individuals make up about 4% of the United States (US) population, which comprises about 9.5 million adults.[1] It may come as a surprise that it was not until 1973 that the Diagnostic and Statistical Manual of Mental Disorders (DSM) began to depathologize homosexuality as a mental illness, and it was not until 1987 that it was fully expunged from the text. The medical community's and government's mismanagement of the HIV/AIDS epidemic in the 1980s also led to lasting stigmatization of the LGBTQ community.[2] Today, immense opportunity remains to make a difference in health.

Care for our patient's communities, not just the LGBTQ community, requires an understanding of intersectionality; this requires a recognition that each person has a unique experience and history with discrimination and a multidimensional awareness attuned to many of the sources of oppression. Discrimination still exists among medical providers and continues to be a barrier to equitable patient care.[3] Today, the majority of otolaryngology training programs provide specific training to better care for LGBTQ community members, yet a minority are able to offer direct patient care experience within some of these communities.[4,5]

While not all trainees are able to care for members of this community during their training, a socially responsive otolaryngologist or trainee can provide excellent and appropriate patient care by becoming educated on contemporary issues for community members and authentically welcoming and listening to their patients. This chapter will discuss a framework for the otolaryngologist to consider the interactions between the patient, provider, and healthcare system specifically for gender and sexual minorities, also referred to as LGBTQ patients. It is important to note that the grouping of "LGBTQ" may not be expansive enough and we intend to describe care for individuals of varying gender and sexuality, including, but not limited to, those who are intersex, questioning, two-spirit, asexual, and more. It is also important to recognize that while these communities are often grouped, they are immensely diverse and even represent different aspects of identification, including sexuality and gender.

Defining terms

The terminologies surrounding gender and sexual identities are geographically, culturally, and temporally evolving. Here, we present a series of relatively standard terms to aid in the understanding of topics surrounding LGBTQ identities, as adapted from the Human Rights Campaign and National LGBT Health Education Center:[6,7]

Lesbian: a woman who experiences emotional, romantic, and/or sexual attraction to women. This term is sometimes also used by nonbinary and femme-identifying individuals as well.

Gay: a person who experiences emotional, romantic, and/or sexual attraction to individuals of the same gender. Men, women, and nonbinary people may use this term to describe themselves.

Bisexual: a person who experiences emotional, romantic, and/or sexual attraction to people of multiple genders, though not necessarily equally, in the same proportions, or at the same time.

Queer: an expansive term previously used as a slur but now reclaimed by the community. It is used to describe a spectrum of identities relating to gender or orientation that do not conform to mainstream notions of heterosexual, cis-gendered identity or expression.

Sex: a label—male or female—assigned based on the type of genitals present at birth.

Gender: a continuum of socially constructed roles, behaviors, internal concepts, and expressions of identity centered around felt masculinity and femininity.

Cisgender or "cis": a term used to describe a gender identity that conforms with societal expectations, including gender expression, of the sex the individual was assigned at birth.

Transgender or "trans": an expansive term used to describe an individual whose gender identity and/or expression differs from cultural expectations of the sex that person was assigned at birth. This term is not linked to sexual orientation.

Gender nonbinary: a gender identity that does not conform exclusively to notions of "man" or "woman," either identifying as both, somewhere in between, or neither at all. This is an umbrella term, and while some nonbinary individuals may identify as trans, not all do.

Gender nonconforming: the extent to which a person's gender identity, role, or expression differs from the cultural norms prescribed for people of a particular sex.

Gender dysphoria: a clinical term describing psychological distress stemming from incongruence between an individual's gender identity and the societal expectations prescribed to their sex assigned at birth.

Health disparities in medicine

Modern medical history in the (US) is fraught with discrimination against the LGTBQ community. The medical community began by labeling gender or sexual minority as a mental illness, with Sigmund Freud explaining it as an arrest of maturation due to developmental trauma.[8] Behaviorists believed it was a learned behavior, despite long-held teaching from the Greco-Romans that sexuality was innate. And the mental health community has worked to recover after pathologizing homosexuality in the DSM, fully removing the classification in 1987. It was no surprise that by the time the HIV/AIDS crisis began in the early 1980s, LGBTQ members were wary of healthcare institutions, delaying testing or treatment for fear of further discrimination. Meanwhile, the early epidemic was attributed exclusively to men who have sex with men (MSM); today, people with heterosexual sex partners represent nearly a quarter of new HIV diagnoses in the (US).[9]

While the repercussions of healthcare discrimination still resonate, and the existence of laws and practices that actively contribute to discrimination still persist, there has been progress. The first gender-affirming surgery was performed in 1965; today, 25% of transgender individuals have received gender-affirming surgery (it bears mentioning that not all transgender individuals seek surgery as part of their transition).[10] The first standards of care for transgender and gender-nonconforming individuals were published in 1979 by the World Professional Association for Transgender Health (WPATH).[11] In 2010, the Obama administration banned discrimination based on sexual orientation and gender identity in programs receiving federal healthcare funding; this order was briefly retracted by the Trump administration, before being reinstated by the Biden administration in 2021.[12,13] Today, 24 states and the District of Columbia prohibit private health insurance from excluding gender-affirming care and the same number must explicitly include such care in state employee health benefits.[14] Despite these protections, more than half of those seeking gender-affirming surgery reported being denied such care, and a quarter were refused coverage of their hormone medication.[15] Alabama, Arizona, Arkansas, and Utah have also introduced new programs to limit or even criminalize best-practice care for transgender youth.[16]

Barriers for LGBTQ individuals in health settings

Gender and sexual minorities have faced historic mistreatment within the healthcare system, which has continued to dramatically affect the care-seeking behavior of these patients into the present day. Many LGBTQ individuals not only fear stigma within the healthcare setting, but research shows providers are often ill-equipped to care for matters related specifically to LGBTQ health. A survey of knowledge, attitudes, and health behaviors of LGBTQ patients administered to 108 oncology providers revealed that less than 50% of providers were able to correctly answer questions about sexual and gender minority health, and that only 28% felt informed on LGBTQ needs.[17] The care gap is strongly felt by patients themselves. Reported barriers to care included lack of provider knowledge and lack of provider effort in inquiring about patient preferences for care.[18] Patients who feel unwelcomed, or that their providers are not able to understand their needs, are less likely to seek care and more likely to receive lesser quality care when they do.

Provider knowledge gaps and social responsiveness may be related to lack of exposure to LGBTQ health issues and internal bias. Research illuminates a pressing lack of education surrounding LGBTQ care among specialists, especially among the surgical fields.[19] This discrepancy in education begins at the earliest stages of training for providers, as medical students and residents across the country report receiving insufficient training for working with LGBTQ patients.[20–22] Moreover, surgeons specifically involved with treating gender dysphoria are reporting deficiencies in their training to treat transgender patients.[19] A survey of residents in a variety of surgical subspecialties related to transgender care revealed that 18% of plastic surgery and 42% of urology programs offered no didactic education, and that 34% and 30%, respectively, did not offer any clinical exposure to working with this patient population.[19] This extends to otolaryngology as well, with a recent survey of 285 residents across 22 programs in the (US) showing that less than one-third of residents report exposure to transgender-related patient care experiences or didactic material, although a majority recognize its importance in training and practice.[5] This lack of formal education and training within otolaryngology is recognized by Chaiet et al., and the authors called for increased competence in caring for LGBTQ populations that starts within residency training itself.[23] The systemic omission of LGBTQ health from medical education is counterproductive to serving these patients and only further exacerbates the health disparities these communities face.

A step toward better health care for our LGBTQ patients is beginning to understand the bias they may face and how our own biases affect our ability to provide optimal care. Stigma, defined as the social devaluation or discrediting associated with a specific characteristic or attribute, can negatively affect care for LGBTQ populations.[24] In fact, stigma and mistrust in the healthcare setting have been shown to specifically affect care-seeking behaviors.[2,24] The stigma that gender and sexual minorities face in clinical environments is ubiquitous and often implicit; Sabin et al. showed pervasiveness of implicit bias among heterosexual providers who favored heterosexual people over gay and lesbian people.[25] In a grim proportion, Quinn et al. showed that 22% of providers assumed their patients were heterosexual on first encounter, an assumption that opens way for the manifestation of these internal biases.[17] LGBTQ patients may alter how much of their identity they share with their providing depending on their own perception of their provider, which directly impacts care and, certainly, patient trust. A study among older LGBTQ patients who were receiving noncancer-related care suggested difficulty in disclosing gender identity and sexual orientation to providers, and those who did not disclose their identities suffered poorer health outcomes across all age.[26,27] Whether through macro or microaggressions, the stigma that LGBTQ individuals face within a clinical environment can quite literally cost lives; it has been documented that transgender patients denied care due to gender identity attempted suicide at a rate almost 50% higher to those who were not denied.[28]

Prior to experiences they may have within the clinical environment itself, gender and sexual minorities face disproportionate barriers to healthcare costs and insurance access. LGBTQ individuals disproportionately live in poverty when compared to heterosexual individuals, especially those who are transgender, with the 2015 US transgender survey reporting 33% of transgender patients did not see a physician due to cost.[29,30] LGBTQ populations are additionally underinsured compared to their heterosexual counterparts. The passage of the Affordable Care Act showed an improvement, as the rate of uninsured LGBTQ individuals with incomes less than 400% of the federal poverty level dropped from 34% to 26% between 2013 and 2014.[31] It is important to note that accessibility, whether related to cost, stigma, or mistrust, is compounded by other barriers to care, including immigration or documentation status, race and ethnicity, accessibility, geographic isolation, or cultural belief frameworks.

Social and disease factors of particular relevance in the LGBTQ community

The intersections of health, disease, gender, and identity affecting the LGBTQ community are understudied, and there exist little data illuminating these overlapping topics within the field of otolaryngology. Many of the issues LGBTQ patients experience in healthcare settings affect their care within otolaryngology as well, though some diseases, conditions, and experiences may be particularly relevant to gender and sexual minorities and require special attention. While nonexhaustive, victims of violence and hate crime, suicide attempts, drug use, HIV infection, cancer, and human papillomavirus (HPV)-related disease highlight specific situations that may be relevant to many LGBTQ patients and call for the attention of sensitive otolaryngologists. It is important to be mindful, however, that while the community at large may demonstrate increased susceptibility for these risk factors, that individual patients may not present with any of these specifications requiring attention, and, the converse is true, that non-LGBTQ patients may also present with any of these conditions.

Harm and physical trauma

Gender and sexual minorities face disproportionate rates of physical trauma, either inflicted by perpetrators of violent hate crime, intimate partner violence, or from self-directed harm. While these situations may not be unique to LGBTQ individuals, evidence suggests that LGBTQ individuals experience these at high rates. According to the US Department of Justice June 2022 Statistical Brief, the rate of violent victimization was more than twice as high for lesbian or gay people when compared to heterosexual people.[32] And, the rate of violence toward transgender people was 2.5 times higher than cisgender people. Domestic violence was eight times higher among bisexual people, and more than twice as high among lesbian or gay people compared to heterosexual people.[32]

Similarly, LGBTQ populations present a starkly increased risk for suicide and self-harm when compared to the overall population. A meta-analysis found there was a significant association between minority stressors (such as LGBTQ bias-based victimization, discrimination, negative family treatment, internalized homo- or transphobia) and suicidal ideation and attempts among LGBTQ adolescents and young adults.[33] It is estimated that over 40% of transgender individuals have attempted self-harm.[34–36]

Within otolaryngology, survivors of physical trauma or suicide attempt may need facial trauma consultation, as well as facial plastic or reconstructive surgery requiring specialized care and follow up. Many of these patients may need advanced care requiring admission to an intensive care unit and will require coordination of care with a variety of support systems that may not conform to normative models of support for cisgender, heterosexual patients. In alignment with previously mentioned trends, many of these patients may have structural, institutional, personal, and/or socioeconomic barriers to receiving care for managing rehabilitative and restorative needs.

Recreational drug use and smoking

Several studies have illuminated increased use of recreational drugs within LGBTQ communities, the complications of which may require attention from specialized otolaryngologic care. One study found that LGBTQ youth were 190% (and the sub-set of females, including lesbian and bisexual, were 400%) more likely to engage in substance use than their heterosexual peers.[37] Bisexual women, lesbian/gay women, and gay men reported higher rates of lifetime use of marijuana, cocaine, inhalants, and hallucinogens than their heterosexual counterparts.[38] Furthermore, there is a higher trend in smoking among LGBTQ populations, which additionally increases incidence and morbidity of a myriad of conditions, including head and neck cancer.[39–41] It is important for otolaryngologists to be sensitive to sexual and gender diversity when assessing patients presenting with these risk factors for disease and perioperative complications.

HIV/AIDS

Although recent evidence suggests that trends may be changing in the demographics of patients with HIV/AIDS, the LGBTQ community has historically been dispropor-tionately affected and may present with an otolaryngologic manifestation.[42,43]

In one study, almost 80% of HIV patients were found to have some otolaryngologic complaint. This may include tumors (e.g., Kaposi's sarcoma, non-Hodgkin's lymphoma), oral lesions (e.g., HSV-1 or herpes zoster, papillomas, oral hairy leukoplakia, candidiasis), adenoid hypertrophy, chronic sinusitis, serous otitis media, or otitis externa.[44,45] It is essential for otolaryngologists to be cognizant of the many manifestations of HIV infection in the head and neck. While the aforementioned diseases, situations, and risk factors are not unique to gender and sexual minorities, they urge the awareness of specialists, notably in otolaryngology.

Cancer

Gender and sexual minorities represent a population historically underrepresented in cancer research and likely represent a modified risk profile for the development of certain forms of cancer, as well as unique factors that influence their outcomes. Several behavioral risk factors for cancer such as high rates of smoking, obesity, and alcohol use have been shown to be more prevalent in female sexual and gender minority populations.[39,46,47] Meanwhile, certain forms of cancer may be more prevalent in MSM populations, as MSM who engage in receptive anal intercourse are at an elevated risk of oncogenic HPV infection and subsequent precursor lesions to anal cancer.[48] In fact, there is evidence to suggest that MSM are at high risk for both HPV and HPV-associated diseases, which would increase risk for HPV-positive oropharyngeal carcinoma.[48] This intersection of sexual practice and oropharyngeal HPV infection has been studied, which has shown the positive association of HPV-related oropharyngeal cancer with number of lifetime sexual partners and stronger associations with sexual behaviors among men.[49] Other data that have demonstrated that oral HPV infection was more common in MSM who had HIV infection, smoking, and more lifetime tongue-kissing and oral sex partners.[50]

The implementation of early vaccination against HPV has provided some encouragement in the prevention of cancer, as it has been shown that vaccination can successfully reduce anal cancer in MSM individuals.[51,52] However, while reductions in anal intraepithelial neoplasia among MSM have been shown, a lack of an identified precursor lesion for oropharyngeal cancer has prevented efficacy studies for this outcome to date within this population.[52,53] While early prevention efforts are important for this subgroup, early awareness of risk and counseling is another key intervention, as Oliver et al. demonstrated that a majority of MSM in their study were not aware that HPV could cause oropharyngeal cancer.[53] Most of these studies exclude transgender women and other people who were assigned male sex at birth, which are another important group to be conscious of when considering these findings. Though the literature suggests that MSM and transgender women may be disproportionately affected by oropharyngeal cancer and other HPV-related diseases of the head and neck, more research is necessary to examine the relationship between gender and sexual minority populations and head and neck pathology.

Gaps exist in our understanding of cancer diagnosis and treatment for LGBTQ individuals, and our understanding of outcomes in this population is similarly limited. In general, cancer surveillance has not included data on sexual and gender minorities.[54] The majority of cancer registries and medical records have not collected information related to sexual orientation and gender identity in the past, limiting the ability to study how disease and risk factors specifically affect these populations.[55] However, there has been slight improvement as of 2015, in which a decision was made by the Department of Health and Human Services to begin to require electronic health record systems with certified technology to include data on gender and sexual orientation, which formally started in 2016.[56]

It is important to bear in mind that disparities in the psychosocial determinants of health affect LGBTQ populations in ways that exacerbate the effects of chronic illness. Sexual and gender minorities are an underserved group facing disproportionate depression, anxiety, and social isolation.[57] Social isolation, particularly nonmarital status, has been associated with poorer outcomes for cancer, including later stage of diagnosis, decreased quality of life, and decreased survival.[58-60] Lack of social support and isolation is of particular concern, with aging studies showing that gay and bisexual men and women are more likely than their heterosexual counterparts to live alone and without children.[61] The variation in household social support structures and disproportionate social isolation for LGBTQ individuals put this population at risk for poorer cancer outcomes.

Gender-affirming care in otolaryngology

Otolaryngologists have come together with other specialists in being able to offer patients an aspect of gender-affirming care. In joining plastic surgery, urology, endocrinology, gynecology, psychiatry, primary care, and other fields, otolaryngology provides valuable expertise in multiple domains among the multidisciplinary team involved in gender affirmation. Specifically, interventions, both medical and surgical, now offer patients the potential to work with otolaryngologists to achieve gender-affirming goals related to voice and facial appearance. These interventions of the head and neck can help lessen the dysphoria associated with differences between gender identity and sex assigned at birth or hormone-related physical characteristics; one's physical body can more closely match their self.

While facial feminizing procedures may target traditionally masculine facial traits, there is no prescribed regimen, and treatments are highly individualized; what may help one person alleviate their gender dysphoria may not be appropriate or desired by another. When desired, gender-affirming surgical care has been shown to improve mental health; decreased mental health burden and attempted suicide have been demonstrated in those who receive gender-affirming surgical care.[62] Facial feminization surgery (FFS) has also been shown to specifically decrease anxiety and depression and improve meaning/purpose and social isolation.[63]

Though we highlight the importance of reducing internal gender dysphoria on a patient's well-being, for many, gender-affirming interventions are also a matter of safety. Unfortunately, being recognized as transgender can be endangering.

Regardless of assigned sex at birth, transgender individuals face disproportionate physical harassment, assault, rape, and murder due to hate crime in the community.[64,65] Many in the transgender and gender-nonconforming community refer to the ability to "pass" for either a socially and societally determined conventional "man" or "woman" as a privilege of safety; those who present with a variety of gender expressions inconsistent with the socially expected role for their sex assigned at birth are at greater risk for being targeted with discrimination and violent crime. For this reason, gender affirmation surgery can improve both gender dysphoria, as well as improve safety.

Many patients presenting for otolaryngologic care along the path of their transition have already taken significant steps and are seeking additional treatment to see their felt self in the mirror. Common gender-affirming interventions offered by otolaryngologists include voice therapy or pitch-altering procedures, as well as bony and soft-tissue recontouring that address incongruent facial features.

According to the 2015 Transgender Survey, however, there is a large demand for gender-affirming therapy that is not being met.[30] Only 11% of respondents identifying as transgender women or gender-nonconforming have undergone voice therapy, and 46% would like to receive therapy. Surgical interventions show a similar gap, with 6% of respondents having been treated with FFS (39% desire surgery), 1% with pitch alteration surgery (16% desire surgery), and 4% with chondrolaryngoplasty, also known as "tracheal shave" surgery (29% desire surgery). It is clear that while the notion of gender-affirming surgery as a medically necessary treatment for gender dysphoria has become more widely recognized, large gaps remain in meeting the needs.

Voice affirmation

The goal of voice therapy is to allow patients to adapt their voices to communicate in a way that is congruent with their gender identity. While some individuals prefer for their voice to be either gender neutral or favor a specific gender identity, some prefer a gender expansive voice to allow for a variety of voice-related gender expressions (i.e., masculine, gender-neutral, feminine). Data show one's voice-gender congruence significantly affects quality of life.[66,67] The study of transgender men showed those whose voices sounded more congruent with their gender reported greater life satisfaction, quality of life, and self-esteem, along with lower levels of anxiety and depression, when compared to those whose voices were less congruent with their gender.[67] A transparent, open, and nonassuming discussion of a patient's voice-related concerns should be conducted before initiating any treatment or intervention, as personal goals for therapy will vary from patient to patient.

Patients may elect to pursue invasive or noninvasive approaches, the latter involving working primarily with speech-language pathologists, voice coaches, singing teachers, and online resources. The targets of speech therapy include pitch, prosody, and vocal resonance to achieve the desired result. Communication therapy may also address voice quality, articulation, speech rate, phrasing, and nonverbal communication. Altering a patient's voice alone may not be enough to offer them full satisfaction; a multimodal approach to voice therapy should be offered to all patients seeking voice-affirming therapy. Surgical interventions to raise pitch may include anterior glottal web formation and cricothyroid approximation, while interventions to lower pitch, though less common, may include thyroplasty.

While much of voice therapy targets tailoring the patient's fundamental frequency, which is correlated with gender perception by listeners, the outcome may not correlate with voice satisfaction or voice-related quality of life.[68] Rather, evidence suggests that voice-related quality of life correlates more strongly with self-ratings of vocal likability, which highlights the notion that the ideal voice for a patient is highly variable and interpersonally distinct; providers should be careful to avoid imposing voice goals.[66]

Facial affirmation

Given the effect of hormones on facial characteristics, alignment of facial appearance with gender identity for those with gender dysphoria offers an enormous opportunity to improve quality of life. Facial plastic surgeons are uniquely situated to leverage their expertise in aesthetics to treat these patients. Commonly performed procedures include contouring the brow and forehead, advancing the hairline, elevating the eyebrows, contouring the mandible, as well as performing rhinoplasty, lip lifts, and chondrolaryngoplasty. Facial implants may also be considered. Work by Spiegel shows feminization of the forehead may have the strongest impact on perception of facial femininity; additionally facial thirds are often addressed in conjunction.[69] While the object of FFS is to feminize facial structure, the surgeon must balance the aesthetic goals with preserving physiologic function and anatomic structural integrity.

Patients pursuing FFS seek an individualized treatment, which requires a thorough and realistic discussion of surgical objectives, as well as limitations. Socially conscious providers should make a large effort not to assume patient goals based on their gender expression or presentation. The preoperative discussion also includes an assessment of what is medically necessary to treat gender dysphoria and what would otherwise be considered cosmetic. Determining the indication requires a thorough understanding of anatomic differences in masculine and feminine facial features, and how these features may be altered to treat gender dysphoria. The otolaryngologist's role is to ask open-ended questions and offer a safe and nonjudgmental space in which a patient may feel comfortable expressing their experiences and preferences. For the otolaryngologist who does not perform gender-affirming therapy, it is critical for them to know what services exist to make appropriate referrals.

Racial minorities, specifically Black and Latinx patients, have been shown to experience increased risk of reoperation and readmission after gender-affirming procedures.[70] This is another example of health disparities, and underscores how clinicians must remain vigilant, and continue to work toward greater equity in outcomes.

The state of insurance coverage for gender-affirming interventions

Despite the evidence of vast improvements in quality of life for transgender and gender-nonconforming individuals, gender-affirming interventions remain largely inaccessible to many patients due to prohibitive cost and lack of insurance coverage.[71,72] These barriers tend to span many areas of gender affirmation surgery but are strongly highlighted in the areas of voice and surgical affirmation. For example, a recent study that determined insurance coverage for gender-affirming voice therapy and surgery, and differences in policies based on state-by-state transgender equality, highlighted limited insurance coverage remains a barrier to comprehensive gender-affirming care.[73] The study showed most insurers demonstrated no established policies for nonsurgical behavioral voice and communication interventions as of 2021. In fact, insurance coverage for these interventions is rare. De Vore et al. found that only 2.7% of commercial insurers had robust policies for voice-related gender-affirming interventions; meanwhile, 75.8% did not provide any coverage, and 13.4% offered no defined policy. The data contrast starkly with coverage for genital ("bottom") and chest ("top") surgery, which are granted favorable coverage by 68%–98% of large commercial insurance companies with preauthorization.[74] In fact, by international standards, voice therapy has been considered to be largely "aesthetic" and thus not given the same consideration of merit for insurance coverage.[75] The poor coverage may represent a more systemic deficit, as voice therapy is less likely to be covered by insurance companies than other types of therapy, even for cisgender patients.[76] Access is exacerbated for transgender patients who face higher rates of unemployment, lower income, and lack of insurance when compared to cisgender patients.[77] Moreover, a paucity of research evaluating efficacy of gender-affirming voice and aesthetic interventions has been used as justification for limiting coverage.[73]

Many of these coverage gaps exist for facial gender affirmation procedures. Gorbea et al. recently conducted a review of coverage of facial gender affirmation surgery by both private and public insurance providers across the (US) and showed that most commercial insurance companies and state Medicaid policies consider the surgery to be "cosmetic" or "aesthetic" instead of medically necessary.[78] The same review highlighted the interprocedural variation in coverage; chondrolaryngoplasty was the most covered procedure (20%), while cheek augmentation, brow lift, cervical rhytidectomy/liposuction, and voice-modifying procedures were the least covered (9%). In contrast, all commercial policies listed genital reconstruction as "medically necessary" and provided robust coverage. Still, most of the gender-affirming procedures were poorly covered. This is partially due to marked heterogeneity in categorization of coverage status for certain procedures with unclear specifications or rationale for labeling certain procedures as cosmetic or medically necessary. In fact, insurance companies do not recognize all gender-affirming surgeries under one umbrella; often, these procedures are coded, billed, and covered differently based on the insurer.

The variation in coverage status even varies geographically, with less coverage for facial gender affirmation surgery in states with less legal support for transgender individuals.[78a] Northeastern states were more likely to have coverage of at least some aspects of facial gender affirmation surgery, with southern states less likely to have coverage with policies that were more likely to lack details about facial gender affirmation surgery altogether.[78] Regardless, the literature consistently comments on the observation that a lack of written criteria for assessing medical necessity of gender affirmation surgery of the head and neck, as well as the lack of consensus of which procedures qualify as such, present principal reasons for poor coverage. These contradict the calls for standards of care and necessity of treatment for gender dysphoria as referenced by the most recent edition of the WPATH Standards of Care, a leading guide for transgender care internationally.[75] These persistent gaps in coverage and inconsistencies with suggested guidelines are especially concerning given the expansion of coverage for gender-affirming surgery in the (US) under the Patient Protection and Affordable Care Act, with Section 1557 citing the exclusion of gender-affirming care by an insurance provider as "unlawful."[79] Further advocacy and lobbying for expansive coverage for both facial and voice-related gender affirmation surgery are essential in providing access to gender dysphoria treatment for transgender and gender-nonconforming populations within the realm of otolaryngology. This is met with a need for standardized criteria for evaluating medical necessity of gender-affirming procedures, as well as more comprehensive and wide-reaching patient education on gender-affirming interventions.

Action steps for improving LGBTQ health

Unconscious bias against LGBTQ identities has been demonstrated among physicians.[17,25] Thus, it is essential that all healthcare providers engage routinely in practices that identify their own biases and assumptions, working to deliver inclusive care. Interacting in a socially conscious and inclusive manner will require a provider to self-educate, use patient-centered, open-ended, and nonheteronormative language, and correct others when mistakes are identified. We present several examples of such practices below, as well as additional particularities that may be important to be conscious of when understanding a patient's context, that extend beyond their LGBTQ identity. It is important to note, however, that though these represent some common situations, this encapsulation is not exhaustive. Seeking to eliminate bias is a consistent effort that may benefit from continued learning using a variety of educational modalities and avenues, be it through in-person safe-space trainings, publicly available online resources, personal reading, or otherwise.[32,80,81]

Patients within the LGBTQ community represent a population with a variety of support systems, family units, housing situations, and social needs. When inquiring about a patient's support system or social context, it is important to use open-ended language when asking questions. For example, using the genderless term "significant other" or "partner" instead of "husband" or "wife," which would carry assumptions about the patient's family, sexuality, or gender. This is an example of removing the assumption of gender from speech. Further, the practice of eliminating bias requires the provider to eliminate assumptions surrounding patients' identities when considering medical workup, diagnosis, and interventions related to sex practices or lifestyle. For example, when relevant, it is important to inquire which sexes a patient engages with in sexual activity before ordering a pregnancy test prior to surgery, rather than simply ordering a pregnancy test for a cis-woman-presenting patient.

Patients may not subscribe to conventional nuclear family or relationship models, regardless of sexuality or gender, and may practice various forms of polyamory or nonmonogamy. Thus, it is important to inquire about living environments and close relationships by using open-ended terms, such as asking who makes up a patient's "support system." This language also removes the assumption that a patient's support system may be a significant other or biological family member, as many individuals form kin-like social relationships with friends and members of the community that are not genetically or romantically related that is termed one's "chosen family." The idea is borne of many queer and transgender individuals needing to leave or being removed from their original homes and family environments due to domestic hostility surrounding their identities; as such, members of the community having found strong, familial bonds and support in others instead. By using nonheteronormative language, the provider decouples the impression of the patient from normative assumptions of nuclear family models, heterosexual relationships, procreation, or cis-gender identity.

A patient's gender or sexual identity may be private or personal, and their expression of this information to the provider represents trust. The process of "coming out," or willingly sharing an identity with others, is a constant process for LGBTQ individuals that gender and sexual minorities may approach with caution. While some people have shared their identities with most or all people in their life, many may have done so to varying extents or not at all. It can be dangerous and unhealthy to disclose someone's gender or sexual identity to another party without their consent, regardless of intent. Instead, if caring for a patient will require a provider to contact or coordinate with other parties in a patient's life, notably family members, friends, or other support systems, it is important to assess the amount of information a patient wishes those parties to know, as with any disclosure of protected health information.

Additionally, it cannot be overemphasized that while a patient presenting to care may be of a gender or sexual minority, it does not mean they are presenting with concerns related to this identity. Additionally, while it is important to keep in mind possible risk factors, it is dangerous to anchor on these during their workup. For example, not all adenoid hypertrophy in adults is related to HIV infection.

Well-intentioned providers with little experience caring for members of the LGBTQ community may have a sense of unease that an unintentional error may offend their patient, harming the patient–provider relationship. The authors would caution that a resulting avoidance likely potentiates discrimination and poor access.

Should a mistake be made by a member of the care team, simply apologizing and being forthcoming are the best ways to establish patient trust. Recognition and sincere apology, followed by forward momentum also avoid the patient needing to assume the role of comforting the clinician. Inclusive and welcoming interactions with LGBTQ patients, regardless of reason for visit, represent an opportunity to form supportive clinical relationships.

Inclusivity in the clinical setting

Normalizing identities of sexual and gender minorities in the clinical environment should extend to all the systemic and structural frameworks of the hospital or clinical setting. This entails giving LGBTQ patients the same opportunity as their peers to indicate their identity, such as having a variety of options for gender and sex declaration on paperwork that goes beyond "male or female." This should include a spectrum of gender identities and option for "intersex," choices to denote personal pronouns and "preferred names," and gender neutral bathrooms. Not only do these interventions make clinical environments more inclusive for LGBTQ patients they also allow health care professionals to better address and serve their needs.[80]

Measures should be taken to ensure that staff on the care team properly address patients to create a culture of inclusivity and reduce bias, even when the patient is not physically or consciously present. These include using proper pronouns and names for patients in all settings, which include but are not limited to interprofessional collaboration, patient handoffs, discussions about patients, referring to patients in discourse while patients are under anesthesia, and to the patient themselves. The important factor is that one should make an active effort to normalize addressing the patient correctly in all settings and to correct others when mistakes are made.

Didactics and education

As formerly discussed, the field of otolaryngology presents large gaps in formal education on and training exposure to treating LGBTQ patients. To increase socially competent training, otolaryngologists at academic institutions or training facilities should work to incorporate didactic material that specifically addresses proper care practices for gender and sexual minorities with a focus on eliminating bias, as well as gender-affirming care within the field's scope. The curriculum should also highlight the intersections between race, income inequality, housing, interactions with law enforcement, violence, and community resilience with LGBTQ identities to provide thorough social contexts for these populations. Though many resources for safe-space training and socially sensitive practices in medicine exist for public use online, the American Academy of Otolaryngology-Head and Neck Surgery presents a video series that may guide education on inclusivity for gender and sexual minority patients particularly within the field of otolaryngology.[81] Equally important is recurring self- and group-education by integrating topics affecting gender and sexual minorities within journal clubs and routine reading. Eliminating bias is a necessary, continuous, and reiterative process that requires longitudinal attention.

Formalized advocacy

Major gaps in insurance coverage for gender-affirming interventions of the head and neck persist, representing a steep access barrier for many transgender and gender-nonconforming patients seeking care.[73] The lack of coverage stems from a lack of standardized criteria for establishing medical necessity of intervention and common designation of gender-affirming procedures as "cosmetic," in addition to intersupplier heterogeneity. As such, further development to determine medical necessity of gender-affirming interventions is needed to better advocate for more expansive coverage, especially in geographic areas with greater disparity.[77] And, as insurers view the lack of literature surveying efficacy of treatments within the field as a justification for limiting coverage, more studies evaluating the success of gender-affirming voice and facial procedures in reducing gender dysphoria are needed.[73] Coverage expansion for chest and genital reassignment surgery has increased in response to increasing bodies of literature and advocacy, and so further lobbying and research should move—in conjunction with institutional advocacy—to push for expanded coverage of gender-affirming care within otolaryngology.

Conclusion

Individuals from the LGBTQ community are a part of our larger communities. They will be seeking otolaryngologic care for a variety of reasons, some which may be related to their LGBTQ identity. Being knowledgeable and sensitive to LGBTQ issues and concerns is a part of the otolaryngologist's role as an equitable caregiver to their community. It is our responsibility to create an inclusive environment where all patients feel welcome to seek care. Remembering the historical (and ongoing) discrimination that members of the LGBTQ community have suffered within the medical system will help our specialty be more conscious of trying to earn the trust of each patient we encounter.

References

1. Gates GJ. LGBT Demographics: Comparisons among Population-Based Surveys. UCLA: The Williams Institute. https://escholarship.org/uc/item/0kr784fx.
2. Mahajan AP, Sayles JN, Patel VA, et al. Stigma in the HIV/AIDS epidemic: a review of the literature and recommendations for the way forward. *AIDS Lond Engl.* 2008;22 (Suppl 2):S67–S79. https://doi.org/10.1097/01.aids.0000327438.13291.62.
3. Shipherd JC, Darling JE, Klap RS, Rose D, Yano EM. Experiences in the veterans health administration and impact on healthcare utilization: comparisons between LGBT and non-LGBT women veterans. *LGBT Health.* 2018;5(5):303–311. https://doi.org/10.1089/lgbt.2017.0179.
4. Goetz TG, Nieman CL, Chaiet SR, Morrison SD, Cabrera-Muffly C, Lustig LR. Sexual and gender minority curriculum within otolaryngology residency programs. *Transgender Health.* 2021;6(5):267–274. https://doi.org/10.1089/trgh.2020.0105.

5. Massenburg BB, Morrison SD, Rashidi V, et al. Educational exposure to transgender patient care in otolaryngology training. *J Craniofac Surg*. 2018;29(5):1252−1257. https://doi.org/10.1097/SCS.0000000000004609.

6. Human Rights Campaign. Glossary of Terms. HRC Foundation, Resources. https://www.hrc.org/resources/glossary-of-terms.

7. National LGBT Health Education Center. Providing Inclusive Services and Care for LGBT People: A Guide for Healthcare Staff. LGBT Health Education. https://www.lgbtqiahealtheducation.org/wp-content/uploads/Providing-Inclusive-Services-and-Care-for-LGBT-People.pdf.

8. Long T, Rodriguez C, Snyder M, Watson R. *Chapter 8: LGBTQ Health and Wellness*. LGBTQ+ Studies: An Open Textbook; 2022.

9. CDC. *HIV Incidence. Center for Disease Control and Prevention*; September 2, 2022. https://www.cdc.gov/hiv/statistics/overview/in-us/incidence.html.

10. Lane M, Ives GC, Sluiter EC, et al. Trends in gender-affirming surgery in insured patients in the United States. *Plast Reconstr Surg Glob Open*. 2018;6(4):e1738. https://doi.org/10.1097/GOX.0000000000001738.

11. Allée K. World Professional Association for Transgender Health. Encyclopedia Britannica. Accessed February 5, 2023. https://www.britannica.com/topic/World-Professional-Association-for-Transgender-Health.

12. Rhodan M. Obamacare Rule Bans Discrimination against Transgender Patients. TIME.

13. Stein S. *White House Reverses Trump Ban on LGBT Health Protections (2)*. Bloomberg Law; May 10, 2021. https://news.bloomberglaw.com/health-law-and-business/biden-administration-reverses-trump-ban-on-lgbt-health-guards.

14. Equality Maps: Healthcare Laws and Policies. Movement Advancement Project. Accessed February 4, 2023. https://www.lgbtmap.org/equality-maps/healthcare_laws_and_policies.

15. James SE, Herman J, Keisling M, Mottet L, Anafi M. *U.S. Transgender Survey (USTS)*. 2015. https://doi.org/10.3886/ICPSR37229.v1. Published online 2019.

16. Ameican Civil Liberties Union. *Mapping Attacks on LGBTQ Rights in U.S. State Legislature*. Legislative Attacks on LGBTQ Rights; February 3, 2023. https://www.aclu.org/legislative-attacks-on-lgbtq-rights.

17. Shetty G, Sanchez JA, Lancaster JM, Wilson LE, Quinn GP, Schabath MB. Oncology healthcare providers' knowledge, attitudes, and practice behaviors regarding LGBT health. *Patient Educ Counsel*. 2016;99(10):1676−1684. https://doi.org/10.1016/j.pec.2016.05.004.

18. Rounds KE, McGrath BB, Walsh E. Perspectives on provider behaviors: a qualitative study of sexual and gender minorities regarding quality of care. *Contemp Nurse*. 2013;44(1):99−110. https://doi.org/10.5172/conu.2013.44.1.99.

19. Morrison SD, Dy GW, Chong HJ, et al. Transgender-related education in plastic surgery and urology residency programs. *J Grad Med Educ*. 2017;9(2):178−183. https://doi.org/10.4300/JGME-D-16-00417.1.

20. Moll J, Krieger P, Moreno-Walton L, et al. The prevalence of lesbian, gay, bisexual, and transgender health education and training in emergency medicine residency programs: what do we know? *Acad Emerg Med*. 2014;21(5):608−611. https://doi.org/10.1111/acem.12368.

21. Obedin-Maliver J, Goldsmith ES, Stewart L, et al. Lesbian, gay, bisexual, and transgender-related content in undergraduate medical education. *JAMA*. 2011;306(9):971−977. https://doi.org/10.1001/jama.2011.1255.

22. Shields R, Lau B, Haider AH. Emergency general surgery needs for lesbian, gay, bisexual, and transgender patients: are we prepared? *JAMA Surg.* 2017;152(7): 617−618. https://doi.org/10.1001/jamasurg.2017.0541.

23. Chaiet SR, Yoshikawa N, Sturm A, Flanary V, Ishman S, Streed CGJ. The otolaryngologist's role in providing gender-affirming care: an opportunity for improved education and training. *Otolaryngol Head Neck Surg.* 2018;158(6):974−976. https://doi.org/10.1177/0194599818758270.

24. Goffman E. *1922−1982. Stigma; Notes on the Management of Spoiled Identity.* Englewood Cliffs, N.J.: Prentice-Hall; 1963:1963. https://search.library.wisc.edu/catalog/999472649302121.

25. Sabin JA, Riskind RG, Nosek BA. Health care providers' implicit and explicit attitudes toward lesbian women and gay men. *Am J Publ Health.* 2015;105(9):1831−1841. https://doi.org/10.2105/AJPH.2015.302631.

26. Brotman S, Ryan B, Cormier R. The health and social service needs of gay and lesbian elders and their families in Canada. *Gerontol.* 2003;43(2):192−202. https://doi.org/10.1093/geront/43.2.192.

27. Durso LE, Meyer IH. Patterns and predictors of disclosure of sexual orientation to healthcare providers among lesbians, gay men, and bisexuals. *Sex Res Soc Policy J NSRC SR SP.* 2013;10(1):35−42. https://doi.org/10.1007/s13178-012-0105-2.

28. Haas A, Rodgers PL, Herman JL. *Suicide Attempts Among Transgender and Gender Non-conforming Adults*; June 10, 2022. Available from: https://williamsinstitute-law-ucla-edu.turing.library.northwestern.edu/research/suicide-attempts-among-transgender-and-gender-non-conforming-adults/.x.

29. Durso L, Baker K, Cray A. *LGBT Communities and the Affordable Care Act: Findings from a National Survey Center for American Progress*; 2013. Available from: https://cdn.americanprogress.org/wp-content/uploads/2013/10/LGBT-ACAsurvey-brief1.pdf.

30. James SE, Herman JL, Rankin S, Keisling M, Mottet L, Anaf M. *The Report of the 2015. U.S. Transgender Survey*; 2015.

31. Baker KD, Cray LE. *Moving the Needle: The Impact of the Affordable Care Act on LGBT Communities.* Center for American Progress; November 17, 2014. https://www.americanprogress.org/issues/lgbt/reports/2014/11/17/101575/moving-the-needle/.

32. Truman J, Morgan R. *Violent Victimization by Sexual Orientation and Gender Identity, 2017−2020.* BJS Statisticians; 2022. https://bjs.ojp.gov/content/pub/pdf/vvsogi1720.pdf.

33. de Lange J, Baams L, van Bergen DD, Bos HMW, Bosker RJ. Minority stress and suicidal ideation and suicide attempts among LGBT adolescents and young adults: a meta-analysis. *LGBT Health.* 2022;9(4):222−237. https://doi.org/10.1089/lgbt.2021.0106.

34. Dickey LM, Singh AA, Walinsky D. Treatment of trauma and nonsuicidal self-injury in transgender adults. *Psychiatr Clin.* 2017;40(1):41−50. https://doi.org/10.1016/j.psc.2016.10.007.

35. Gooren LJ. Clinical practice. Care of transsexual persons. *N Engl J Med.* 2011;364(13): 1251−1257. https://doi.org/10.1056/NEJMcp1008161.

36. Winter S, Diamond M, Green J, et al. Transgender people: health at the margins of society. *Lancet Lond Engl.* 2016;388(10042):390−400. https://doi.org/10.1016/S0140-6736(16)00683-8.

37. Marshal MP, Friedman MS, Stall R, et al. Sexual orientation and adolescent substance use: a meta-analysis and methodological review. *Addict Abingdon Engl.* 2008;103(4): 546−556. https://doi.org/10.1111/j.1360-0443.2008.02149.x.

38. Schuler MS, Stein BD, Collins RL. Differences in substance use disparities across age groups in a national cross-sectional survey of lesbian, gay, and bisexual adults. *LGBT Health.* 2019;6(2):68−76. https://doi.org/10.1089/lgbt.2018.0125.

39. King BA, Dube SR, Tynan MA. Current tobacco use among adults in the United States: findings from the National Adult Tobacco Survey. *Am J Publ Health.* 2012;102(11):e93−e100. https://doi.org/10.2105/AJPH.2012.301002.

40. Jethwa AR, Khariwala SS. Tobacco-related carcinogenesis in head and neck cancer. *Cancer Metastasis Rev.* 2017;36(3):411−423. https://doi.org/10.1007/s10555-017-9689-6.

41. Jemal A, Bray F, Center MM, Ferlay J, Ward E, Forman D. Global cancer statistics. *CA Cancer J Clin.* 2011;61(2):69−90. https://doi.org/10.3322/caac.20107.

42. Hillel A, O'Mara W, Nemechek A, Mushatt DM. Head and neck manifestations in HIV infection. *J La State Med Soc.* 2004;156(5):245−253.

43. Hall HI, Song R, Tang T, et al. HIV trends in the United States: diagnoses and estimated incidence. *JMIR Public Health Surveill.* 2017;3(1):e8. https://doi.org/10.2196/publichealth.7051.

44. Prasad HKC, Bhojwani KM, Shenoy V, Prasad SC. HIV manifestations in otolaryngology. *Am J Otolaryngol.* 2006;27(3):179−185. https://doi.org/10.1016/j.amjoto.2005.09.011.

45. Rzewnicki I, Olszewska E, Rogowska-Szadkowska D. HIV infections in otolaryngology. *Med Sci Monit Int Med J Exp Clin Res.* 2012;18(3):RA17−21. https://doi.org/10.12659/msm.882505.

46. Althuis MD, Fergenbaum JH, Garcia-Closas M, Brinton LA, Madigan MP, Sherman ME. Etiology of hormone receptor-defined breast cancer: a systematic review of the literature. *Cancer Epidemiol Biomark Prev Publ Am Assoc Cancer Res Cosponsored Am Soc Prev Oncol.* 2004;13(10):1558−1568.

47. Cochran SD, Mays VM. Risk of breast cancer mortality among women cohabiting with same sex partners: findings from the National Health Interview Survey, 1997-2003. *J Womens Health.* 2012;21(5):528−533. https://doi.org/10.1089/jwh.2011.3134.

48. Machalek DA, Poynten M, Jin F, et al. Anal human papillomavirus infection and associated neoplastic lesions in men who have sex with men: a systematic review and meta-analysis. *Lancet Oncol.* 2012;13(5):487−500. https://doi.org/10.1016/S1470-2045(12)70080-3.

49. Chaturvedi AK, Graubard BI, Broutian T, et al. NHANES 2009−2012 findings: association of sexual behaviors with higher prevalence of oral oncogenic human papillomavirus infections in U.S. men. *Cancer Res.* 2015;75(12):2468−2477. https://doi.org/10.1158/0008-5472.CAN-14-2843.

50. Read TRH, Hocking JS, Vodstrcil LA, et al. Oral human papillomavirus in men having sex with men: risk-factors and sampling. *PLoS One.* 2012;7(11):e49324. https://doi.org/10.1371/journal.pone.0049324.

51. Herrero R, Quint W, Hildesheim A, et al. Reduced prevalence of oral human papillomavirus (HPV) 4 years after bivalent HPV vaccination in a randomized clinical trial in Costa Rica. *PLoS One.* 2013;8(7):e68329. https://doi.org/10.1371/journal.pone.0068329.

52. Palefsky JM, Giuliano AR, Goldstone S, et al. HPV vaccine against anal HPV infection and anal intraepithelial neoplasia. *N Engl J Med.* 2011;365(17):1576−1585. https://doi.org/10.1056/NEJMoa1010971.

53. Oliver SE, Gorbach PM, Gratzer B, et al. Risk factors for oral human papillomavirus infection among young men who have sex with men-2 cities, United States, 2012–2014. *Sex Transm Dis*. 2018;45(10):660–665. https://doi.org/10.1097/OLQ.0000000000000845.

54. Bowen DJ, Boehmer U. The lack of cancer surveillance data on sexual minorities and strategies for change. *Cancer Causes Control*. 2007;18(4):343–349. https://doi.org/10.1007/s10552-007-0115-1.

55. Howlader N, Ries LAG, Mariotto AB, Reichman ME, Ruhl J, Cronin KA. Improved estimates of cancer-specific survival rates from population-based data. *J Natl Cancer Inst*. 2010;102(20):1584–1598. https://doi.org/10.1093/jnci/djq366.

56. Thompson HM, Kronk CA, Feasley K, Pachwicewicz P, Karnik NS. Implementation of gender identity and assigned sex at birth data collection in electronic health records: where are we now? *Int J Environ Res Publ Health*. 2021;18(12). https://doi.org/10.3390/ijerph18126599.

57. *Institute of Medicine (US) Committee on Lesbian, Gay, Bisexual, and Transgender Health Issues and Research Gaps and Opportunities. The Health of Lesbian, Gay, Bisexual, and Transgender People: Building a Foundation for Better Understanding*. National Academies Press (US); 2011. https://doi.org/10.17226/13128. https://www.ncbi.nlm.nih.gov/books/NBK64806/.

58. Hinyard L, Wirth LS, Clancy JM, Schwartz T. The effect of marital status on breast cancer-related outcomes in women under 65: a SEER database analysis. *Breast Edinb Scotl*. 2017;32:13–17. https://doi.org/10.1016/j.breast.2016.12.008.

59. Torbrand C, Wigertz A, Drevin L, et al. Socioeconomic factors and penile cancer risk and mortality; a population-based study. *BJU Int*. 2017;119(2):254–260. https://doi.org/10.1111/bju.13534.

60. Fleisch Marcus A, Illescas AH, Hohl BC, Llanos AAM. Relationships between social isolation, neighborhood poverty, and cancer mortality in a population-based study of US adults. *PLoS One*. 2017;12(3):e0173370. https://doi.org/10.1371/journal.pone.0173370.

61. Wallace SP, Cochran SD, Durazo EM, Ford CL. The health of aging lesbian, gay and bisexual adults in California. *Policy Brief UCLA Cent Health Policy Res*. 2011;(PB2011-2):1–8.

62. Bränström R, Pachankis JE. Reduction in mental health treatment utilization among transgender individuals after gender-affirming surgeries: a total population study. *Am J Psychiatr*. 2020;177(8):727–734. https://doi.org/10.1176/appi.ajp.2019.19010080.

63. Caprini RM, Oberoi MK, Dejam D, et al. Effect of gender-affirming facial feminization surgery on psychosocial outcomes. *Ann Surg*. July 4, 2022. https://doi.org/10.1097/SLA.0000000000005472.

64. Wirtz AL, Poteat TC, Malik M, Glass N. Gender-based violence against transgender people in the United States: a call for research and programming. *Trauma Violence Abuse*. 2020;21(2):227–241. https://doi.org/10.1177/1524838018757749.

65. Stotzer R. Violence against transgender people: a review of United States data. *Aggress Violent Behav*. 2009;14(3):170–179.

66. Hancock AB, Krissinger J, Owen K. Voice perceptions and quality of life of transgender people. *J Voice*. 2011;25(5):553–558. https://doi.org/10.1016/j.jvoice.2010.07.013.

67. Watt SO, Tskhay KO, Rule NO. Masculine voices predict well-being in female-to-male transgender individuals. *Arch Sex Behav*. 2018;47(4):963–972. https://doi.org/10.1007/s10508-017-1095-1.

68. McNeill EJM, Wilson JA, Clark S, Deakin J. Perception of voice in the transgender client. *J Voice*. 2008;22(6):727–733. https://doi.org/10.1016/j.jvoice.2006.12.010.
69. Spiegel JH. Facial determinants of female gender and feminizing forehead cranioplasty. *Laryngoscope*. 2011;121(2):250–261. https://doi.org/10.1002/lary.21187.
70. Tran BNN, Epstein S, Singhal D, Lee BT, Tobias AM, Ganor O. Gender affirmation surgery: a synopsis using American college of surgeons national surgery quality improvement program and national inpatient sample databases. *Ann Plast Surg*. 2018;80 (4 Suppl 4):S229–S235. https://doi.org/10.1097/SAP.0000000000001350.
71. Puckett JA, Cleary P, Rossman K, Newcomb ME, Mustanski B. Barriers to gender-affirming care for transgender and gender nonconforming individuals. *Sex Res Soc Policy J NSRC SR SP*. 2018;15(1):48–59. https://doi.org/10.1007/s13178-017-0295-8.
72. El-Hadi H, Stone J, Temple-Oberle C, Harrop AR. Gender-affirming surgery for transgender individuals: perceived satisfaction and barriers to care. *Plast Surg Oakv Ont*. 2018;26(4):263–268. https://doi.org/10.1177/2292550318767437.
73. DeVore EK, Gadkaree SK, Richburg K, et al. Coverage for gender-affirming voice surgery and therapy for transgender individuals. *Laryngoscope*. 2021;131(3):E896–E902. https://doi.org/10.1002/lary.28986.
74. Ngaage LM, Knighton BJ, Benzel CA, et al. A review of insurance coverage of gender-affirming genital surgery. *Plast Reconstr Surg*. 2020;145(3):803–812. https://doi.org/10.1097/PRS.0000000000006591.
75. Coleman E, Bockting W, Botzer M, et al. Standards of care for the health of transsexual, transgender, and gender-nonconforming people. *Int J Transgenderism*. 2012;13(4):165–232 (Version 7).
76. Portone C, Johns 3rd MM, Hapner ER. A review of patient adherence to the recommendation for voice therapy. *J Voice*. 2008;22(2):192–196. https://doi.org/10.1016/j.jvoice.2006.09.009.
77. Koma W, Rae M, Neuman T, Kates J, Dawson L. *Demographics, Insurance Coverage, and Access to Care Among Transgender Adults*; October 21, 2020. https://www.kff.org/health-reform/issue-brief/demographics-insurance-coverage-and-access-to-care-among-transgender-adults/. Accessed June 8, 2022.
78. Gorbea E, Gidumal S, Kozato A, Pang JH, Safer JD, Rosenberg J. Insurance coverage of facial gender affirmation surgery: a review of Medicaid and commercial insurance. *Otolaryngol Head Neck Surg*. 2021;165(6):791–797. https://doi.org/10.1177/0194599821997734.
78a. Gadkaree SK, DeVore EK, Richburg K, et al. National variation of insurance coverage for gender-affirming facial feminization surgery. *Facial Plast Surg Aesthetic Med*. 2021;23(4):270–277. https://doi.org/10.1089/fpsam.2020.0226.
79. The Federal Register. *Nondiscrimination in Health Programs and Activities; a Rule by the Health and Human Services Department*. Center for Medicaid and Medicare Services; 2022.
80. Squires A. *How to Make Your Practice a Safe Space: LGBTQ+ Allyship and Healthcare*. *Pediatric EHR Solutions*; 2018. https://blog.pcc.com/how-to-make-your-practice-a-safe-space-lgbtq-allyship-and-healthcare.
81. Taylor DJ, Denneny JC. AAO-HNS Implicit Bias Video Series. American Academy of Otolaryngology-Head and Neck Surgery. https://www.entnet.org/about-us/diversity-equity-inclusion/implicit-bias-video-series/.

Transgender care in otolaryngology

6

Samuel A. Floren[1], Amber Maria Sheth[2], Scott Randolph Chaiet[1]

[1]*Division of Otolaryngology—Head and Neck Surgery, University of Wisconsin School of Medicine and Public Health, Madison, WI, United States;* [2]*Department of Surgery, University of Wisconsin School of Medicine and Public Health, Madison, WI, United States*

Introduction

There are many classifications to describe transgender individuals. Sexual and gender minorities (SGMs) are a diverse and heterogenous group of minoritized people with similar lived experiences and disparities, many of whom are encompassed in the lesbian, gay, bisexual, transgender, queer, intersex, and asexual (LGBTQIA) community (Table 6.1). The word transgender has been described as an umbrella term. Notably, this can include a variety of gender identity terms which are gender minorities. There are some 1.3 million adults (0.5%) and 300,000 youth (1.4%, ages 13 and older) in the United States (US) who identify as transgender.[1] A more inclusive label is transgender and gender diverse (TGD) individuals, all whose intrinsic sense of self (gender) is different than their assigned sex at birth, which will be used in this chapter. Up to 14% of TGD people expressed discomfort with being described as transgender; other terms to describe their gender identity include gender nonbinary/nonconforming and genderqueer.[2]

TGD individuals face difficult societal disparities and medical discrimination. Many of these are outside of the scope of this otolaryngology-centric chapter. However, many societal injustices influence the way in which we interact with patients in our clinics, such as discrimination experienced at work, lack of access to gender-appropriate bathrooms, etc.

It is incumbent on providers to understand disparities to promote more healthy and equitable health care. To this end, the American Academy of Otolaryngology—Head and Neck Surgery (AAO-HNS) states that "culturally effective care is predicated on cultural sensitivity and cultural competence."[3] The AAO-HNS policy continues that it "will support diversity in all of its forms, encompassing but not limited to age, disability status, economic circumstance, ethnicity, gender, race, religion, and sexual orientation." Further, the Hippocratic Oath states specifically to "do no harm or injustice to [our patients]." It is the Academy's policy, a sacred oath, and our ethical obligation to practice culturally competent and medically sound care to all our patients inclusive of SGMs.

Healthcare Disparities in Otolaryngology. https://doi.org/10.1016/B978-0-443-10714-6.00014-6

85

Table 6.1 Important definitions.

Sex	Outward characteristics assigned at birth, often based on genital anatomy or karyotype
Gender identity	The gender with which one intrinsically identifies (inwardly focused)
Gender expression	The outward expression of one's gender by mannerisms, dress, etc. (outwardly focused)
Sexual/romantic orientation	The kind of person one is attracted to
Heterosexual	One who is attracted to someone of the opposite gender identity
Cisgender	One whose gender identity and sex are congruent
LGBTQIA	An acronym for "lesbian, gay, bisexual, transgender, queer, intersex, asexual/agender" that has come to symbolize the marginalized gender and sexual minorities

Original.

The role of otolaryngology in the treatment of gender dysphoria

Gender dysphoria is the experience by individuals of incongruence between one's experienced or expressed gender and their assigned gender, lasting at least six months.[4] The treatment of gender dysphoria may require intervention by many medical and surgical disciplines, but only for those suffering from dysphoria. Treatment is frequently multidisciplinary and will help affirm a patient in their own gender identity; authors have called for the incorporation of gender-affirming care teams and patient care conferences, similar to "tumor boards," in order to help individualize care to patients needs and goals.[5] There are many disciplines that can be beneficial including (but not limited to) endocrinology, urology, plastic surgery, gynecology, facial plastic surgery, laryngology, speech and language pathology, mental health, and psychiatry.

Although there are many TGD patients who require gender-affirming medical and surgical intervention for the treatment of gender dysphoria, there is also a cohort that is not interested in actively pursuing anatomic or hormonal treatment for gender affirmation. This leads to a heterogenous collection of patient's goals of care, to which the care team needs to be understanding and sensitive. Approximately half of TGD patients (54%) have received either surgery or hormonal therapy, with only 25% having ever undergone transition-related surgery.[2]

Otolaryngologists can play a key role for TGD patients that wish to pursue treatment of gender dysphoria. Some of the gender-affirming interventions offered by otolaryngologists include facial surgery and pitch-altering voice surgery (in conjunction with voice therapy with our speech and language pathologist colleagues). For feminizing facial surgery, historically known as facial feminization surgery (FFS), there are a variety of surgeries offered, including but not limited to contouring of the frontal bone, scalp advancement (for lowering the hairline), brow lift, rhinoplasty, cheek augmentation, lip augmentation, genioplasty (chin shaping), and mandible changes.[6] Further surgical interventions include chondrolaryngoplasty, for the reduction of prominent thyroid cartilage,[7] and feminization laryngoplasty, to raise the fundamental frequency of a patient's voice.[8] Additionally, speech and language pathologists provide voice therapy to help patients have a gender-congruent voice that may or may not be accompanied by surgical intervention.[9]

Masculinizing hormone therapy often increases facial hair, deepens the voice, and causes fat redistribution to a more stereotypical masculine facial structure. Therefore, fewer patients will seek masculinizing facial surgery.[10] Interventions include forehead augmentation, cheek volume changes including buccal fat reduction, rhinoplasty, mandibular angle augmentation, chin augmentation, and thyroid cartilage augmentation. A 2019 review of scholarly works surrounding facial masculinization found a relative paucity of academic works compared to the facial feminization literature, and only 2 of 15 articles that included outcome analyses.[11]

Of the 1.3 million TGD in the US, there is a large demand for surgical intervention. In the US Transgender Study (USTS) in 2015, 39% of transgender women/nonbinary patients desired feminizing surgery of the face or neck and even more (46%) desired gender-related voice therapy.[12] Surgery or therapy to masculinize the face or voice was not assessed in transgender men.

Otolaryngologists share the unique privilege of providing gender-affirming care that will both be seen by the patient every time they look in a mirror and that can also have a substantial impact on how the patient is perceived by others, including visual or auditory recognition of femininity and masculinity. While TGD patients have diverse health needs that go beyond interventions to treat gender dysphoria, otolaryngology as a specialty has an important role in providing gender-affirming care.

Efficacy of gender-affirming care

Gender-affirming care is a spectrum of care that involves social, behavioral, and medical interventions for the purpose of affirming someone's gender identity as it contrasts with their sex assigned at birth.[12a] This can range from behavioral counseling and voice therapy to medical and hormonal treatment to reconstructive surgery.

In an analysis of survey respondents to the USTS, researchers discovered that transgender individuals who had undergone gender-affirming surgery within the previous two years had significantly lower psychological distress, suicidal ideation, and tobacco smoking than their matched peers who had not undergone surgery. Yet despite its benefits, 59.2% of all respondents reported desire to but not undergoing gender confirmation surgery of any type.[13] A study specific to FFS compared cisgender females to female transgender individuals with and without gender-affirming surgery, finding those who underwent gender-affirming facial surgery had statistically significant improvement in their mental health quality of life. Additionally, it importantly showed no difference in the improvement between patients who underwent gender reassignment surgery and those who underwent FFS.[14]

Indeed, the literature seems to point to the benefit of gender-affirming care in reducing gender dysphoria. This cements the otolaryngologist's role in understanding the milieu of this care and our place in it. However, there is a discrepancy between the demand of otolaryngologic specific gender-affirming care and delivery of the care. Per the 2015 USTS results regarding respondents assigned male at birth, 46% desire gender-related voice therapy (while only 11% have received it), 39% desire facial feminization (while only 4% have received it), 29% desire chondrolaryngoplasty (while only 4% have received it), and 16% desired pitch-altering phonosurgery (while only 1% have received it). Both barriers in coverage of affordable surgical care and access to providers contribute to these gaps. However, more recent data point to increased utilization of surgical services in gender-affirming care.[15]

In conjunction with the need for more insurance coverage, based on the evidence of its benefit to reduce gender dysphoria, there is increased urgency for the otolaryngologist with an understanding of gender-affirming care to improve access to care. And, while many otolaryngologists will not perform gender-affirming surgery, it does not lessen the need to understand its indications, speak knowledgably about the treatments provided to treat gender dysphoria, and participate in advocacy; this can include referrals to regional surgeons or speech and language pathologists engaging in gender-affirming care.

TGD disparities background

TGD individuals have been the subject of historic and ongoing discrimination that spans a lack of civil rights from the federal legal level to discrimination at the individual level. Transphobia describes the pattern of discrimination, both systemic and individual, against TGD people and contributes to their status as a marginalized population. While a full discussion of the history and current issues affecting TGD people is beyond the scope of this chapter, a brief overview of disparities affecting the TGD population as studied by the 2015 USTS will be included.

Moreover, the inclusion of this data is not to reduce the experiences of TGD populations to statistics alone, but rather to convey the scope of inequities facing this community. Imperative to approaching these statistics is an understanding that intersecting systems of oppression result in worse outcomes for TGD people who hold other marginalized identities, such as racial, ethnic, or ability status.[16] Additionally, the TGD community is one of current and historic strength and resilience, with literatureshowing improved mental health outcomes when surrounded by supportive friends and family.[17]

TGD people face high levels of mistreatment and violence,[18] ranging from rejection by family members,[19] mistreatment and harassment in the school environment,[20] workplace mistreatment,[21] and sexual assault.[22] Additionally, according to the USTS, 46% of respondents reported experiencing verbal harassment and

9% reported physical violence against them in the year prior due to their gender identity. Given the hostile legal, societal, and interpersonal landscape for TGD individuals, it is sadly unsurprising that mental health conditions are highly prevalent in this population. In the USTS, 40% of respondents reported at least one suicide attempt in their lifetime, compared with the national attempted suicide rate of 4.6% in the general population.

Identities are intersectional, and TGD people who are also people of color are disproportionately impacted by confluent systems of transphobia and racism. Respondents to the USTS who identified as transgender people of color were more than three times as likely to be living in poverty compared to the general population. Respondents who were undocumented immigrants were more likely to be facing severe economic hardship compared to other respondents and had high rates of physical violence perpetrated against them. Transgender people who have disabilities also face significant impacts of discrimination, as indicated by 45% of USTS respondents with disabilities indicating that they were living in poverty.

In all, these statistics describe a system of societal disparities experienced by TGD people. Together, these form the social determinants of health for TGD people, and as such are important for any medical provider to understand. While no single patient is their community's statistic, understanding the background of disparities experienced by the TGD community can help the physician consider the challenges that may impact a TGD patient's initial presentation, ability to interact with the healthcare system, and treatment course.

Health disparities and barriers to gender-affirming care

TGD patients face a variety of challenges within the healthcare system. Barriers include upstream determinants such as access to care and experiences in the delivery of care. Broadly, as mentioned earlier in this chapter, TGD people are more likely to be living in poverty than their cisgender counterparts, which has downstream impacts on healthcare access. When compared with cisgender persons, TGD patients are less likely to be insured, limiting their access to general and gender-affirming care.[23] Additionally, TGD patients are more likely to struggle with tobacco use, a risk factor of upper aerodigestive tract cancers and surgical site complications.[24] In addition to intersectional identities, poverty is also more common among TGD persons as a whole relative to cis-straight persons.[25] Perhaps most notable, TGD patients are significantly less likely to seek medical care and more likely to be discriminated in the clinical setting (with this effect being more pronounced in American Indian and Middle Eastern populations).[12]

Healthcare providers should be aware of the experiences TGD patients have in our clinical spaces. In 2015, 23% of USTS respondents reported avoiding medical care due to fear of being mistreated as a transgender person. And when they did obtain medical care, 33% of those who saw a healthcare provider had at least one negative experience related to being transgender, such as being verbally harassed or refused treatment because of their gender identity. Additionally, higher percentages of transgender people of color and transgender people with disabilities reported negative experiences in the healthcare setting. These struggles are compounded by limitations of access and the obstacle of insurance coverage specific to gender-affirming care. Despite legislation in 2014 preventing insurance companies from discriminating coverage based on transgender status, insurance companies continue to have highly variable policies with regard to gender-affirming treatment, resulting in yet another hurdle to their care.[26] Insurance companies may also require additional steps including psychological evaluation, compounding the barriers to care.

Structural barriers to accessing gender-affirming surgery result in negative health effects, with a nearly 50% increase in attempted suicide rate by TGD patients who were denied medical care because of their gender status (from 41% to 60%) compared to peers who were not denied care. This violates our first duty of "do no harm."[27] While much of these data are for gender-affirming care, and not specific to otolaryngologic care, all providers have a responsibility to be aware of the systemic and upstream barriers to accessing care for the TGD population, and where possible reduce these barriers.

Gap in physician education

Education of the otolaryngology physician workforce is sorely lacking.[5] Less than one third (29.7%) of current otolaryngology trainees (residents or fellows) are exposed to transgender didactic education or gender-affirming care. This contrasts with plastic surgery and urology,[28] who are exposed at higher rates of 82% and 70%, respectively.

More TGD-based curricula need to be incorporated into otolaryngology training and residency programs. In a recent survey of otolaryngology program directors, respondents reported that where it existed, curricula around the care of SGM individuals revolved primarily around medical care rather than cultural sensitivity best practices.[29] Cited barriers to implementation of SGM educational topics in otolaryngology residency programs were lack of experienced faculty and lack of time.

Misgendering

It is important that everyone practicing in the medical care of TGD patients utilize cultural sensitivity best practices with avoidance of misgendering through appropriate personal pronouns. Misgendering is when someone is referred to by a gender to which they do not identify. In the case of an accidental misgendering, one should acknowledge and briefly apologize for the mistake, but ongoing misgendering is a form of discrimination. Introducing oneself with one's own pronouns can demonstrate attention to inclusivity and create a welcoming environment both with patients and colleagues. However, no one is obligated to share their pronouns. The surgeon can also be an advocate as a leader among medical professionals by using the correct pronouns for patients and reminding others of a patient's pronouns if misgendering occurs. This matter of cultural sensitivity requires a lifelong practice in humility and sensitivity.

While innocuous to some, misgendering can have a significant negative effect on patient care. One qualitative study found that misgendering (among other trans-exclusionary microaggressions) can lead transgender individuals to take their peers' medical advice over that of their physicians.[30] Another study found that misgendering led to a breach of trust in the patient–physician relationship, resulting in the patient needing to educate the physician.[31] Resources exist to help avoid this form of discrimination, most notably electronic medical records (EMRs), which can provide clinicians and office staff the patient's preferred pronouns and preferred names.[32] However, resources are only valuable and useful if used. Otolaryngologists can be leaders in knowing how to effectively leverage the EMR to correctly document a patient's gender, and to strive for inclusive gender pronoun use for in-person interactions with all individuals in the office.

TGD providers

Important to understanding diversity within otolaryngology is recognizing our own field. There is great value in celebrating TGD otolaryngologists, speech language pathologists, healthcare professionals, and staff. Unfortunately, providers also face discrimination. A survey of LGBTQIA physicians found 22% had been socially ostracized and 65% had heard derogatory comments about LGBTQIA individuals at work.[33] Medical students face similar issues, where 60% of transgender and gender-expansive individuals concealed their gender identity, with over 40% citing fear of discrimination as their motivation.[34] Our role in cultural sensitivity and antidiscriminatory behavior must also be carried into the remainder of the workplace and is important to create an inclusive environment for all colleagues.

Conclusion

The population prevalence of TGD people is increasing,[35] and societal norms are moving toward greater civil rights for transgender people. Medical and surgical innovation has brought gender-affirming therapies to TGD individuals such as facial gender-affirming surgery.

There are upstream disparities and determinants of health for the TGD population, but otolaryngologists are positioned to have a positive impact in this health care. Otolaryngologists have a responsibility to provide culturally sensitive trans care and to set the tone for culturally sensitive care to our TGD patients. We recognize the fast-paced nature of evolving terminology and social norms, but even small changes toward inclusivity can have a large impact on reducing barriers to health care such as correcting misgendering. Otolaryngologists will likely have TGD patients at some point in their practice and are uniquely seated as part of the gender-affirming multidisciplinary team to provide education, advocacy, referral services, or surgical care for our patients.

References

1. Herman JL, Flores AR, O'Neill KK. *How Many Adults and Youth Identify as Transgender in the United States?* The Williams Institute, UCLA School of Law; 2022.
2. James SE, Herman JL, Rankin S, Keisling M, Mottet L, Anafi M. *The Report of the 2015 U.S. Transgender Survey.* Washington, DC: National Center for Transgender Equality; 2016.
3. Diversity, Equity, and Inclusion. *American Academy of Otolaryngology-Head and Neck Surgery*; 2023. Retrieved February 16, 2023, from https://www.entnet.org/about-us/diversity-equity-inclusion.
4. American Psychiatric Association. *Diagnostic and Statistical Manual of Mental Disorders.* 5th ed. Arlington, VA: American Psychiatric Publishing; 2013.
5. Massenburg BB, Morrison SD, Rashidi V, et al. Educational exposure to transgender patient care in otolaryngology training. *J Craniofac Surg.* July 2018;29(5):1252—1257. https://doi.org/10.1097/SCS.0000000000004609. PMID: 29771846.
6. Altman K. Facial feminization surgery: current state of the art. *Int J Oral Maxillofac Surg.* August 2012;41(8):885—894. https://doi.org/10.1016/j.ijom.2012.04.024. Epub 2012 Jun 6. PMID: 22682235.
7. Tang CG, Debbaneh PM, Kleinberger AJ. Chondrolaryngoplasty. *Otolaryngol Clin.* August 2022;55(4):871—884. https://doi.org/10.1016/j.otc.2022.04.009. Epub 2022 Jun 21. PMID: 35750521.
8. Brown SK, Chang J, Hu S, et al. Addition of wendler glottoplasty to voice therapy improves trans female voice outcomes. *Laryngoscope.* July 2021;131(7):1588—1593. https://doi.org/10.1002/lary.29050. Epub 2020 Aug 26. PMID: 32846023.
9. Quinn S, Oates J, Dacakis G. The effectiveness of gender affirming voice training for transfeminine clients: a comparison of traditional versus intensive delivery schedules. *J Voice.* April 7, 2022;S0892—1997(22). https://doi.org/10.1016/j.jvoice.2022.03.001. Epub ahead of print. PMID: 35400554.
10. Harris J, Premaratne I, Spector J. Facial masculinization from procedures to payment: a review. *LGBT Health.* October 2021;8(7):444—453. https://doi.org/10.1089/lgbt.2020.0128. Epub 2021 Aug 16.
11. Sayegh F, Ludwig D, Ascha M, et al. Facial masculinization surgery and its role in the treatment of gender dysphoria. *J Craniofac Surg.* 2019;30(5):1339—1346. https://doi.org/10.1097/SCS.0000000000005101.
12. National Center for Transgender Equality. *US Transgender Survey*; 2015. http://www.ustranssurvey.org/.
12a. Boyle P. What Is Gender-Affirming Care? Your Questions Answered AAMC. https://www.aamc.org/news-insights/what-gender-affirming-care-your-questions-answered. [Accessed 27 September 2022].

13. Almazan AN, Keuroghlian AS. Association between gender-affirming surgeries and mental health outcomes. *JAMA Surg*. 2021;156(7):611−618. https://doi.org/10.1001/jamasurg.2021.0952.
14. Ainsworth TA, Spiegel JH. Quality of life of individuals with and without facial feminization surgery or gender reassignment surgery. *Qual Life Res*. September 2010;19(7):1019−1024. https://doi.org/10.1007/s11136-010-9668-7. Epub 2010 May 12. PMID: 20461468.
15. Lane M, Ives GC, Sluiter EC, et al. Trends in gender-affirming surgery in insured patients in the United States. *Plast Reconstr Surg Glob Open*. April 16, 2018;6(4), e1738. https://doi.org/10.1097/GOX.0000000000001738. PMID: 29876180; PMCID: PMC5977951.
16. Crenshaw K. Mapping the margins: intersectionality, Identity politics, and violence against women of color. *Stanford Law Rev*. 1991;43:1241−1299.
17. Puckett JA, Matsuno E, Dyar C, Mustanski B, Newcomb ME. Mental health and resilience in transgender individuals: what type of support makes a difference? *J Fam Psychol*. December 2019;33(8):954−964. https://doi.org/10.1037/fam0000561. Epub 2019 Jul 18. PMID: 31318262; PMCID: PMC7390536.
18. Wirtz AL, Poteat TC, Malik M, Glass N. Gender-based violence against transgender people in the United States: a call for research and programming. *Trauma Violence Abuse*. 2020;21(2):227−241. https://doi.org/10.1177/1524838018757749.
19. Koken JA, Bimbi DS, Parsons JT. Experiences of familial acceptance-rejection among transwomen of color. *J Fam Psychol*. December 2009;23(6):853−860. https://doi.org/10.1037/a0017198. PMID: 20001144; PMCID: PMC2840628.
20. Movement Advancement Project and GLSEN. *Separation and Stigma: Transgender Youth and School Facilities*; April 2017. http://lgbtmap.org/transgender-youth-school.
21. Davis NB, Yeung ST. Transgender equity in the workplace: a systematic review. *Sage Open*. 2022;12(1). https://doi.org/10.1177/21582440221082863.
22. Grant JM, Mottet LA, Tanis J, Harrison J, Herman JL, Keisling M. *Injustice at Every Turn: A Report of the National Transgender Discrimination Survey*. Washington: National Center for Transgender Equality and National Gay and Lesbian Task Force; 2011.
23. *AAMC Advisory Committee on Sexual Orientation, Gender Identity, and Sex Development. Implementing Curricular and Institutional Climate Changes to Improve Health Care for Individuals Who Are LGBT, Gender Nonconforming, or Born with DSD*. Association of American Medical Colleges; 2014:280.
24. Azagba S, Latham K, Shan L. Cigarette, smokeless tobacco, and alcohol use among transgender adults in the United States. *Int J Drug Pol*. 2019;73:163−169. https://doi.org/10.1016/j.drugpo.2019.07.024.
25. Badgett M, Choi S, Wilson BD. *LGBT Poverty in the United States: A Study of Differences between Sexual Orientation and Gender Identity Groups*. UCLA: The Williams Institute; 2019. Retrieved from https://escholarship.org/uc/item/37b617z8.
26. Ngaage LM, Xue S, Borrelli MR, et al. Gender-affirming health insurance reform in the United States. *Ann Plast Surg*. August 1, 2021;87(2):119−122. https://doi.org/10.1097/SAP.0000000000002674. PMID: 33470627.
27. Haas AP, Rodgers PL, Herman JL. Suicide Attempts Among Transgender and Gender Non-conforming Adults. Published January 2014 https://williamsinstitute.law.ucla.edu/research/suicide-attempts-among-trans gender-and-gender-non-conforming-adults/. Accessed September 24, 2017.
28. Morrison SD, Dy GW, Chong HJ, et al. Transgender-related education in plastic surgery and urology residency programs. *J Grad Med Educ*. 2017;9:178−183.

29. Goetz TG, Nieman CL, Chaiet SR, Morrison SD, Cabrera-Muffly C, Lustig LR. Sexual and gender minority curriculum within otolaryngology residency programs. *Transgend Health.* 2021;6(5):267−274. https://doi.org/10.1089/trgh.2020.0105. Published 2021 Oct 4.

30. Haire BG, Brook E, Stoddart R, Simpson P. Trans and gender diverse people's experiences of healthcare access in Australia: a qualitative study in people with complex needs. *PLoS One.* 2021;16(1), e0245889. https://doi.org/10.1371/journal.pone.0245889. Published 2021 Jan 28.

31. Persson Tholin J, Broström L. Transgender and gender diverse people's experience of non-transition-related health care in Sweden. *Int J Transgenderism.* 2018;19(4): 424−435. https://doi.org/10.1080/15532739.2018.1465876.

32. Thadikonda KM, Gast KM, Chaiet SR. Sexual orientation and gender identity and surgery. In: Telem DA, Martin CA, eds. *Diversity, Equity and Inclusion. Success in Academic Surgery.* Cham: Springer; 2021. https://doi.org/10.1007/978-3-030-55655-6_11.

33. Eliason MJ, Dibble SL, Robertson PA. Lesbian, gay, bisexual, and transgender (LGBT) physicians' experiences in the workplace. *J Homosex.* 2011;58(10):1355−1371.

34. Mansh M, White W, Gee-Tong L, et al. Sexual and gender minority identity disclosure during undergraduate medical education: "in the closet" in medical school. *Acad Med.* 2015;90(5):634−644.

35. Nolan IT, Kuhner CJ, Dy GW. Demographic and temporal trends in transgender identities and gender confirming surgery. *Transl Androl Urol.* June 2019;8(3):184−190. https://doi.org/10.21037/tau.2019.04.09. PMID: 31380225; PMCID: PMC6626314.

Health disparities related to aging: the growing need for geriatric otolaryngology

7

Michael Collins[1], Patrick Adamcyzk[1], Kourosh Parham[2]

[1]*University of Connecticut School of Medicine, Farmington, CT, United States;* [2]*Department of Surgery, Division of Otolaryngology, Head and Neck Surgery, University of Connecticut School of Medicine, Farmington, CT, United States*

Introduction

Eliminating health disparities across the United States (US) has been a focal point of the US Department of Health and Human Services' *Healthy People* initiatives for the past few decades. Over that time course, the associated goals of each initiative have evolved as growing bodies of evidence have illuminated the multifactorial nature of health disparities faced by Americans. In Healthy People 2000, the second iteration of the initiative, the primary goal was to simply reduce disparities among Americans.[1] In the most recent initiative, Healthy People 2030, the objective has updated to "eliminate health disparities, achieve health equity, and attain health literacy to improve the health and well-being of all."[2] While evolving research dedicated to understanding how disparities play a role in health outcomes is extremely important, numerous definitions of what may be considered a disparity have emerged. Most succinctly, health disparities may be defined as "clinically and statistically significant differences in health outcomes or health care use between socially distinct vulnerable and less vulnerable populations that are not explained by the effects of selection bias."[3,4] Vulnerable populations often face discrimination due to perceived differences in social status, often identified by others as differences in race, ethnicity, age, literacy, sexual orientation, and socioeconomic status. Across the spectrum of medicine, detection of contributors has been successful, yet fully understanding the context-dependent nature of disparities is lacking.[4]

Within otolaryngology, disparities affecting patients in and out of the hospital are being explored. For example, both African American and Hispanic patients are significantly less likely to visit an outpatient otolaryngologist than Caucasian patients and reported lower average cost per emergency department visit. Further, uninsured and lower-income patients with less educational attainment are significantly less likely to receive outpatient otolaryngology care when compared to privately insured and higher-income patients with higher educational attainment.[5] It is documented that across the spectrum of otolaryngology, racial and ethnic minority

Healthcare Disparities in Otolaryngology. https://doi.org/10.1016/B978-0-443-10714-6.00008-0

status, insurance status, and lower socioeconomic status greatly impact point of presentation, disease progression, treatment course, and overall health outcome.[5–16] However, little research has explored geriatric status as a major health disparity in otolaryngology, indicating the great need for further study.

Aging is a ubiquitous human trait, affecting every person regardless of race, ethnicity, gender identity, sexual orientation, and socioeconomic status. As humans get older, advanced age is "associated with changes in dynamic biological, physiological, environmental, psychological, behavioral, and social processes."[17] Many age-related changes are normal and benign, from graying hair to skin changes. However, advanced age may result in decline in senses, diminished activities of daily living (ADLs), and greater susceptibility to disease processes not seen in younger age groups.[17] Importantly, age is thought to be the greatest indicator of overall health due to the accumulation of exposures to external health risks in conjunction with lifestyle choices made throughout one's lifetime. In essence, older age is intersectional; it reflects the culmination of disparities experienced by patients throughout their lifetimes.[18,19] Through the lens of demographics, economic insecurity, frailty, cognitive decline, health literacy, and geography (Fig. 7.1), otolaryngologists may further understand the intersectionality of older age and make more informed proactive and reactive treatment decisions.

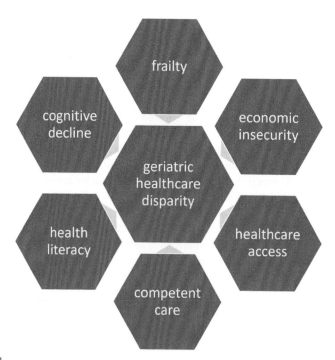

FIGURE 7.1

Factors contributing to geriatric health disparity.

Demographic shifts

Careful attention to factors that influence geriatric care is critical in large part because of the demographic shift that has been underway over the past several decades, captured by US Census data.[20] Those age 65 and over grew from 35.0 million in 2000, to 49.2 million in 2016, representing 12.4% and 15.2% of the total population, respectively. Forces behind this growth included improved health care, in general, as well as the graying of the baby boomers born after World War II between 1946 and 1964. By comparison, while the 65 and over population made up 15.2% of the population, 22.8% of the population were pediatric. For the first time in US history, older adults are projected to outnumber children by 2035. This trend is not expected to change course. By 2060, less than 1/5 of the US population will be under the age of 18, whereas nearly a quarter will be 65 or older, almost 95 million Americans (Fig. 7.2).

Economic insecurity

Economic insecurity is defined as "the anxiety produced by the possible exposure to adverse economic events and by the anticipation of the difficulty to recover from them."[21] Such adverse economic events span an enormous spectrum, from loss of employment to unforeseen medical expenditures, to even normal aging.[22] Economic insecurity within the geriatric population is multifaceted, and understanding key contributors to a patient's economic insecurity facilitates provision of the most comprehensive care.

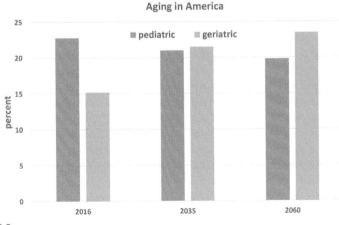

FIGURE 7.2

The anticipated demographic shifts that will alter the health care landscape.

Among senior households, 78% are financially insecure and do not have the economic ability to sustain them through their lives.[23] This estimation was made through the development and application of the Senior Financial Stability Index (SFSI) measuring housing costs, home equity, assets, budget, and health expenditures. Health expenditures within the geriatric population, specifically, represent an enormous hurdle for senior households facing a greater burden of chronic illness and increased susceptibility to acute medical events requiring hospitalization and continued follow-up. According to the CDC, 85% of seniors have at least one chronic disease, and 60% of older individuals have at least two, reflecting a complex care issue when considering care options for patients at greater financial risk.[24]

The culmination of chronic disease within the geriatric population further exacerbates the economic burden with increased frailty and decreased ability to attain gainful employment. Geriatric patients have little ability to mitigate the financial erosion caused by managing one or more medical comorbidities.[25] Currently, 41% of all senior households spend more than 15% of their income on healthcare expenses, putting them at risk of medication noncompliance, medical device noncompliance, and loss to follow-up.[23,25] Out-of-pocket medical expenditures within the geriatric population are significant; geriatric patients comprise the vast majority of total Medicare beneficiaries, and Medicare maintains high cost-sharing requirements.[25,26] Coupled with Medicare not covering routine health-maintenance visits such as vision care, hearing exams, and hearing aids, the ability of many geriatric patients to manage a plethora of health issues may well be impossible.[25]

Within geriatric otolaryngology, the need for cost-effective care is growing. As life expectancy within the US continues to grow, the demand for otolaryngology-based procedures and office visits will rise in lockstep.[27] Between 1960 and 2015, life expectancy of Americans grew from 69.7 to 79.4 years.[28] While such an increase can be attributed to public health efforts increasing awareness about tobacco use, alcohol consumption, and the benefits of increased physical activity, the US is expected to gain more years in average life expectancy in the coming decades. By 2060, the average American is expected to live 85.6 years, underscoring the greater need for both geriatric-competent physicians in the field of otolaryngology and more macrolevel financial accommodations for the increased demand in services.[27,28] Current estimates indicate that geriatric patients will comprise 29.8% of all otolaryngology visits by 2030, a steep rise from 17.9% in 2010. Among all diagnoses made in patients above the age of 65 seeing an otolaryngologist, 73% are otology related.[29] Given that Medicare does not cover hearing aids or exams for the fitting hearing aids, undue financial burden is placed on geriatric patients in financial distress and discourages such patients from pursuing needed treatment means.

Those with private insurance are now able to receive some coverage which is helpful, but since Medicare is the main payer for healthcare services in the geriatric population, the gap is substantial. For geriatric patients with functional hearing loss, an average bundled cost of $2500 for hearing aids would be considered a catastrophic expense, pushing 4% of that population into poverty.[30] However, consideration should be given to the macrolevel implications of allowing untreated hearing loss to persist in the geriatric population. Untreated hearing loss has been directly associated with increased risk of cognitive decline, dementia, risk of falls, increased emergency department use, hospitalizations, and reduced quality of life (QOL).[31] Further, untreated hearing loss has been shown to increase 30-day readmission rates, increased inpatient and outpatient visits, and increased length of stay (LOS) at 2, 5, and 10 years following initial diagnosis of hearing loss. This creates an average additional cost to the healthcare system of $22,434 over a 10-year period, relative to patients with no evidence of hearing impairment.[31] Compared to an upfront cost ranging from $1000 to $4000 to proactively treat patients with functional hearing loss and provide hearing aids, major savings may be made by providing some level of cost reduction.[31,32]

One evolving avenue by which enormous savings may be realized is through the provision of over-the-counter (OTC) hearing aids, which were made possible with the passage of The OTC Hearing Aid Act of 2017 and the subsequent FDA approval in August 2022. Despite the contentious political landscape surrounding the issue, it has been suggested that providing an OTC pathway by which patients unable to afford traditional hearing aids may be assist with expanding access.[33,34] Importantly, the implementation of such legislation would not render the position of audiologists and otolaryngologists in providing hearing aids obsolete; instead, it has been argued that the opposite is expected.[34] Greater affordability, resulting in a much larger patient pool requiring counseling and guidance on the proper use of their hearing aids, could allow for complementary legislation to cover services rendered by audiologists to come to fruition. Reimbursing services provided by audiologists, independent of the sale of a hearing aid, would allow audiologists to shift their focus to patient-centered counseling and teaching rather than the sale of hearing aids. Efforts are being made to improve the current hearing ecosystem that is currently leaving many untreated with the Build Back Better Act. Signed into law in August 2022, the Build Back Better Act includes the expansion of Medicare's hearing benefit which will revamp the current market and create a competitive environment for hearing aids and increase the demand for audiological rehabilitative services.[34,35] Independent of the costs associated with increased readmission rates, hospitalizations, and broader healthcare usage, the robust link between hearing loss and the development of dementia underscores the need to consider the broader implications of allowing hearing loss to go untreated. Hearing loss is considered to be one of the strongest modifiable risk factors for dementia, with hearing aid usage being the greatest protective factor from decline.[36] In 2020, Alzheimer's and other dementias were responsible for $305 billion in total economic costs. By 2050, this is expected to rise to more than $1.1 trillion, indicating the imperative need to employ robust protective measures to diminish system-wide costs.[37]

With a rapidly expanding geriatric population, as understanding of other age-related otolaryngologic problems grows and improved treatments become available, nonotologic disorders of aging, such as voice, swallowing, head and neck cancer, and facial plastics, are expected to rise in proportion. As of 2021, the global market for services rendered by otolaryngologists was $16.15 billion dollars. By 2030, the market is expected to reach $27.95 billion with a forecasted compounded annual growth rate (CAGR) of 6.30%. Importantly, North America and, more specifically the US, comprises the greatest market for such services.[38] Thus, the cost burden is likely to expand beyond what is currently in place.

Frailty

"Frailty [is] a biologic syndrome of decreased reserve and resistance to stressors, resulting from cumulative declines across multiple physiologic systems, and [causes] vulnerability to adverse outcomes."[39] The frail patient may experience age-associated declines in muscle mass, weight, balance, endurance, walking ability, and activity level. However, multiple age-associated deficits must be present in order to deem a patient as frail. While numerous frailty indices are currently used in clinical practice and some controversy exists among clinicians regarding the most accurate measure of frailty, addressing frailty and its implications will play an integral role in treating geriatric patients.

Frailty, as a phenotype, predisposes affected patients to numerous negative clinical outcomes and consistently increases the risk of mortality. About 15% of geriatric nonnursing home patients meet criteria for frailty, and 45% are prefrail, warranting specific treatment considerations in older adults, regardless of perceived independence. Further, frailty may be considered a complex accumulation of life experience and hardship, with women, racial and ethnic minorities, persons in assisted-living settings, persons of lower socioeconomic status, and even persons in certain geographic locations experiencing increased rates of frailty. Importantly, the prevalence of frailty rapidly rises with age. Only 9% of patients aged 65–69 are considered frail, compared to 38% of patients aged 90 and older, highlighting the impact of age. Frailty is now used in various clinical settings as a screening measure for perioperative surgical risk assessment due to the increased burden of chronic disease among frail patients and decreased physiological compensatory ability to endogenous and exogenous stressors.[40]

In examining the incidence of postoperative complications following minor procedures, nonfrail, prefrail, and frail patients experienced complication rates of 3.9%, 7.3%, and 11.4%, respectively. The incidence of postoperative complications following major procedures in nonfrail, prefrail, and frail patients was 19.5%, 33.7%, and 43.5%, respectively. After adjustment for known risks and patient-specific factors, frailty remained an independent risk factor for postoperative complications. Frailty has also been shown to be strong predictor of LOS. Across both minor and major surgical procedures, frailty remains an independent predictor of greater LOS, with 65%–89% increases in LOS, respectively, relative to nonfrail patients.[41]

With an aging and increasingly frail population, otolaryngologists must adapt to the needs of an older population at greater risk of perioperative morbidity and mortality. In examining the utility of a modified frailty index (mFI) in otolaryngology, the mFI was found to be a more robust predictor of morbidity and mortality in patients compared to ASA score, age, or wound class (Table 7.1).

In procedures with low rates of morbidity and mortality, frailty significantly alters the postoperative landscape with mortality increasing from 0.1% to 11.9% and a 26.2% risk of Clavien–Dindo grade IV complications.[42] The Clavien–Dindo classification is a validated postoperative assessment tool with applications to numerous surgical fields, underscoring the need for clinical consideration (Table 7.2).[43]

Such findings are further reinforced when examining the efficacy of the Hospital Frailty Risk Score (HFRS) in the setting of head and neck cancer surgery. Frail patients, compared to their nonfrail counterparts experienced increased 30-day readmission rates (18% vs. 9.5%, $P < 0.01$), increased LOS (8.2 vs. 6.8, $P = 0.02$), and increased total cost of perioperative care ($275,000 vs. $188,000, $P < 0.01$).[44] Within head and neck cancer, frailty accurately predicts type and severity of complication. More specifically, frail patients experience increased rates of medical and Clavien–Dindo grade III or higher complications, independent of age and comorbidity.[45] Frail patients undergoing thyroid cancer surgery echo a similar perioperative course with a threefold increase in susceptibility to in-hospital mortality and surgical complications, in addition to a fivefold increase in medical complications.[46] Ultimately, frailty is a strong predictor of morbidity and mortality that must be considered when treating geriatric patients. Frailty has been shown across the spectrum of otolaryngology to drastically reshape the perioperative treatment journey with increased LOS, readmissions rates, complication rates, and overall mortality. Assessing preoperative frailty is vital for patient risk stratification, counseling, and optimization of treatment decisions.[42–47]

Table 7.1 The modified frailty index—criteria.

Modified frailty index (mFI)—criteria
History of diabetes mellitus
Functional status 2 (not independent)
History of chronic obstructive pulmonary disease or pneumonia
History of congestive heart failure
History of percutaneous coronary intervention, stenting, or angina
History of hypertension requiring medication
History of peripheral vascular disease or ischemic rest pain
History of impaired sensorium
History of transient ischemic attack or cerebrovascular accident
History of cerebrovascular accident with neurological deficit

Table 7.2 The Clavien–Dindo classification for postoperative assessment.

Grades	Definition
Grade I	Any deviation from the normal postoperative course without the need for pharmacological treatment or surgical, endoscopic and radiological interventions. Allowed therapeutic regimens are: drugs as antiemetics, antipyretics, analgetics, diuretics, and electrolytes and physiotherapy. This grade also includes wound infections opened at the bedside.
Grade II	Requiring pharmacological treatment with drugs other than such allowed for grade I complications. Blood transfusions and total parenteral nutrition are also included.
Grade III	Requiring surgical, endoscopic, or radiological intervention
-IIIa	Intervention not under general anesthesia
-IIIb	Intervention under general anesthesia
Grade IV	Life-threatening complication (including CNS complications)[a] requiring IC/ICU management
-IVa	Single organ dysfunction (including dialysis)
-IVb	Multiorgan dysfunction
Grade V	Death of a patient

[a] *brain hemorrhage, ischemic stroke, subarachnoid bleeding, but excluding transient ischemic attacks (TIAs); IC, intermediate care; ICU, intensive care unit (The Clavien-Dindo Classification | AssesSurgery GmbH. The Clavien-Dindo Classification. https://www.assessurgery.com/clavien-dindo-classification/. Accessed September 18, 2022).*

Cognitive decline

Cognitive decline, or diminished memory, problem-solving ability, or speed processing, is a hallmark trait of the geriatric patient population that is associated with increased age.[47,48] Importantly, cognitive impairment among the geriatric population spans an enormous spectrum from mild cognitive impairment (MCI), wherein individuals maintain the ability to independently perform most ADLs, to more severe forms of dementia such as Alzheimer's disease, Parkinson's disease, and many more, in which patients significantly lose their ability to perform ADLs.[49] However, the importance of considering the mental faculties of geriatric patients cannot be overstated due to their demonstrated evidence in patient outcomes.

On a superficial level, two-third of all Americans experience some form of cognitive decline at an average of 70. However, numerous modifiable and unmodifiable risk factors exist and contribute to the development of cognitive impairment, including sex, racial and ethnic background, social advantage, and educational attainment. Across all forms of dementia, women experience a lifetime risk of 37% compared to that of men at 24%. Notably, the most advantaged groups (white individuals and/or those with higher educational attainment) experience delayed onset of cognitive impairment that is generally present only at the very end of life. This is in stark contrast to more disadvantaged groups (Black individuals and/or those with lower educational attainment) in which there is earlier onset, greater number of years impaired, and overall greater lifetime risk.[50] While stratifying risk of cognitive impairment by racial and ethnic background and educational attainment may speak to larger social issues within the US, it necessitates an increased index of suspicion by clinicians when approaching treatment in the geriatric population.

Across the spectrum of medicine, an exhaustive amount of research has demonstrated the link between patient outcomes and cognitive impairment. Medical and surgical patients with dementia are at greater risk of urinary tract infections, pressure ulcers, delirium, and pneumonia. Further, diminished cognition has also been shown to be the most significant risk factor for urinary and fecal incontinence, with 36% and 2% new incontinence, respectively, upon discharge. While patients with dementia experience an increased propensity to develop delirium out-of-hospital, dementia patients are more susceptible to new onset delirium during hospitalization. Of note, dementia has been associated with at least one episode of delirium within three days of admission, increased risk of ICU admission, and in-hospital death in patients aged $\geq$65 years.[51]

The cognitively impaired patient is also at greater risk of falls, a serious public health concern in the geriatric population. Postural stability, or the coordination of motor and sensory systems, is required for divided attention, planning movements, and responding to environmental stimuli. Research has indicated the key regulatory role that cognition plays in gait and balance. Impaired cognition has been identified in clinical practice guidelines as a fall risk factor despite limited measures to quantify the impairment, as well as which dimensions of cognition should be evaluated for the risk of falling.[52] In the community and hospital, cognitive deficits have been associated with increased fall risk, recurrent falls, as well as falls due to behavioral problems.[52,53] While falls have not been consistently demonstrated to be associated with measures of global cognition, poor performance on the Mini Mental Status Exam (MMSE, <27) has been strongly linked to fall-related injuries in the community. With each point decrease on the MMSE, fall risk has been shown to increase by approximately 20% in adults in the community.[53] Falls within the hospital, specifically, are critically important due to risk of fracture and other injury, as well as the broader economic implications of increased LOS and delayed recovery.[52]

Within the realm of impaired cognition, polypharmacy is a particularly relevant consideration in the treatment of geriatric patients. Polypharmacy is defined as the "the concomitant use of 5 or more medications" and may be considered appropriate or inappropriate, depending on the extent of patient comorbidities and treatment needs.[53] Inappropriate polypharmacy refers to OTC medications, supplements with little to no evidence-backed science, inappropriate prescription medications, and their associated interactions and side effects that ultimately diminish benefits and increase risks. Broadly, inappropriate polypharmacy has numerous clinical consequences including adverse drug reactions, depression, frailty, disability, increased health care use, postoperative complications, and mortality. Consideration of the type of medication and its potential side effects and interactions is also crucial for facilitating the most comprehensive care. It is estimated that 13.9% of all dementia patients are prescribed CNS-active polypharmacy, or "overlapping prescription fills for 3 or more medications from the following drug classes: antidepressants, antipsychotics, antiepileptics, benzodiazepines, nonbenzodiazepine benzodiazepine receptor agonist hypnotics, and opioids."[54] An excess of the above drug classes may be responsible for increased falls, further diminished cognition, and mortality.[55] In older adults, an estimated 30% of hospital visits are related to polypharmacy and therefore may be considered preventable.[56] In the inpatient setting, polypharmacy and dependence for at least one ADL has been shown to be associated with adverse drug reactions in patients with dementia.[52] This may be a result of inability to communicate and/or recognize side effects. The relationship between dementia and adverse clinical events (i.e., hypertensive crisis, electrolyte disorders, infection, etc.) has been demonstrated that a single event increases the risk of death by a factor of 10. MCI, conversely, has been shown to be associated with adverse events, but no relationship has been shown with mortality.[52]

Within geriatric otolaryngology, the implications of cognitive impairment are imperative to consider when educating, counseling, and selecting treatment means. Otolaryngologists can further provide meaningful treatment that alleviates common etiologies that occur alongside dementia, including hearing loss, falls, and dysphagia.[57] Hearing loss, specifically, presents a crucial point in the development of dementia that may allow for intervention by otolaryngologists. Hearing loss is independently associated with all-cause dementia after adjustment for age, sex, race, education, smoking, diabetes, and hypertension. Risk of all-cause dementia further increases log-linearly with hearing loss severity, reflecting a key point in the development of dementia that may allow for harm reduction and prevention.[58] While a direct link between dementia and hearing loss has yet to be identified and a number of theories seeking to explain the relationship have been proposed, otolaryngologists should use such data to make informed treatment decisions. Cochlear implants present one solution to potentially alleviate the burden of dementia on patients with hearing loss. Notably, Medicare coverage for cochlear implantation is reasonable, but treatment is generally reserved for patients with more advanced stage hearing loss with failure to gain benefit from hearing aids.[59] In examining patients 18 months postcochlear implantation, speech perception, QOL, communication, and executive function improvements have been observed in nontertiary educated males.[60] Hearing aids, as previously discussed, present a potential avenue by which the development of dementia may be alleviated, despite the economic pitfalls many patients face with acquiring them. The use of hearing aids has been shown to delay the diagnosis of dementia, Alzheimer's disease, anxiety, depression, and falls.[61] While further research is needed regarding the use of augmented-hearing devices and the development of dementia, current treatment means should be employed to preserve QOL and delay decline in cognition in at-risk patients.

Dysphagia, commonly known as difficulty swallowing, may be considered a complex problem of the "behavioral, sensory, and preliminary motor acts in preparation for the swallow, as well as cognitive awareness of the upcoming eating situation, visual recognition of food, and all of the physiologic responses to the smell and presence of food."[62] Dysphagia may be the result of one or multiple of the above mechanisms and is a common symptom in individuals with neurologic disease. It is estimated that the prevalence of dysphagia among dementia patients when clinically and instrumentally assessed is 32%—45% and 84%—93%, respectively.[63] Geriatric dysphagia is multifactorial with numerous targets along the digestive tract. The oral phase is highlighted by diminished salivation and diminished dental health. Importantly, Medicare does not provide dental health coverage, contributing to the decline in overall health.[64] Specifically, dysphagia is a known risk factor for malnutrition and pneumonia and requires specialized treatment means in afflicted individuals.[65,66] In patients with dementia, the odds of hospitalization due to pneumonia are reported to be 1.50[67] and 1.88[68] times relative to control groups, and the odds of pneumonia-associated mortality are increased by twofold.[69] Otolaryngologists may improve QOL, prevent unnecessary hospitalization, and extend life through counseling and making appropriate intervention in patients with dysphagia, when indicated. Appropriate intervention includes surgery for conditions such as cricopharyngeal hypertrophy or Zenker's diverticulum, the prevalence of which increases with age. Evidence indicates that both swallowing rehabilitation interventions, alternative nutritional intake, and prophylactic measures may decrease the risk of malnutrition and pneumonia in the geriatric individuals.[66]

Health literacy

An individual's capability to retrieve and understand basic health information to make informed judgments, or health literacy,[70] is an influential component in health outcomes within many areas of medicine. Insufficiencies in skills associated with health literacy (i.e., reading, writing, communication, computation, application of health knowledge, and, recently, digital technology) are common. Only 12% of US adults are proficiently health literate.[71] The remainder of these Americans struggle with everyday health information seen in health care facilities, retail outlets, media, etc.[72] Health disparities, because of health literacy disparities, have manifested themselves in many of the most prevalent diseases including heart failure, diabetes, and COVID-19. Noteworthy is that not all groups of individuals are equally affected. One socially disadvantaged group facing particularly low levels of health literacy is geriatrics. Adults aged 65 and above have shown to be less health literate than all younger age groups. Even within the geriatric group, such disparities continue to be present, disproportionately affecting racial and ethnic minorities.[73] Health disparities, because of inadequate health literacy, have materialized themselves in numerous domains of medicine for the elderly. It is essential to highlight and address these disparities for an increasingly older population. In geriatric otolaryngology, as noted above, age-related hearing loss, also known as presbycusis, offers a cogent context for consideration of disparities in health literacy.

Presbycusis is a condition witnessed frequently by otolaryngologists. Within the US, one-third of people aged 65 to 74 are estimated to have hearing loss. Almost half of those older than 75 years of age have difficulty hearing.[73] These numbers are predicted to increase. Individuals over 70 with hearing loss are anticipated to rise from 44 million in 2020 to 73 million by 2060.[74] Hearing loss is further complicated by low rates of acceptance and help-seeking behavior seen among the elderly,[75] as well as a lack of awareness of their condition, given the low screening rate and gradual nature of the disorder.[76] These factors all reduce a patient's retrieval of health information regarding presbycusis, limiting their health literacy.

It is believed that greater emphasis on specific and targeted medical evaluations and treatments is essential in the identification of mental health implications associated with hearing loss and hearing loss itself.[77] Otolaryngologists, through an increased understanding of hearing loss, mental health issues, and the interplay between the two, could provide great benefit to this demographic. They could potentially conduct adapted evaluation. Through this, they would aid in the identification of a disorder that would have otherwise gone unnoticed, ultimately providing education, treatment, and referral. In such a model, otolaryngologists would be able to provide their older patients with information about a condition that was previously absent, but necessary, to make informed health judgments. The anticipated increase in patient health literacy, stemming from these adjusted evaluations, may help address the inadequacies and disparities in hearing loss awareness and mental health treatment that geriatrics within otolaryngology face.

Along with the prevalence, comorbidities, and lack of awareness of hearing loss, stark inequities are faced by the geriatric community in the adoption and use of hearing aids, the main treatment related to presbycusis, even after hearing loss is identified. These disparities are not seen when comparing this population to their younger counterparts. In fact, when comparing individuals who could have benefited from hearing devices between the two groups, geriatrics were 24% more likely to have used hearing devices. Rather, disparities are seen within the 30% of geriatrics who have used hearing aids.[78] One study found geriatric Black and Mexican American individuals to be 58% and 78% less likely, respectively, than White individuals to report regular hearing aid use.[79] Geriatric health literacy disparities continue to play a role in presbycusis, as it is one rationale attributed to these inequities as well.

As a group with notably low health literacy, geriatrics may find navigating the healthcare path to hearing aids even more complicated than it already is. This journey begins with multiple entry points (i.e., otolaryngologists, primary care providers, audiologists, hearing aid specialists, and others).[80] Then, multiple visits for audiologic assessment, device fitting, counseling, and medical evaluation take place. Should a geriatric patient manage to successfully traverse this involved system, which is often unguided, and receive their device, they continue to face health literacy-related challenges. Obstacles can be seen when attempting to read and interpret hearing aid user guides. These guides were found to have a mean reading level grade of 9.6,[81] higher than the recommended range of 6—8.[82] Such discrepancies coincide with reports of poor directivity as a reason for the nonuse of hearing aids. Not needing hearing aids and hearing well enough were also reasons cited for the lack of adherence to hearing aids.[83] Findings like this potentially indicate that the importance of hearing loss treatment was not adequately understood by the patients. The significance of these disparities is further highlighted with early discoveries demonstrating the reduction in dementia risk with hearing aid use.[84] Inadequate hearing health has the potential to have detrimental outcomes. Given health literacy's role in the awareness, adoption, and adherence of hearing aids in the geriatric community, it is critical that geriatric health literacy remains an issue at the forefront of improvement efforts.

Substantial system level changes are necessary to resolve the disparities seen in health literacy. These efforts are seen with the Affordable Care Act of 2010, the Department of Health and Human Services' National Action Plan to Improve Health Literacy, and the Plain Writing Act of 2010.[85] These macrolevel approaches do not mean that health care providers are unable to make a substantial impact beginning at a smaller scale. With little work done on geriatric otolaryngology health disparity as it relates to health literacy, we must look at other disciplines of medicine for such examples. Two community pharmacies, for instance, were found to be highly successful when battling low immunization rates due to lack of awareness of a vaccine. With infections being one of the leading causes of morbidity and mortality in geriatrics,[86] extensive implementation could have profound effects.

Interestingly, many parallels regarding vaccination and hearing aid usage, and their relationship to health literacy, exist. For one, hearing aids and immunization are both preventative measures to phenomena progressively affecting individuals as they age, presbycusis and immunosenescence.[87] Both contain inequities in the administration of these preventative measures, disproportionately affecting geriatric racial and ethnic minorities.[88] And in both, these inequities have been linked to health literacy.[89] It is these commonalities that may suggest that the efforts performed by these community pharmacies may be effective within otolaryngology as well.

One of these efforts included the marketing strategy of personal selling. This tactic resulted in patient commitments to receive a specific vaccine 10 times greater when compared to a similar pharmacy who only implemented passive promotion using signage and informational brochures.[90] Perhaps personal selling of hearing aids may have a place in otolaryngology clinics for geriatrics identified with hearing loss. This could be one effort in combating low hearing aid treatment rates. Another pharmacy significantly improved vaccination rates of the same vaccine using automated telephone messages.[91] Likewise, automated phone calls may also have a place in otolaryngology, reminding individuals of the importance of adhering to their hearing aids.

Limited work is present in geriatric otolaryngology on health literacy. It will remain key to learn from other disciplines of medicine and their mitigative techniques. These areas house potential concepts that can be incorporated within otolaryngology.

Healthcare access and quality

Healthcare access is the appropriately timed use of health resources for optimal health outcomes.[92] Not receiving timely care in the US is prevalent. Over one-third of adults avoid medical evaluation that they deem imperative.[93] Such instances of inaccessibility have had profound effects in a broad spectrum of medical disciplines. These effects include poor glycemic control,[94] worse cancer outcomes,[95,96] and substandard oral health.[97] Disparity in access to health care among nonelderly Americans is greatly attributed to the absence of health insurance.[98–100] In 2020, 11.5% of those younger than 65 were uninsured. The elderly, on the other hand, have significantly higher rates of health insurance coverage, in part due to Medicare. The same year, geriatrics saw an only 0.7% rate of being uninsured and a 49% rate of Medicare-associated coverage.[101] Such rates may lead to the incorrect belief that the elderly do not face the same challenge of health care inaccessibility as their younger equivalents. The contrary is seen, almost one quarter of older adults reported avoiding necessary medical care.[102] Cultural, social, economic, and geographic factors all contribute to the disparities seen when gauging the elderly population's access to health care. Following access, it is critical that this population receives tailored care accommodating their uniquely vulnerable characteristics.

Culture

As the US becomes increasingly diverse, accommodation of the associated increase in cultural differences will be necessary in the health care setting. These cultural differences include mistrust of the healthcare system and stigma of receiving health care, both of which impact healthcare access.

Trust is a critical component in relationships, including the one between a patient and the provider. Mistrust between these two parties has shown to be a variable contributing to many aspects of healthcare inaccessibility. Not trusting one's own physician, for example, is associated with a decrease in the utilization of preventative health resources.[103] Mistrust maintains its contribution to healthcare inaccessibility even after initial contact, playing a role during the healthcare visit. Patients with low levels of trust were more likely to report that a needed or requested service was not provided. Even weeks after physician contact, trust's effects do not diminish. Low levels of trust are associated with patients not following doctor's advice and not reporting symptom improvement after two weeks.[103]

Given trust's prominent role in healthcare accessibility, it is worrisome to note that 16% of the public exhibits mistrust of their doctor. This high rate of mistrust is primarily observed in the younger population.[104] The higher levels of trust geriatrics have in their healthcare providers can be explained by their increased number of both interactions with providers and opportunities to develop effective interpersonal relationships.[105,106] Concerning, however, are the disparities within the geriatric group. Within this group, minority patients have been found to have substantially lower levels of healthcare trust when compared to white patients.[105-107]

The historical mistreatment of minorities by the medical community provides many reasons for the lack of trust seen among this group. This includes the USPHS Syphilis Study at Tuskegee. In this study, Black men with syphilis, who did not provide informed consent, were left to suffer with a progressing disease, despite widely available treatments.[108] Such historical mistreatment can be extended to otolaryngology when discussing the "tonsil riots" of 1906. These riots were a result of tonsillectomies being performed on lower-income immigrant children at school, with little to no parental awareness.[109] Mistreatment of minority individuals is not limited to the past and remains prevalent in many areas of medicine. Minority individuals continue to be prescribed analgesics at lower rates when compared to White individuals.[110,111] This marginalized group also is less likely to be recommended for bypass surgery.[112] And within otolaryngology, Black individuals with head and neck cancer are more likely to present with a metastatic cancer, less likely to receive definitive treatment, and have a decreased likelihood of survival from the head and neck cancer.[113]

Undoing the mistrust caused by decades of unjust health care to minorities will require changes in many aspects of the healthcare system. Enhanced racial and ethnic diversity among physicians is one step that has shown to ameliorate these disparities[114] and should continue to be taken.[115] This is particularly pertinent within the field of otolaryngology, which currently trails behind other surgical specialties in the representation of minority individuals.[116] Another step includes the physician's behavior during the patient visit. Reassurance, encouragement of questions, elaboration of test results, nonjudgmental behaviors, and inquiring about a patient's desires were all actions patients cited as successful in constructing a trusting, extended term relationship with a provider.[117] Such behaviors are particularly important during new patient–provider relationships, and other scenarios where patient anxiety and vulnerability may be elevated. This includes scenarios where patients are being treated for head and neck cancers, hearing loss, and swallowing disorders, among others. These efforts will undoubtedly work to increase the trust seen between minority individuals within the geriatric community and otolaryngologists. Such a reduction will be one step in addressing the many barriers to healthcare access this population faces.

Distribution

Distribution of physicians plays a prominent role in healthcare accessibility in rural areas. Approximately 9% of physicians practice in the rural setting, despite 14% of the population living there.[118,119] Disproportionately affected by this poor distribution are the 1 in 5 geriatric individuals living in these areas.[120] Not only is this distribution disparity seen in the context of population size, but also in terms of healthcare need. Increased rates of smoking, physical inactivity, and chronic diseases are seen in rural communities when compared to urban communities.[121] Distribution of otolaryngologists coincides with these findings.[122] Only 38.2% of otolaryngologists serve nonmetropolitan areas that represent 55.3% of the population.[123]

Compounding the health impact from the poor distribution of health care is the poorer quality of care seen in the rural setting.[124] This manifests itself within many areas of otolaryngology. Head and neck cancer patients, for example, have lower rates of survival during treatment at small-bed, rural, or nonteaching hospitals.[125] Additionally, patients presenting with early stages of laryngeal cancer in a rural setting saw decreased rates of laryngeal preservation techniques as first treatment.[126] Outside of cancer treatment, rural community adult members have reported insufficient access to qualified providers as a considerable hurdle when seeking audiologic care.[127]

Despite these disparities and the expected rise in the number of geriatric individuals living in rural areas,[128] there have been 139 rural hospital closures since 2010. This trend does not appear to be stopping, with 2019 being the worst year for closures.[129]

Provider competency and healthcare quality

Identification of variables that influence geriatric health disparity needs to be followed by efforts to address these variables. It has been effectively demonstrated that improved care of the geriatric patient, particularly the vulnerable elders, improves elder health outcomes. Thus, provider competency in provision of geriatric care needs to be addressed. Optimizing surgical care for older adults is critical, as patients 65 years and older account for more than 40% of all inpatient operations. This older population has displayed distinct challenges in this area. Older adults have shown to have higher rates of mortality following surgical intervention.[130] Postoperatively, they are also more likely to experience complications, including delirium and falls.[131] Falls are the leading cause of fatal and nonfatal injuries for adults aged 65 and older.[132] Delirium accounts for up to a $150 billion annual cost to the US.

A major initiative to address geriatric disparities was launched by the American College of Surgeons (ACS) in collaboration with the American Geriatrics Society. This evidence-based initiative became part of the National Surgical Quality Program Initiative covering pre- and perioperative care of the geriatric patient.[133,134] This was followed by the Geriatric Surgery Verification program that was designed to systematically evaluate surgical care and outcomes for the aging adult population by participating hospitals.[135] Surgical specialties have paralleled the ACS effort by creating care pathways, specifically targeting the common geriatric problems such as hip fractures.[136] Within otolaryngology, there are few examples of systematic effort to improve the quality of geriatric care. The one exception is the American

Academy of Otolaryngology—Head and Neck Surgery quality improvement project which was launched with the development of the age-related hearing loss measures intended for clinicians to evaluate the patient perception, structure, process, and outcomes of care.[137]

In parallel with quality improvement initiatives, empowering the next generation of otolaryngologists, who will be faced with managing the otolaryngologic needs of a growing geriatric population, needs to take place. While age-based subspecialization (e.g., pediatric otolaryngology) may come to mind as one strategy to position our specialty to face the coming challenge, this is not a preferred solution. The limitations of such an approach are highlighted by difficulty of geriatric fellowships to fill all of their spots and train enough geriatricians to meet the growing needs. An alternative model of next gen empowerment is to integrate geriatric training into the otolaryngology residency curriculum. This model would capitalize on each subspecialty within otolaryngology to make geriatric-focused contributions driven by insight, experience, and the limited, but growing amount of data that is being generated. This is the strategy that has been adopted by the American Board of Otolaryngology—Head and Neck Surgery as it updates the otolaryngology job task analysis.

Conclusion

The geriatric population faces numerous age-associated issues that must be addressed to provide the most comprehensive care. Economic insecurity, cognitive decline, frailty, inadequate health literacy, and lack of access are ubiquitous among geriatric patients, and greater awareness is required to alleviate such disparities. Further research and initiatives in otolaryngology—head and neck surgery and allied fields will be necessary to define strategies and programs that may lift patient burden, promote positive health outcomes, and extend longevity of life.

References

1. Healthy People—HP2020 Overview of Health Disparities. https://www.cdc.gov/nchs/healthy_people/hp2020/health-disparities.htm. Accessed August 4, 2022.
2. Health Equity in Healthy People 2030. https://www.health.gov/healthypeople/priority-areas/health-equity-healthy-people-2030. Accessed August 4, 2022.
3. Kilbourne AM, Switzer G, Hyman K, Crowley-Matoka M, Fine MJ. Advancing health disparities research within the health care system: a conceptual framework. *Am J Publ Health.* 2006;96(12):2113—2121. https://doi.org/10.2105/AJPH.2005.077628.
4. Unequal Treatment: How to Move from Detecting to Understanding. Bulletin—The official member magazine of the American Academy of Otolaryngology-Head and Neck Surgery. https://www.bulletin.entnet.org/aao-hnsf-2021/article/21259132/unequal-treatment-how-to-move-from-detecting-to-understanding-and-reducing-health care-disparities-within-otolaryngology. Accessed August 4, 2022.

5. Ruthberg JS, Khan HA, Knusel KD, Rabah NM, Otteson TD. Health disparities in the access and cost of health care for otolaryngologic conditions. *Otolaryngol Head Neck Surg*. 2020;162(4):479−488. https://doi.org/10.1177/0194599820904369.

6. https://bulletin.entnet.org/aao-hnsf-2021/article/21403373/out-of-committee-outcomes-research-and- -medicine-growing-the-evidence-base-for-healthcare-disparities-and-soc ial-determinants-of-health-research-in-otolaryngologyhead-and-neck-surgery.

7. Chen AY, Halpern M. Factors predictive of survival in advanced laryngeal cancer. *Arch Otolaryngol Head Neck Surg*. 2007;133(12):1270−1276. https://doi.org/10.1001/archotol.133.12.1270.

8. Shavers VL, Harlan LC, Winn D, Davis WW. Racial/ethnic patterns of care for cancers of the oral cavity, pharynx, larynx, sinuses, and salivary glands. *Cancer Metastasis Rev*. 2003;22(1):25−38. https://doi.org/10.1023/a:1022255800411.

9. Olarte LS, Megwalu UC. The impact of demographic and socioeconomic factors on major salivary gland cancer survival. *Otolaryngol Head Neck Surg*. 2014;150(6):991−998. https://doi.org/10.1177/0194599814526556.

10. Schrank TP, Han Y, Weiss H, Resto VA. Case-matching analysis of head and neck squamous cell carcinoma in racial and ethnic minorities in the United States–possible role for human papillomavirus in survival disparities. *Head Neck*. 2011;33(1):45−53. https://doi.org/10.1002/hed.21398.

11. Saini AT, Genden EM, Megwalu UC. Sociodemographic disparities in choice of therapy and survival in advanced laryngeal cancer. *Am J Otolaryngol*. 2016;37(2):65−69. https://doi.org/10.1016/j.amjoto.2015.10.004.

12. Zandberg DP, Liu S, Goloubeva O, et al. Oropharyngeal cancer as a driver of racial outcome disparities in squamous cell carcinoma of the head and neck: 10-year experience at the University of Maryland Greenebaum Cancer Center. *Head Neck*. 2016; 38(4):564−572. https://doi.org/10.1002/hed.23933.

13. Megwalu UC, Ma Y. Racial disparities in oropharyngeal cancer survival. *Oral Oncol*. 2017;65:33−37, 10.1016/j. evidencebased oraloncology.2016.12.015.

14. Shin JY, Yoon JK, Shin AK, Blumenfeld P, Mai M, Diaz AZ. Association of insurance and community-level socioeconomic status with treatment and outcome of squamous cell carcinoma of the pharynx. *JAMA Otolaryngol Head Neck Surg*. 2017;143(9): 899−907. https://doi.org/10.1001/jamaoto.2017.0837.

15. Inverso G, Mahal BA, Aizer AA, Donoff RB, Chuang SK. Health insurance affects head and neck cancer treatment patterns and outcomes. *J Oral Maxillofac Surg*. 2016;74(6): 1241−1247. https://doi.org/10.1016/j.joms.2015.12.023.

16. Megwalu UC. Impact of county-level socioeconomic status on oropharyngeal cancer survival in the United States. *Otolaryngology-Head Neck Surg (Tokyo)*. 2017;156(4): 665−670. https://doi.org/10.1177/0194599817691462.

17. Understanding the Dynamics of the Aging Process | National Institute on Aging. https://www.nia.nih.gov/about/aging-strategic-directions-research/understanding-dynamics-ag ing. Accessed July 3, 2022.

18. Health Inequalities in Old Age. United Nations. https://www.un.org/development/desa/ageing/wp-content/uploads/sites/24/2018/04/Health-Inequalities-in-Old-Age.pdf. Accessed July 3, 2022.

19. WORLD REPORT ON AGEING AND HEALTH. World Health Organization. https://apps.who.int/iris/bitstream/handle/10665/186463/9789240694811_eng.pdf. Accessed July 5, 2022.

20. *The Population 65 Years and Older*. United States Census Bureau; 2016. www.census. gov/library/visualizations/interactive/population-65-years.html. Accessed July 6, 2022.

21. Bossert W, D'Ambrosio C. Measuring economic insecurity. *Int Econ Rev*. 2013;54(3): 1017−1030.

22. What triggers economic insecurity and who is most at risk? | DISD. United Nations. www.un.org/development/desa/dspd/2021/04/economic-insecurity/. Accessed June 11, 2022.

23. Wheary J, Shapiro T, Meschede T. Living Longer on Less The New Economic (In)Security of Seniors. Demos. www.demos.org/research/living-longer-less-new-economic-insecurity-seniors. Published January 28, 2009. Accessed June 12, 2022.

24. Supporting Older Patients with Chronic Conditions | National . National Institute on Aging. www.nia.nih.gov/health/supporting-older-patients-chronic-conditions. Accessed July 6, 2022.

25. Fong JH. Out-of-pocket health spending among Medicare beneficiaries: which chronic diseases are most costly? *PLoS One*. 2019;14(9):e0222539. https://doi.org/10.1371/journal.pone.0222539.

26. 2022 Medicare Parts A & B Premiums and Deductibles/2022 . Medicare.gov. https://www.cms.gov/newsroom/fact-sheets/2022-medicare-parts-b-premiums-and-deductibles 2022-medicare-part-d-income-related-monthly-adjustment. Accessed July 8, 2022.

27. Chiu BL, Pinto JM. Aging in the United States: opportunities and challenges for otolaryngology-head and neck surgery. *Otolaryngol Clin North Am*. 2018;51(4): 697−704. https://doi.org/10.1016/j.otc.2018.03.001.

28. Living Longer: Historical and Projected Life Expectancy in the United States Census Bureau. https://www.census.gov/content/dam/Census/library/publications/2020/demo/p25-1145.pdf. Accessed July 3, 2022.

29. Creighton Jr FX, Poliashenko SM, Statham MM, Abramson P, Johns 3rd MM. The growing geriatric otolaryngology patient population: a study of 131,700 new patient encounters. *Laryngoscope*. 2013;123(1):97−102. https://doi.org/10.1002/lary.23476.

30. Jilla AM, Johnson CE, Huntington-Klein N. *Hearing Aid Affordability in the United States, Disability and Rehabilitation*. Assistive Technology; 2020. https://doi.org/10.1080/17483107.2020.1822449.

31. Reed NS, Altan A, Deal JA, et al. Trends in health care costs and utilization associated with untreated hearing loss over 10 years. *JAMA Otolaryngol Head Neck Surg*. 2019; 145(1):27−34. https://doi.org/10.1001/jamaoto.2018.2875.

32. Hearing aid prices—How much do hearing aids cost? Healthy Hearing. https://www.healthyhearing.com/help/hearing-aids/prices. Accessed July 23, 2022.

33. Senators press FDA to finalize OTC hearing aids, accuse industry of MEDTECHDIVE. https://www.medtechdive.com/news/senators-warren-grassley-otc-hearing-aids-accuse-industry/626662/. Accessed July 27, 2022.

34. Lin FR, Reed NS. Over-the-counter hearing aids: how we got here and necessary next steps. *J Am Geriatr Soc*. 2022;70(7):1954−1956. https://doi.org/10.1111/jgs.17842.

35. The Build Back Better Framework | The White House. The White House. https://www.whitehouse.gov/build-back-better/. Accessed July 30, 2022.

36. Livingston G, Huntley J, Sommerlad A, et al. Dementia prevention, intervention, and care: 2020 report of the Lancet Commission. *Lancet*. 2020;396(10248):413−446. https://doi.org/10.1016/S0140-6736(20)30367-6.

37. Health and Economic Costs of Chronic Diseases | CDC. Centers for Disease Control and Prevention. https://www.cdc.gov/chronicdisease/about/costs/index.htm. Accessed June 27, 2022.

38. Ear Nose Throat (ENT) Treatment Market Size to Hit US$ 27.95 Bn. GlobeNewsWire. https://www.globenewswire.com/news-release/2022/02/15/2385574/0/en/Ear-Nose-Throat-ENT-Treatment-Market-Size-to-Hit-US-27-95-Bn-by-2030.html. Published February 15, 2022. Accessed July 28, 2022.

39. Fried LP, Tangen CM, Walston J, et al. Frailty in older adults: evidence for a phenotype. *J Gerontol A Biol Sci Med Sci.* 2001;56(3):M146–M156. https://doi.org/10.1093/gerona/56.3.m146.

40. Bandeen-Roche K, Seplaki CL, Huang J, et al. Frailty in older adults: a nationally representative profile in the United States. *J Gerontol A Biol Sci Med Sci.* 2015;70(11): 1427–1434. https://doi.org/10.1093/gerona/glv133.

41. Makary MA, Segev DL, Pronovost PJ, et al. Frailty as a predictor of surgical outcomes in older patients. *J Am Coll Surg.* 2010;210(6):901–908. https://doi.org/10.1016/j.jamcollsurg.2010.01.028.

42. Adams P, Ghanem T, Stachler R, Hall F, Velanovich V, Rubinfeld I. Frailty as a predictor of morbidity and mortality in inpatient head and neck surgery. *JAMA Otolaryngol Head Neck Surg.* 2013;139(8):783–789. https://doi.org/10.1001/jamaoto.2013.3969.

43. Clavien PA, Barkun J, de Oliveira ML, et al. The Clavien-Dindo classification of surgical complications: five-year experience. *Ann Surg.* 2009;250(2):187–196. https://doi.org/10.1097/SLA.0b013e3181b13ca2.

44. Voora RS, Qian AS, Kotha NV, et al. Frailty index as a predictor of readmission in patients with head and neck cancer. *Otolaryngology-Head Neck Surg (Tokyo).* 2022; 167(1):89–96. https://doi.org/10.1177/01945998211043489.

45. Goldstein DP, Sklar MC, de Almeida JR, et al. Frailty as a predictor of outcomes in patients undergoing head and neck cancer surgery. *Laryngoscope.* 2020;130(5): E340–E345. https://doi.org/10.1002/lary.28222.

46. Xu D, Fei M, Lai Y, Shen Y, Zhou J. Impact of frailty on inpatient outcomes in thyroid cancer surgery: 10-year results from the U.S. national inpatient sample. *J Otolaryngol Head Neck Surg.* 2020;49(1):51. https://doi.org/10.1186/s40463-020-00450-5. Published 2020 Jul 22.

47. Park HL, O'Connell JE, Thomson RG. A systematic review of cognitive decline in the general elderly population. *Int. J. Geriat. Psychiatry.* 2003;18:1121–1134. https://doi.org/10.1002/gps.1023.

48. Klimova B, Valis M, Kuca K. Cognitive decline in normal aging and its prevention: a review on non-pharmacological lifestyle strategies. *Clin Interv Aging.* 2017;12: 903–910. https://doi.org/10.2147/CIA.S132963. Published 2017 May 25.

49. Mild Cognitive Impairment (MCI) | Symptoms & Treatments | alz.org. Alzheimer's Association. https://www.alz.org/alzheimers-dementia/what-is-dementia/related_conditions/mild-cognitive-impairment. Accessed June 26, 2022.

50. Hale JM, Schneider DC, Mehta NK, Myrskylä M. Cognitive impairment in the U.S.: lifetime risk, age at onset, and years impaired [published correction appears in SSM Popul Health. 2020 Dec 10;12:100715]. *SSM Popul Health.* 2020;11:100577. https://doi.org/10.1016/j.ssmph.2020.100577. Published 2020 Mar 31.

51. Fogg C, Griffiths P, Meredith P, Bridges J. Hospital outcomes of older people with cognitive impairment: an integrative review [published online ahead of print, 2018

Jun 26]. *Int J Geriatr Psychiatr.* 2018;33(9):1177—1197. https://doi.org/10.1002/gps.4919.

52. Muir SW, Gopaul K, Manuel M, Montero O. The role of cognitive impairment in fall risk among older adults: a systematic review and meta-analysis. *Age Ageing.* May 2012;41(3):299—308. https://doi.org/10.1093/ageing/afs012.

53. Cheng CM, Chang WH, Chiu YC, et al. Association of polypharmacy with mild cognitive impairment and cognitive ability: a nationwide survey in Taiwan. *J Clin Psychiatry.* 2018;79(6):17m12043. https://doi.org/10.4088/JCP.17m12043. Published 2018 Sep. 25.

54. Maust DT, Strominger J, Kim HM, et al. Prevalence of central nervous system—active polypharmacy among older adults with dementia in the US. *JAMA.* 2021;325(10): 952—961. https://doi.org/10.1001/jama.2021.1195.

55. Is Polypharmacy Risky for People with Dementia? | Alzheimer. Alzheimer's Drug Discovery Foundation. www.alzdiscovery.org/news-room/announcements/is-polypharmacy-risky-for-people-with-dementia. Accessed June 26, 2022.

56. Chippa V, Roy K. Geriatric Cognitive Decline and Polypharmacy—StatPearls—NCBI. National Library of Medicine. www.ncbi.nlm.nih.gov/books/NBK574575/. Accessed July 8, 2022.

57. Otolaryngology Patients with Dementia: A Growing Care Need and Opportunity. bulletin—The official member magazine of the American Academy of Otolaryngology-Head and Neck Surgery. bulletin.entnet.org/home/article/22236746/otolaryngology-patients-with-dementia-a-growing-care-need-and-opportunity. Published June 10, 2022. Accessed June 28, 2022.

58. Lin FR, Metter EJ, O'Brien RJ, Resnick SM, Zonderman AB, Ferrucci L. Hearing loss and incident dementia. *Arch Neurol.* 2011;68(2):214—220. https://doi.org/10.1001/archneurol.2010.362.

59. Krogmann R, Al Khalili Y. Cochlear Implants—StatPearls—NCBI Bookshelf. National Library of Medicine. www.ncbi.nlm.nih.gov/books/NBK544280/. Accessed July 8, 2022.

60. Sarant J, Harris D, Busby P, et al. The effect of cochlear implants on cognitive function in older adults: initial baseline and 18-month follow up results for a prospective international longitudinal study. *Front Neurosci.* 2019;13:789. https://doi.org/10.3389/fnins.2019.00789. Published 2019 Aug 2.

61. Mahmoudi E, Basu T, Langa K, et al. Can hearing aids delay time to diagnosis of dementia, depression, or falls in older adults? *J Am Geriatr Soc.* 2019;67(11):2362—2369. https://doi.org/10.1111/jgs.16109.

62. Logemann JA. Effects of aging on the swallowing mechanism. *Otolaryngol Clin North Am.* 1990;23(6):1045—1056.

63. Affoo RH, Foley N, Rosenbek J, Kevin Shoemaker J, Martin RE. Swallowing dysfunction and autonomic nervous system dysfunction in Alzheimer's disease: a scoping review of the evidence. *J Am Geriatr Soc.* 2013;61(12):2203—2213. https://doi.org/10.1111/jgs.12553.

64. Dental services - Your Medicare Coverage. Medicare.gov. https://www.medicare.gov/coverage/dental-services. Accessed June 28, 2022.

65. Sura L, Madhavan A, Carnaby G, Crary MA. Dysphagia in the elderly: management and nutritional considerations. *Clin Interv Aging.* 2012;7:287—298. https://doi.org/10.2147/CIA.S23404.

66. Espinosa-Val MC, Martín-Martínez A, Graupera M, et al. Prevalence, risk factors, and complications of oropharyngeal dysphagia in older patients with dementia. *Nutrients.* 2020;12(3):863. https://doi.org/10.3390/nu12030863. Published 2020 Mar 24.

67. Zhao Y, Kuo TC, Weir S, Kramer MS, Ash AS. Healthcare costs and utilization for Medicare beneficiaries with Alzheimer's. *BMC Health Serv Res.* 2008;8:108. https://doi.org/10.1186/1472-6963-8-108. Published 2008 May 22.

68. Phelan EA, Borson S, Grothaus L, Balch S, Larson EB. Association of incident dementia with hospitalizations. *JAMA.* 2012;307(2):165−172. https://doi.org/10.1001/jama.2011.1964.

69. Foley NC, Affoo RH, Martin RE. A systematic review and meta-analysis examining pneumonia-associated mortality in dementia. *Dement Geriatr Cogn Disord.* 2015; 39(1−2):52−67. https://doi.org/10.1159/000367783.

70. Institute of medicine (US) committee on health literacy. In: Nielsen-Bohlman L, Panzer AM, Kindig DA, eds. *Health Literacy: A Prescription to End Confusion.* Washington (DC): National Academies Press (US); 2004.

71. Smith B, Magnani JW. New technologies, new disparities: the intersection of electronic health and digital health literacy. *Int J Cardiol.* 2019;292:280−282. https://doi.org/10.1016/j.ijcard.2019.05.066.

72. Kutner M, Greenberg, et al. *The Health Literacy of America's Adults: Results from the 2003 National Assessment of Adult Literacy*; 2006. https://nces.ed.gov/pubs2006/2006483.pdf.

73. NIDCD fact sheet hearing and balance. U.S. DEPARTMENT OF HEALTH AND HUMAN SERVICES • National Institutes of Health. https://www.nidcd.nih.gov/sites/default/files/Documents/health/hearing/AgeRelatedHearingLoss.pdf. Accessed September 19 2022.

74. Goman AM, Reed NS, Lin FR. Addressing estimated hearing loss in adults in 2060. *JAMA Otolaryngol Head Neck Surg.* 2017;143(7):733−734. https://doi.org/10.1001/jamaoto.2016.4642.

75. Mackenzie CS, Scott T, Mather A, Sareen J. Older adults' help-seeking attitudes and treatment beliefs concerning mental health problems. *Am J Geriatr Psychiatr.* 2008; 16(12):1010−1019. https://doi.org/10.1097/JGP.0b013e31818cd3be.

76. Malani P, Kullgren J, Solway E, et al. *National poll on healthy aging: hearing loss among older adults - screening and testing*; 2021. Published online March 2, https://doi.org/10.7302/245.

77. Cosh S, Helmer C, Delcourt C, Robins TG, Tully PJ. Depression in elderly patients with hearing loss: current perspectives. *Clin Interv Aging.* 2019;14:1471−1480. https://doi.org/10.2147/CIA.S195824. Published 2019 Aug 14.

78. Quick Statistics About Hearing. NIDCD. Accessed August 11, 2022. https://www.nidcd.nih.gov/health/statistics/quick-statistics-hearing.

79. Nieman CL, Marrone N, Szanton SL, Thorpe Jr RJ, Lin FR. Racial/ethnic and socioeconomic disparities in hearing health care among older Americans. *J Aging Health.* 2016; 28(1):68−94. https://doi.org/10.1177/0898264315585505.

80. Donahue A, Dubno JR, Beck L. Guest editorial: accessible and affordable hearing health care for adults with mild to moderate hearing loss. *Ear Hear.* 2010;31(1):2−6. https://doi.org/10.1097/AUD.0b013e3181cbc783.

81. Caposecco A, Hickson L, Meyer C. Hearing aid user guides: suitability for older adults. *Int J Audiol.* 2014;53(Suppl 1):S43−S51. https://doi.org/10.3109/14992027.2013.832417.

82. Ridpath J. Nih.gov. Published 2009. Accessed August 14, 2022. https://www.nhlbi.nih. gov/files/docs/ghchs_readability_toolkit.pdf.

83. McCormack A, Fortnum H. Why do people fitted with hearing aids not wear them? *Int J Audiol.* 2013;52(5):360−368. https://doi.org/10.3109/14992027.2013.769066.

84. Bucholc M, McClean PL, Bauermeister S, et al. Association of the use of hearing aids with the conversion from mild cognitive impairment to dementia and progression of dementia: a longitudinal retrospective study. *Alzheimers Dement (NY).* 2021;7(1):e12122. https://doi.org/10.1002/trc2.12122. Published 2021 Feb 14.

85. Koh HK, Berwick DM, Clancy CM, et al. New federal policy initiatives to boost health literacy can help the nation move beyond the cycle of costly 'crisis care. *Health Aff.* 2012;31(2):434−443. https://doi.org/10.1377/hlthaff.2011.1169.

86. Gorina Y, Hoyert D, Lentzner H, Goulding M. Trends in causes of death among older persons in the United States. *Aging Trends.* 2005;(6):1−12.

87. Sadighi Akha AA. Aging and the immune system: an overview. *J Immunol Methods.* 2018;463:21−26. https://doi.org/10.1016/j.jim.2018.08.005.

88. Elekwachi O, Wingate LT, Clarke Tasker V, et al. A review of racial and ethnic disparities in immunizations for elderly adults. *J Prim Care Community Health.* 2021;12. https://doi.org/10.1177/21501327211014071, 21501327211014071.

89. Lu PJ, Euler GL, Jumaan AO, Harpaz R. Herpes zoster vaccination among adults aged 60 years or older in the United States, 2007: uptake of the first new vaccine to target seniors. *Vaccine.* 2009;27(6):882−887. https://doi.org/10.1016/j.vaccine.2008.11.077.

90. Bryan AR, Liu Y, Kuehl PG. Advocating zoster vaccination in a community pharmacy through use of personal selling. *J Am Pharmaceut Assoc.* 2013;53(1):70−77. https:// doi.org/10.1331/JAPhA.2013.11097.

91. Hess R. Impact of automated telephone messaging on zoster vaccination rates in community pharmacies. *J Am Pharmaceut Assoc.* 2013;53(2):182−187. https://doi.org/ 10.1331/JAPhA.2013.12222.

92. Committee on monitoring access to personal health care services, institute of medicine, national Academy of sciences. In: Millman M, ed. *Access to Health Care in America.* National Academies Press; 1993.

93. Kannan VD, Veazie PJ. Predictors of avoiding medical care and reasons for avoidance behavior. *Med Care.* 2014;52(4):336−345. https://doi.org/10.1097/MLR.000000000 0000100.

94. Zhang X, Bullard KM, Gregg EW, et al. Access to health care and control of ABCs of diabetes. *Diabetes Care.* 2012;35(7):1566−1571. https://doi.org/10.2337/dc12-0081.

95. Erickson BK, Martin JY, Shah MM, Straughn Jr JM, Leath 3rd CA. Reasons for failure to deliver National Comprehensive Cancer Network (NCCN)-adherent care in the treatment of epithelial ovarian cancer at an NCCN cancer center. *Gynecol Oncol.* 2014; 133(2):142−146. https://doi.org/10.1016/j.ygyno.2014.02.006.

96. Smith EC, Ziogas A, Anton-Culver H. Delay in surgical treatment and survival after breast cancer diagnosis in young women by race/ethnicity. *JAMA Surg.* 2013;148(6): 516−523. https://doi.org/10.1001/jamasurg.2013.1680.

97. Northridge ME, Kumar A, Kaur R. Disparities in access to oral health care. *Annu Rev Publ Health.* 2020;41:513−535. https://doi.org/10.1146/annurev-publhealth-040119-094318.

98. Kreider AR, French B, Aysola J, Saloner B, Noonan KG, Rubin DM. Quality of health insurance coverage and access to care for children in low-income families. *JAMA Pediatr.* 2016;170(1):43−51. https://doi.org/10.1001/jamapediatrics.2015.3028.

99. Diamant AL, Hays RD, Morales LS, et al. Delays and unmet need for health care among adult primary care patients in a restructured urban public health system. *Am J Publ Health.* 2004;94(5):783–789. https://doi.org/10.2105/ajph.94.5.783.

100. Taber JM, Leyva B, Persoskie A. Why do people avoid medical care? A qualitative study using national data. *J Gen Intern Med.* 2015;30(3):290–297. https://doi.org/10.1007/s11606-014-3089-1.

101. Cha AE, Cohen RA. National Health Statistics Reports. Cdc.gov. Accessed September 1, 2022. https://www.cdc.gov/nchs/data/nhsr/nhsr169.pdf.

102. Leyva B, Taber JM, Trivedi AN. Medical care avoidance among older adults. *J Appl Gerontol.* 2020;39(1):74–85. https://doi.org/10.1177/0733464817747415.

103. Thom DH, Kravitz RL, Bell RA, Krupat E, Azari R. Patient trust in the physician: relationship to patient requests. *Fam Pract.* 2002;19(5):476–483. https://doi.org/10.1093/fampra/19.5.476.

104. The American Board of Internal Medicine Foundation commissioned NORC to conduct surveys of trust in the U.S. health care system General Public Survey. Norc.org. Published 2021. Accessed September 23, 2022. https://www.norc.org/PDFs/ABIM%20Foundation/20210520_NORC_ABIM_Foundation_Trust%20in%20Healthcare_Part%201.pdf.

105. Halbert CH, Armstrong K, Gandy Jr OH, Shaker L. Racial differences in trust in health care providers. *Arch Intern Med.* 2006;166(8):896–901. https://doi.org/10.1001/archinte.166.8.896.

106. Musa D, Schulz R, Harris R, Silverman M, Thomas SB. Trust in the health care system and the use of preventive health services by older black and white adults. *Am J Publ Health.* 2009;99(7):1293–1299. https://doi.org/10.2105/AJPH.2007.123927.

107. Watkins YJ, Bonner GJ, Wang E, Wilkie DJ, Ferrans CE, Dancy B. Relationship among trust in physicians, demographics, and end-of-life treatment decisions made by african American dementia caregivers. *J Hospice Palliat Nurs.* 2012;14(3):238–243. https://doi.org/10.1097/njh.0b013e318243920c.

108. Tuskegee study - Timeline - CDC - NCHHSTP. Cdc.gov. Published May 3, 2021. Accessed August 11, 2022. https://www.cdc.gov/tuskegee/timeline.htm.

109. Alrassi J, Cochran J, Rosenfeld RM. Tonsil riots and vaccine hesitancy: a 100-year legacy of medical mistrust. *Otolaryngol Head Neck Surg.* 2022;166(6):1144–1146. https://doi.org/10.1177/01945998211037707.

110. Singhal A, Tien YY, Hsia RY. Racial-ethnic disparities in opioid prescriptions at emergency department visits for conditions commonly associated with prescription drug abuse. *PLoS One.* 2016;11(8):e0159224. https://doi.org/10.1371/journal.pone.0159224. Published 2016 Aug 8.

111. Berger AJ, Wang Y, Rowe C, Chung B, Chang S, Haleblian G. Racial disparities in analgesic use amongst patients presenting to the emergency department for kidney stones in the United States. *Am J Emerg Med.* 2021;39:71–74. https://doi.org/10.1016/j.ajem.2020.01.017.

112. Dovidio JF, Eggly S, Albrecht TL, Penner LA, Penner &. Racial Biases in Medicine and Healthcare Disparities. https://doi.org/10.4473/TPM23.4.5.

113. Mahal BA, Inverso G, Aizer AA, Bruce Donoff R, Chuang SK. Impact of African-American race on presentation, treatment, and survival of head and neck cancer. *Oral Oncol.* 2014;50(12):1177–1181. https://doi.org/10.1016/j.oraloncology.2014.09.004.

114. LaVeist TA, Pierre G. Integrating the 3Ds–social determinants, health disparities, and health-care workforce diversity. *Publ Health Rep*. 2014;129 Suppl 2(Suppl 2):9−14. https://doi.org/10.1177/00333549141291S204.

115. Medical school enrollment more diverse in 2021. AAMC. Published December 6, 2021. Accessed August 8, 2022. https://www.aamc.org/news-insights/press-releases/medical-school-enrollment-more-diverse-2021.

116. Ukatu CC, Welby Berra L, Wu Q, Franzese C. The state of diversity based on race, ethnicity, and sex in otolaryngology in 2016. *Laryngoscope*. 2020;130(12): E795−E800. https://doi.org/10.1002/lary.28447.

117. Dang BN, Westbrook RA, Njue SM, Giordano TP. Building trust and rapport early in the new doctor-patient relationship: a longitudinal qualitative study. *BMC Med Educ*. 2017;17(1):32. https://doi.org/10.1186/s12909-017-0868-5. Published 2017 Feb 2.

118. Rosenblatt RA, Hart LG. Physicians and rural America. *West J Med*. 2000;173(5): 348−351. https://doi.org/10.1136/ewjm.173.5.348.

119. United States Department of Agriculture Rural America at a glance - USDA. https://www.ers.usda.gov/webdocs/publications/80894/eib-162.pdf. Accessed September 2, 2022.

120. US Census Bureau. In some states, more than half of older residents live in rural areas. Published online 2021. Accessed September 16 2022. https://www.census.gov/library/stories/2019/10/older-population-in-rural-america.html.

121. Matthews KA, Croft JB, Liu Y, et al. Health-related behaviors by urban-rural county classification — United States, 2013. *Morb Mortal Wkly Rep - Surveillance Summ*. 2017;66(5):1−8. https://doi.org/10.15585/mmwr.ss6605a1.

122. Urban MJ, Wojcik C, Eggerstedt M, Jagasia AJ. Rural-urban disparities in otolaryngology: the state of Illinois: rural otolaryngology disparities. *Laryngoscope*. 2021; 131(1):E70−E75. https://doi.org/10.1002/lary.28652.

123. Vickery TW, Weterings R, Cabrera-Muffly C. Geographic distribution of otolaryngologists in the United States. *Ear Nose Throat J*. 2016;95(6):218−223.

124. UnitedHealth Group. Modernizing Rural Health Care: Coverage, quality and Innovation. Modernizing Rural Health Care: Coverage, quality and innovation. https://www.unitedhealthgroup.com/content/dam/UHG/PDF/2011/UNH-Working-Paper-6.pdf. Published July 2011. Accessed August 28, 2022.

125. Allareddy V, Konety BR. Characteristics of patients and predictors of in-hospital mortality after hospitalization for head and neck cancers. *Cancer*. 2006;106(11): 2382−2388. https://doi.org/10.1002/cncr.21899.

126. Mackley HB, Teslova T, Camacho F, Short PF, Anderson RT. Does rurality influence treatment decisions in early stage laryngeal cancer? *J Rural Health*. 2014;30(4): 406−411. https://doi.org/10.1111/jrh.12069.

127. Powell W, Jacobs JA, Noble W, Bush ML, Snell-Rood C. Rural adult perspectives on impact of hearing loss and barriers to care. *J Community Health*. 2019;44(4): 668−674. https://doi.org/10.1007/s10900-019-00656-3.

128. Skoufalos A, Clarke JL, Ellis DR, Shepard VL, Rula EY. Rural aging in America: proceedings of the 2017 connectivity summit. *Popul Health Manag*. 2017;20(S2):S1−S10. https://doi.org/10.1089/pop.2017.0177.

129. Rural Hospital Closures. Sheps Center. Published June 22, 2020. Accessed July 7, 2022. https://www.shepscenter.unc.edu/programs-projects/rural-health/rural-hospital-closures/.

130. Gajdos C, Kile D, Hawn MT, Finlayson E, Henderson WG, Robinson TN. Advancing age and 30-day adverse outcomes after nonemergent general surgeries. *J Am Geriatr Soc*. 2013;61(9):1608−1614. https://doi.org/10.1111/jgs.12401.
131. Inouye SK, Westendorp RG, Saczynski JS. Delirium in elderly people. *Lancet*. 2014; 383(9920):911−922. https://doi.org/10.1016/S0140-6736(13)60688-1.
132. Bergen G, Stevens MR, Burns ER. Falls and fall injuries among adults aged ≥65 Years - United States, 2014. *MMWR Morb Mortal Wkly Rep*. 2016;65(37):993−998. https://doi.org/10.15585/mmwr.mm6537a2. Published 2016 Sep. 23.
133. Chow WB, Rosenthal RA, Merkow RP, et al. Optimal preoperative assessment of the geriatric surgical patient: a best practices guideline from the American College of Surgeons national surgical quality improvement program and the American geriatrics society. *J Am Coll Surg*. 2012;215(4):453−466. https://doi.org/10.1016/j.jamcollsurg.2012.06.017.
134. Mohanty S, Rosenthal RA, Russell MM, Neuman MD, Ko CY, Esnaola NF. Optimal perioperative management of the geriatric patient: a best practices guideline from the American College of Surgeons NSQIP and the American geriatrics society. *J Am Coll Surg*. 2016;222(5):930−947. https://doi.org/10.1016/j.jamcollsurg.2015.12.026.
135. Berian JR, Rosenthal RA, Baker TL, et al. Hospital standards to promote optimal surgical care of the older adult: a report from the coalition for quality in geriatric surgery. *Ann Surg*. 2018;267(2):280−290. https://doi.org/10.1097/SLA.0000000000002185.
136. Lian T, Brandrud A, Mariero L, Nordsletten L, Figved W. 60% Reduction of reoperations and complications for elderly patients with hip fracture through the implementation of a six-item improvement programme. *BMJ Open Qual*. 2022;11(3):e001848. https://doi.org/10.1136/bmjoq-2022-001848.
137. Gurgel RK, Briggs SE, Dhepyasuwan N, Rosenfeld RM. Quality improvement in otolaryngology-head and neck surgery: age-related hearing loss measures. *Otolaryngol Head Neck Surg*. 2021;165(6):765−774. https://doi.org/10.1177/01945998211000442.

Understanding rural–urban disparities in otolaryngology

Ashok A. Jagasia, Matthew J. Urban

Department of Otorhinolaryngology—Head and Neck Surgery, Rush University Medical Center,
Rochester, MN, United States

Introduction

Social determinants of health (SDOH) as defined by the CDC are the "conditions in the places where people live, learn, work, and play that affect a wide range of health risks and outcomes."[1] Factors such as gender, race, housing, education, food, and social economic status are but a few of the nonbiological elements that are critical to both individual and population health. Geography uniquely interplays with all of these SDOH in shaping the environments where people live, learn, work, and play. There has been extensive research demonstrating the significant health disparities among rural communities in the US. Rural regions experience inequities in cancer care,[2] higher rates of suicide,[3] higher infant mortality,[4] and higher premature and all-cause mortality.[5,6] Geographic isolation along with lower social economic status limit access to healthcare specialists and subspecialists. This is further compounded by specific health insurance plans that are dictated by employers or the extent of poverty, which may not be accepted by many providers or even tertiary medical centers. While there has been much effort in many different areas including health policies and programs created by Federal as well as State agencies to address these health disparities, much work remains to be done.

The effects of SDOH on otolaryngology care have been increasingly recognized. Large reviews have characterized SDOH in otolaryngology specific to pediatric otolaryngology,[7,8] head and neck cancer,[9–11] rhinology,[12–14] laryngology,[15] and otology.[16–18] However, while studies on socioeconomic status, education, and ethnic disparities are relatively well represented, rurality is often left out of these reviews completely[8–14,16] or only narrowly addressed.[7,15,18] In fact, a recent scoping review broadly characterized the literature on rural otolaryngology care and noted numerous gaps and potential areas for further investigation.[19]

Despite the paucity of literature, otolaryngologists are uniquely positioned to provide care to rural populations. As a regional anatomic specialist, the otolaryngologist has the expertise to offer high-impact medical and surgical treatments, while maintaining a breadth of understanding across multiple organ systems and disease processes. Otolaryngologists treat patients of all ages, and ear, nose, and throat

Healthcare Disparities in Otolaryngology. https://doi.org/10.1016/B978-0-443-10714-6.00001-8

complaints are among the most common reasons for rural patients to visit a physician.[20,21] In addition, many otolaryngologic diseases require prompt treatment and close surveillance, such as head and neck cancers. Otolaryngologists are also trained in emergency care and are masters of the airway.

Although there is a clear need for specialized ear, nose, and throat care in rural environments, the US otolaryngology workforce remains preferentially located in urban and suburban environments.

This chapter primarily aims to: (1) merge the existing scientific literature with examples from the authors' clinical experiences to broadly highlight rural disparities in otolaryngology disease and treatment and (2) present potential interventions that may help to close the healthcare gap for rural patients. The senior author (AAJ), also on staff at a tertiary medical center, has been providing care to the rural communities of Central Illinois for the last six years, averaging about 3000 patient visits and 500 surgical cases per year. This text will focus on rural care in the domestic US as ear, nose, and throat initiatives in international and developing countries present a number of unique challenges and opportunities that are outside the scope of this chapter. The authors hope that this work helps to stimulate discussion and future action to extend high quality otolaryngology specialized care to as many patients as possible who are currently underserved in rural regions across the country.

Quantifying disparities

Quantifying rural healthcare disparities is particularly challenging because of the heterogeneity among populations and regions. Determining which regions are "rural" is important to study access to care, but inexact and inconsistent as definitions have changed over time. The US Census Bureau defines rural as "any population, housing, or territory NOT in an urban area."[22] This definition is not precise, but designed to capture regions that are sparsely populated with some geographic isolation from an urban center. In 2010, the US Census expanded its definition of urban areas to include "urban clusters": suburbanized regions or densely settled areas near small towns.[23] The National Center for Health Statistics (NCHS) now classifies each US county 1−6 based on rurality (Table 8.1). By defining rural regions based on both population and geography, there can be a more accurate assessment of these populations' access to healthcare. As an example, the authors recently characterized the otolaryngology workforce by geography in Illinois.[24] Illinois is centrally located, has a high percentage of farmland, and mirrors the greater US in many of the US Census Bureau's demographic and economic characteristics.[25] Fig. 8.1 notes the distribution of the 276 board-certified practicing otolaryngologists in Illinois in 2019.[24] Graphically, the rural (NCHS class V/VI) counties in blue on the left panel are largely devoid of practicing otolaryngologists (pins on the right panel). Note that much of the center and southeastern portion of the state is classified as rural, while southwestern Illinois contains a rim of "urban" counties (and a number of corresponding practicing otolaryngologists). Many of these southwestern "urban"

Table 8.1 National Center for Health Statistics (NCHS) county rural urban classification system.

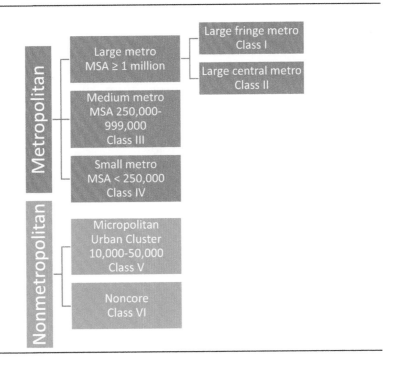

counties are also sparsely populated. For instance, Bond County, IL is 100% rural by population density (as determined by US Census), but classified as Class 2 (urban) in the NCHS scheme based on its proximity to St. Louis. Degree of geographic isolation is generally not well characterized among studies of rural disparities. More than a third of the studies in the rural otolaryngology literature examine a single rural community or hospital, complicating comparisons between populations which may vary a great deal in geographic access to healthcare resources.[19] The US Census Bureau emphasizes that nonmetro is not the same as rural, because metro is defined at the county level and there are many rural areas within urban counties.[20] However, while imperfect, the Census county-based Rural–Urban continuum codes are widely available and were commonly used by studies that sought to characterize more than a single rural population. The NCHS characterization accounts for important variables such as proximity to metropolitan areas and commuting patterns which better account for the true conditions experienced by individual patients. Database studies in particular unanimously characterized rurality as binary for the purpose of analysis, as it is difficult or impossible to distinguish different degrees of rurality. Admittedly, no perfect classification system exists, and there is

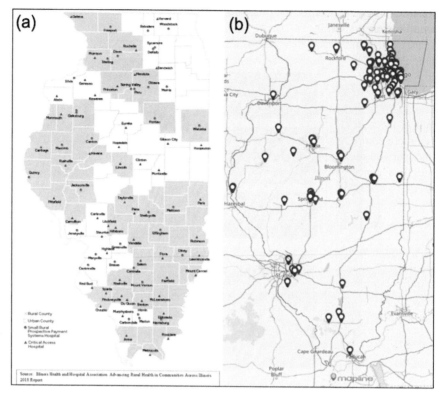

FIGURE 8.1

(A) Graphic representation of urban and rural counties in Illinois. See text for citation. (B) Distribution of academy-registered otolaryngologists in Illinois (generated using Mapline, Provo, UT).

significant heterogeneity at the county level, but more sophisticated classification schemes such as the NCHS can improve research quality and identification of rural populations in need.

Access to care

Although widely agreed that rural access to otolaryngology care must be improved, there are only two studies to date characterizing the urban—rural population distribution of otolaryngologists. The above-cited study of Illinois identified a significant per-capita deficiency in otolaryngologists for NCHS nonmetropolitan counties (class V/VI).[24] In fact, only 7.2% of Illinois counties with a rural population greater than 40% housed any otolaryngologist primary practice locations, while 82% of counties with a rural population less than 40% housed at least one otolaryngologist.[24] This is clearly a massive disparity. Illinois otolaryngologists tended to practice in a roughly similar population density in counties composed of large cities, small cities, and suburbs, yet there was a near total paucity of practicing ENTs in rural counties, despite a significant population size.[24] Fig. 8.2 represents otolaryngologists per capita by county in Illinois as a function of rural population percentage (US Census). Note, there is a precipitous drop in practicing otolaryngologists as the rural population reaches 40%–50%. The per capita data confirm the access to care discrepancies, but the study's geographical data were even more compelling. Metropolitan counties in Illinois averaged 0.94 otolaryngologists per 100 square miles, while nonmetropolitan/rural counties were more than 30 times less concentrated with only 0.03 otolaryngologists per 100 square miles. NCHS class VI counties (Table 8.1) encompassed the largest land area in the state at greater than 18,000 square miles with a population of greater than 600,000 and zero practicing otolaryngologists.[24] Although average travel and wait times to seek specialized care are difficult to calculate, the gaps are certainly striking.

A similar study by Winters et al. examined practicing otolaryngologists in seven southeastern states in the US in 2014.[26] They found fewer otolaryngologists per capita in rural counties for all seven states with the largest gap in Oklahoma (urban: 1 otolaryngologist per 29,545 vs. rural: 1 otolaryngologist per 70,738). They also noted a higher percentage of Medicaid and uninsured patients in rural counties.

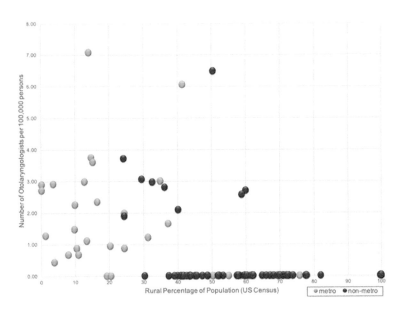

FIGURE 8.2

Otolaryngologists/100,000 persons versus rural percentage of population for each county in Illinois. National Center for Health Statistics (NCHS) class for each county is represented with color scheme and legend.

Although only a handful of states have been formally studied, the trends likely hold true across the country. While some patients may have the means, financial and family constraints often limit the ability of rural patients to travel for care, particularly for those with chronic disease where recurring visits are required. For instance, a 2014 study found that rural patients with larynx cancer were less likely to be treated with organ preservation radiation and more likely to undergo a surgical resection.[27] The hardship of repeated travel, particularly for rural patients of low socioeconomic status, is particularly high.

Travel time, costs, family status, and occupation all factor into treatment decisions, but are not the only reasons that patients in rural settings struggle to find access to otolaryngology care. Fig. 8.3 is a fishbone diagram summarizing causes and subcauses of limited access to otolaryngology care. There are notable contributing factors in all four categories: people, policies, plant (environment), and processes (both formal and informal). People living in rural areas may be concerned about the social stigma of seeking care due to culture, poor health literacy, or mistrust. Federal, state, and local government policies may incentivize providers to practice in rural settings with educational grant funding or debt forgiveness, but these programs are often targeted to primary care rather than specialists. Transportation is a challenge not only due to physical distance but also because of a lack of public transportation and poor road conditions. Also, smaller budgets and narrow margins at rural/critical access hospitals may limit the clinical technology available and thus the scope of the otolaryngologist's practice. For instance, a study in 2013 found that rural patients with melanoma were less likely to undergo sentinel lymph node biopsy than urban counterparts.[28] Like many subspecialists, otolaryngologists require certain specialized equipment in order to offer the most up-to-date and in-depth care. Lastly, formal and informal processes are critical to the gaps in care. Workforce

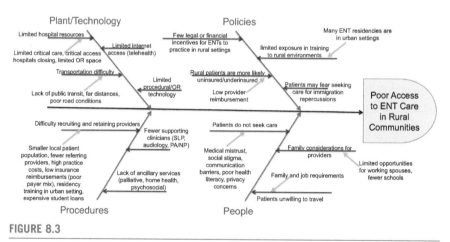

FIGURE 8.3

Rural otolaryngology care disparities cause analysis.

shortages occur not only because of difficulty in attracting providers but also because high practice costs and low reimbursements are driving existing providers away from rural regions with high uninsured and Medicaid populations. The formal process of graduate medical education also occurs almost exclusively at urban tertiary care centers for otolaryngologists. Very few training programs offer exposure to rural otolaryngology other than patients who travel to urban centers for tertiary level care.

Recognizing these existing barriers is an important first step to implementing solutions that can improve access for rural patients. However, physical access to care is only one of the many place-based characteristics which influence health, although it is by far the most commonly researched across specialties. Only a small minority of studies account for the interplay of rurality and race, education, poverty, or religion, which are critical to health disparities in this population. These factors must be considered at both an individual and community level. Rural populations are also changing. Over time, an increase in demographic and economic diversity within rural communities has further complicated their healthcare needs. Cosby et al. examined US mortality trends by geography over the last 50 years and found that while the urban poor had the highest mortality rates in the 1970s and 1980s, mortality rates for rural patients in poverty have surpassed the aforementioned group and continue to grow disparate.[5] Changing rural populations, along with the exacerbation of disparities by the recent COVID-19 pandemic for certain marginalized groups, emphasizes the importance of research in this area.[29] Although improving rural access to an otolaryngologist will not remedy all the abovementioned disparities, it is certainly a start to improving the overall health of this important population.

Subspecialty analysis

Otolaryngology is an extremely diverse field with fellowships and advanced training across a number of specialized areas. In order to organize and analyze the rural care disparities in otolaryngology, the authors will split the field into eight subspecialties: otology/neurotology, pediatrics, head and neck surgery, endocrine surgery, laryngology, facial plastic surgery, rhinology, and sleep surgery. Table 8.2 and much of the literature analysis in this section was adapted from the authors' 2022 rural otolaryngology scoping review.[19] Table 8.2 is a condensed summary of the existing literature related to rural care across all eight of the above subspecialties. Each will be discussed individually.

Otology

As evident in Table 8.2, the majority of rural literature in otolaryngology addresses topics in otology, particularly hearing loss. Almost 90% of otology-related studies which met inclusion on the recent scoping review pertained to hearing loss.[19] There were a few notable trends which are highlighted in Table 8.2.[19] Rural patients have

Table 8.2 Literature summary for rural otolaryngology disparities by specialty and topic based on 2022 scoping review.

ENT specialty	Topic/Condition	Findings	Author, year
Adult sleep	Obstructive sleep apnea	Higher cost for hospital admission at rural centers after obstructive sleep apnea surgery	Kezerian, 2010
Facial plastic surgery and trauma	Missed injuries	16% trauma patients at rural center with missed head and neck injuries	Aaland, 1996
	Injury patterns	Increased proportion of maxilla and orbit fractures versus mandible at rural center	Smith, 2012
		Animal-related causes are a significant etiology of pediatric temporal bone fractures specific to rural patients	Ort, 2004
		Increasing rural trauma referrals over 10-year period	Roden, 2012
Pediatrics	Tonsillectomy	Lower rates of tonsillectomy versus urban children	Yan, 2021
		Higher rates of tonsillectomy versus urban children	Cooper, 2020
Rhinology	Allergic rhinitis	Rhinitis more prevalent in urban environments	Song, 2015; Turkeltaub, 1991
		No trends in prevalence for urban/rural environments	Nathan, 1997
	CRS	Higher cost to treat CRS in rural areas	Pai, 2000
	FESS	Higher costs and less image guidance utilization in rural FESS	Thomas, 2019; Bhattacharyya, 2014
	AFRS	Higher rate of craniofacial involvement in rural populations	Miller, 2014
	TSR	Low volume centers are more likely to be rural; have higher costs and longer hospital stays	Mckee, 2018

Table 8.2 Literature summary for rural otolaryngology disparities by specialty and topic based on 2022 scoping review.—*cont'd*

ENT specialty	Topic/Condition	Findings	Author, year
Head and neck cancer	Survival	Rural patients have worse HNC survival outcomes than urban patients	Hashibe, 2018; Clarke, 2020; Papenberg, 2020
		No difference in HNC survival	Pagedar, 2019
		Rural patients have better oral cavity cancer survival outcomes	Harris, 2020
	Risk factors and prevalence	High rates of smoking, problem alcohol use, and pesticide exposure in rural regions may be associated with higher HNC and thyroid cancer	Howren, 2021; Zuniga, 2018; Papenberg, 2020
		Trends in HNC incidence are disparately worsening in rural areas versus urban areas	Pagedar, 2019–12
		Lower rates of larynx and oral cavity cancer in rural Minnesota	Schreinemacher, 1999
		Higher rate of larynx cancer in rural areas	Zuniga, 2018
	Diagnosis/ screening	Rural patients were less likely to be diagnosed at a young age compared to urban patients	Mukherjee, 2020
		A media campaign targeted at rural patients increased the likelihood that patients underwent a head and neck exam for screening	Logan, 2015
	Treatment	Rural patients with melanoma less likely to receive a sentinel lymph node biopsy	Shah, 2013
		Rural patients with larynx cancer are less frequently treated with primary radiation	Mackley, 2014
		Patients further from treatment centers were more likely to receive appropriate treatment	Ringstrom, 2018

Continued

Table 8.2 Literature summary for rural otolaryngology disparities by specialty and topic based on 2022 scoping review.—*cont'd*

ENT specialty	Topic/Condition	Findings	Author, year
		Hospitalization	HNC patients hospitalized at rural centers had lower costs and LOS, but also increased mortality	Adjei Boakye, 2019; Allareddy, 2006
Endocrine	Thyroid cancer	Thyroid cancer incidence increasing in rural areas faster than urban areas	Hanley, 2015
		Enhanced detection programs are less ubiquitous in rural areas, resulting in a lower incidence of thyroid cancer	Li, 2013; McDow, 2020
		No survival advantage for PTC patients traveling to metropolitan centers	White, 2017
		Decreased risk of developing PTC for adults who grew up in rural environment	Clarke, 2015
		Lower survival for thyroid cancer in rural areas	McDow, 2020
	Thyroid nodules	FNAB in rural settings are comparable to urban settings in accuracy and can reduce surgical intervention	Haas, 1993; Guo, 2017; Thang, 2017
	Thyroidectomy/ Parathyroidectomy	Similar rate of complications for thyroid and parathyroid surgery a rural environment	Richmond, 2007; Al-Qurayshi, 2017
		Rural region is associated with increased costs for thyroid surgery	Biron, 2015
		Low volume surgeons more likely to perform parathyroidectomy at rural hospitals	Al-Qurayshi, 2017
Laryngology	Dysphagia	Rurality did not predict poststroke dysphagia or feeding tube	Bonilha, 2014; George, 2014
	Voice	Rural patients were less likely to undergo stroboscopy	Cohen, 2014

Table 8.2 Literature summary for rural otolaryngology disparities by specialty and topic based on 2022 scoping review.—*cont'd*

ENT specialty	Topic/Condition	Findings	Author, year
Otology/ Neurotology	Noise and hearing protection	Rural residents have unique exposure to high noise levels including gun firing, farm equipment, and animals	Kramer, 1982; Rosemberg, 2015; McCullagh, 2020; Holt, 1993
		The rate of use of hearing protection is low in rural patients	Rosemberg, 2015
		Educational interventions can increase long-term use of hearing protection	Marlenga, 2011
		An educational intervention did not increase intent to use hearing protection in 4th graders	McCullagh, 2020
	Hearing loss (HL) prevalence	Hearing loss is similar between rural and urban adults, similar incidence of congenital HL at urban and rural hospitals	Ives, 1995; Bush, 2015
		Hearing loss is more prevalent in rural adults (particularly men) versus urban adults	Hay-McCutcheon, 2017; Ciletti, 2008; Karlovich, 1988; Kramer, 1982
		Hearing impairment is nearly universal in rural residents	Flamme, 2005
	Hearing testing	Barriers to treatment of congenital hearing loss in rural patients include lower education level of parents, less awareness of results of newborn hearing screening upon hospital discharge, increased distance to treatment centers, and less awareness of treatment options	Bush, 2015
		Rural practices are less likely to provide hearing testing for pediatric patients	Bush, 2015
		Rural children are less likely to have follow-up	Bush, 2014; Cunningham, 2017

Continued

Table 8.2 Literature summary for rural otolaryngology disparities by specialty and topic based on 2022 scoping review.—*cont'd*

ENT specialty	Topic/Condition	Findings	Author, year
	Hearing amplification, cochlear implants (CIs)	after a failed newborn hearing screening and have longer delays in diagnosis	
		Longer distances to CI centers are associated with delays in pediatric hearing amplification and CI placement	Bush, 2013
		Rural patients with congenital hearing loss have a delay in diagnosis, time to amplification, and time to CI	Bush, 2014
		Rural children are less likely to communicate with their CIs	Easterbrooks, 2000
		Barriers to acquiring hearing aids in rural adults include lack of providers, increased distance traveled to acquire devices, and high cost of hearing aids	Powell, 2019; Chan, 2017; Hay-McCutcheon, 2020
		Rural adults have increased latency between time of hearing loss and acquiring a hearing aid	Chan, 2017; Hixon, 2016
		Rural veterans live further from VAs offering audiologic and surgical CI care	Shayman, 2019
	Otologic infections	Rural patients prescribed ototopical antibiotics had no difference in proportion of ENT versus non-ENT prescribers. Rural prescribers were more likely to prescribe brand-name agents	Crowson, 2015
		Urban patients were slightly more likely to receive amoxicillin within three days of diagnosis of acute otitis media	McEwen, 2003

Table 8.2 Literature summary for rural otolaryngology disparities by specialty and topic based on 2022 scoping review.—*cont'd*

ENT specialty	Topic/Condition	Findings	Author, year
Healthcare systems		Otorrhea after tube placement more prevalent among urban children, followed by rural and suburban in that order	Ah-Tye, 2001
	Cholesteatoma	Rural patients more likely to have residual post-op cholesteatoma and have more surgeries; no difference in recurrence, complications, and improvement in air-bone gap	Kennedy, 2020
	Telemedicine	Live ENT telemed clinic provides cost savings, high satisfaction and validity, and shorter referral times for rural patients	Philips, 2019; Seim, 2018
	Access to care	Fewer per capita ENT in rural counties, which may be improved by urban physician outreach	Urban, 2021; Winters, 2011; Gruca, 2014
		Rural patients had less health-related internet use	Pagedar, 2018
		Rural patients had higher no-show rate	Fiorillo, 2018

AFRS, *allergic fungal rhinosinusitis;* CI, *cochlear implant;* CRS, *chronic rhinosinusitis;* ENT, *otolaryngology;* FESS, *functional endoscopic sinus surgery;* FNAB, *fine needle aspiration biopsy;* HL, *hearing loss;* HNC, *head and neck cancer;* LOS, *length of stay;* PTC, *papillary thyroid carcinoma;* TSR, *transsphenoidal resection.*

high rates of noise exposure from unique sources including farm equipment, animals, and firearms.[30–32] Noise exposure, age, demographics, poverty, and limited access to hearing health care all contribute to a high incidence of hearing loss. Therefore, most studies reporting on the prevalence of acquired hearing loss found that the prevalence was higher in rural populations,[33–36] while a study by Ives et al. found a prevalence comparable to the national average.[37] Prevalence of congenital hearing loss expectedly did not vary between rural and urban populations.[38]

Much less has been published regarding hearing interventions in US rural communities. Two randomized controlled trials (RCTs) have examined noise exposure education interventions in children. McCullagh et al. demonstrated an increase in knowledge but no change in intent to use hearing protection.[39] Marlenga et al. found increased hearing protection use but failed to demonstrate a difference in noise-induced hearing loss.[40] Prevention programs have been effective in other communities and can likely be applied in a rural setting. Additionally, there are numerous unique barriers to receiving care for both congenital and acquired hearing loss in rural pediatric and adult populations,[41–44] resulting in delays to care.[45–51] Many of these barriers are reflected in the above fishbone diagram (Fig. 8.3). Specifically, Easterbrooks et al. demonstrated that rural Georgian students with cochlear implants are less likely to use their implants for communication than their urban counterparts and postulated a main barrier to use was the lack of integrated speech therapists and parental support.[52] Interventions for acute or sudden hearing loss have not been formally studied in a rural setting, but in the senior author's experience, the availability of specialty interventions such as intratympanic steroid injections is severely restricted for rural patients of Central Illinois. The senior author (AAJ) recently encountered a patient with severe diabetes and profound sudden hearing loss in his rural clinic. She did not have access to audiologic evaluation and was not a candidate for oral steroid treatment. Although equipment in the rural setting was limited, partnership with an urban tertiary care center allowed for the patient to receive prompt audiologic evaluation and treatment with an intratympanic steroid injection. Her hearing was promptly restored to her premorbid condition, and despite long travel distances, she was very satisfied with otherwise inaccessible specialty care.

A small number of studies have pertained to otologic conditions other than hearing loss.[53,54] Kennedy et al. found that rural patients are more likely to have residual cholesteatomas postoperatively.[55] Cholesteatoma is an example of a disease which may be diagnosed by a primary care doctor, but it is typically managed surgically in a tertiary or quaternary setting to prevent severe sequela. Because recurrence is not uncommon (50% in rural patients in the cited study), close monitoring with nearby otologic surgical services is critical to high quality treatment of this disease. In this work, the authors suggested more aggressive consideration for canal wall down procedures in order to facilitate follow-up closer to the patient's home.[55] Similar disparities have been identified in other disease process, for instance, McEwen et al. found that urban patients were slightly more likely to receive amoxicillin within three days of diagnosis of acute otitis media.[56]

Head and neck surgery

After otology, head and neck cancer is the second most commonly studied subspecialty in terms of rural inequality in care. Because of the risk of mortality, technologic advances in care, need for surveillance, and potential for screening and prevention, outreach to provide high quality head and neck cancer care for more isolated populations is of particular importance. Roughly 20% of the rural literature in our recent scoping review pertained to head and neck surgery.[19] While practice patterns were most commonly studied in otology, outcomes were most commonly studied in head and neck cancer. There were five studies presenting disparities in survival (Table 8.2). Three studies showed worse survival outcomes for rural head and neck cancer patients,[57–59] one study found no significant difference in survival,[60] and one study identified the opposite trend with improved outcomes for rural cancer patients.[61] Again, distance to primary care, a lack of access to high volume centers, insurance status, and fewer public transportation options were cited as potential reasons for those studies showing later stage presentation and worse overall survival. Clarke et al. also noted significantly lower survival in rural Black patients in comparison to rural White patients.[58] However, barriers in physical access to care did not uniformly reduce care quality. A number of studies across subspecialties referenced the "referral bias" or "distance bias" phenomena, where patients who travel farther have improved disease outcomes. For oral cavity cancer, Ringstrom et al. found a higher likelihood of "ideal" treatment for patients traveling further[62] and Harris et al. found improved overall survival for rural patients.[61] White et al. found improved quality of care for patients traveling from rural areas for the treatment of papillary thyroid cancer.[63] The theory behind "referral bias" is that patients who travel may be more highly motivated, or more likely to end up at high volume centers, which have repeatedly demonstrated improved outcomes particularly for cancer care.

Beyond outcomes, three studies were published on disparities in rural cancer treatment[27,28,62] and two examined disparities in screening.[64,65] Ringstrom et al. and Mackley et al. found that rural patients who were further from radiation centers were less likely to receive primary radiation for oropharynx[62] and larynx[27] cancer, respectively. Four studies were published on risk factors and prevalence.[66–69] A study of 1990 data by Schrienemachers et al. found a lower rate of oral cavity and larynx cancers in agricultural Minnesota,[69] while newer studies[66,68] have demonstrated increasing rural incidence of head and neck cancers. Finally, two studies evaluated disparities in hospital outcomes of head and neck cancer patients with one study identifying lower costs and shorter length of stay in rural hospitals,[70] but another study noting increased mortality for hospitalized head and neck cancer patients.[71] Of note, the majority of the head and neck cancer studies of rural populations are based on large databases, and in contrast to otology, only a few studies characterized a solitary rural population.

Pediatric otolaryngology

Pediatric otolaryngology is a particularly broad discipline with overlap across the above-named specialties. Table 8.2 splits studies related to pediatrics into their associated subspecialties. Upon recent review, pediatric hearing loss comprised the largest segment of literature (12/15 pediatric related studies).[72] One study examined patterns in rural pediatric temporal bone fractures,[73] and two studies were published on rural disparities in pediatric obstructive sleep apnea (OSA) and tonsillectomy. Yan et al. identified longer wait times and driving distances resulting in significantly lower rates of tonsillectomy and adenoidectomy for rural children in South Carolina.[74] Contrarily, Cooper et al. queried inpatient and ambulatory surgery databases for eight states and found that rates of tonsillectomy were higher in nonmetropolitan areas, particularly for White children.[75] Cooper et al. postulated that these trends might reflect overuse in the rural demographic, particularly in children presenting with recurrent tonsillitis.[75] The American Academy of Otolaryngology clinical practice guidelines provide recommendations for when to consider tonsillectomy, but each patient is considered individually. Although access to a surgeon would seemingly limit the number of tonsillectomy procedures for rural children, difficulty accessing reliable transportation, limited parental time-off work, or mistrust in the healthcare system altogether may sway rural families toward surgery rather than observation and repeated courses of antibiotics for recurrent tonsillitis.

Rhinology

Since the expansion of endoscopic surgery to the sinonasal cavity in the 1980s, there has been an explosion of technology and indications for endoscopic sinus surgery (ESS). Rapid expansion in image-guided technology and the adaptation of this technology to facilitate extended endonasal approaches has become a mainstay at tertiary care centers but is less frequently utilized in rural and community settings. McKee et al. found that high volume centers in transsphenoidal pituitary surgery were less likely to be in rural settings but did not identify a higher readmission rate or length of stay for rural patients.[76] Bhattacharyya et al. found that rural settings were significantly less likely to utilize intraoperative image guidance technology than urban settings.[77] Additionally, Thomas et al. recently reported that ESS was significantly more expensive at rural and community facilities, potentially secondary to lower overall volume.[78] Like many other areas of otolaryngology, rhinology is a field of continual innovation in both technology and techniques. Cutting-edge interventions are much more likely to be available in urban high-volume centers, while access is often much more limited for rural patients. Even basic rhinologic services may be unavailable in many US rural settings. The senior author recently evaluated a patient in his rural clinic who presented with a constellation of long-standing nonspecific symptoms including fatigue, muscle, weakness, joint pain but also nasal obstruction. Nasal endoscopy demonstrated crusting and, although serology had been inconclusive, nasal biopsy confirmed granulomatosis with polyangiitis (previously Wegener's granulomatosis). The patient had a prolonged period of suffering from these symptoms without a diagnosis because of limited access to a basic rhinologic examination.

Endocrine surgery

Thyroid and parathyroid disease manifest as both simple and complex constellations that may be managed primarily medically or often surgically. Sometimes disease processes may require referral to a high-volume or specialized center, while other conditions are aptly managed in the community. In the literature, epidemiology and practice patterns were the most commonly studied rural disparities in endocrine surgery. Like head and neck cancer, database studies were the most common study design. Four studies compared the incidence of thyroid cancer in rural versus urban environments[79–82] with mixed results. Although two studies[80,82] agreed that incidence was increasing more rapidly in metropolitan areas due to access to advanced diagnostics, one study[79] refuted this. Access to high resolution ultrasound and molecular testing (more frequently implemented in urban academic centers and teaching hospitals) may improve early detection of small tumors and thus increase thyroid cancer incidence. Although well-differentiated thyroid cancer has a favorable prognosis in general, early treatment of small tumors may afford a survival advantage for these patients. Rural patients may not be aware of these newer screening modalities, and primary care doctors without access to these resources might be less likely to refer patients to a center with advanced diagnostic capabilities.

Three studies assessed thyroidectomy and parathyroidectomy in a rural setting. According to two National Inpatient Sample (NIS) database studies, low volume surgeons were more likely to operate in rural locations,[83] have a higher rate of complications,[83] and costs were higher after thyroidectomy at a rural center.[84] White et al. published that rural patients who traveled to academic centers for the treatment of papillary thyroid carcinoma (PTC) were more likely to receive standard of care treatment, although they were unable to detect a difference in overall survival.[63] Richmond et al. refuted the notion that thyroidectomies performed at rural centers suffered from a higher complication rate by publishing a retrospective cohort from their solo rural practice.[85] The remaining three studies pertained to fine needle aspiration (FNA) of thyroid nodules, noting that FNA is both feasible and accurate in a rural setting.[86–88] Le et al. introduced an ultrasound-guided biopsy program to a remote 19-bed critical access hospital instituted by the radiology department.[88] The hospital lacked on-site pathology services and specimens required transportation to an affiliated institution; however, there was a 94% success rate at initial biopsy and greater than 80% of patients received benign FNA results and were able to maintain their usual care at the small community hospital saving travel time and costs for many individuals.[88] Patients with suspicious FNA findings were transferred to the affiliated tertiary institution for surgical resection. A close partnership between a well-equipped tertiary care center and rural hospital can not only consolidate resources for those necessitating escalation of care but also reduce travel expenses and maintain care at the rural site for many patients and their families.

Laryngology

Laryngology is a broad field ranging from precise microsurgical techniques to open cancer surgery. The literature on rural laryngology is limited, with only two studies on rural disparities in swallow and one on voice.[89–91] Two studies failed to find an association between rurality and poststroke dysphagia.[89,90] However, Cohen et al. noted lower rates of stroboscopy in rural areas.[91] Stroboscopy is critical for evaluation and treatment decisions for a variety of vocal pathologies. Provider training, cost, and availability of technology impact the availability of this important diagnostic tool for rural patients. High quality voice and swallow care requires close integration with specialized speech and language pathologists (SLPs). Although no studies have examined rural access to SLP services, patients who are geographically isolated from providers also do not have these supporting services, which are integral to a comprehensive care plan.

Facial plastic and reconstructive surgery

Facial plastic surgeons are trained to treat both cosmetic and reconstructive concerns in the head and neck region for patients of all ages. Facial plastic surgery is an integral component of otolaryngology training programs and encompasses a broad range of pathology and procedures from microvascular reconstruction to repair of congenital deformity to rejuvenation of the aging face. We performed a broad literature search of rural facial plastic surgery including both cosmetic and reconstructive procedures, but the publications identified were all related to rural facial trauma. A few studies characterized epidemiologic trends (changing injury patterns over time[73,92,93]), while Aaland et al.[94] found a low rate of missed injuries at a rural trauma center compared to the literature norms (Table 8.2). The majority of these studies characterized the experience of a single rural trauma hospital. Otolaryngologists must recognize that rural environments pose unique risks for facial trauma including injuries from agricultural equipment and livestock along with increased frequency and unique mechanisms for motor vehicle collisions.[93] While nasal bone fractures and mandible fractures are traditionally recognized as the most common facial fractures, Smith et al. found that orbital fractures were most common in reviewing a single rural center over two years.[93] Additionally, longer transport times may result in a higher proportion of patients arriving intubated or obtunded confounding initial neurologic and vision examinations.[93] Surgeons may need to consider long travel distances in determining treatment plans for patients with facial fractures and may favor open approaches with internal fixation rather than closed approaches that may require prolonged intermaxillary fixation to establish dental occlusion. No studies in the literature examined practice patterns in this regard, and it is potentially an area for future research.

With the exception of trauma, there were no studies characterizing rural facial cosmetic or reconstructive surgery. A recent study from a plastic surgery group at the Mayo Clinic found that skin cancer, head and neck reconstruction, and head and neck aesthetic surgery comprised more than 1/3 of the practice volume of rural plastic surgeons.[95] The need for facial plastic and reconstructive specialists is clear, but there is no data characterizing practice patterns or disease disparities. Presently, there are no otolaryngologist-facial plastic surgeons practicing within the Central Illinois region. Patients requiring nasal reconstruction, surgical intervention for facial nerve paralysis, or complex repair of facial defects related to cutaneous malignancies have to be routinely referred to tertiary medical centers. In addition, there are no otolaryngologists who treat nasal valve collapse, a commonly diagnosed condition affecting a relatively large population of patients. In the senior author's practice, it is common for patients to present with persistent nasal obstruction after previous septoplasty and inferior turbinate reduction by a local otolaryngologist due to underlying nasal valve collapse. Providing nasal valve repair in the rural setting has allowed the senior author to improve symptoms for many of these patients while avoiding tertiary referral and travel costs.

Sleep surgery

Sleep surgery is one of the newest divisions of specialized in-depth training for otolaryngologists. OSA is a common, chronic disease that is ideally managed in a multidisciplinary setting. Positive airway pressure is currently the gold standard to treat OSA; however, low adherence rates limit its use. Sleep surgery has emerged as an adjunct/alternative to positive airway pressure, and newer procedures such as upper airway stimulation devices have shown promising results. Very few studies have examined adult sleep surgery in rural patient populations, but obesity and older age are two risk factors for OSA which are highly prevalent in rural communities. In our recent scoping review, only one study which met inclusion criteria related to adult sleep surgery.[19] Kezirian et al. identified higher costs for inpatient sleep apnea surgeries performed in rural centers.[96] They noted that urban high volume centers are likely more cost effective. The majority of their cohort was treated with palate surgery, and newer procedures such as the upper airway stimulation devices were not tracked. It is likely that these procedures are performed in a much more limited capacity in rural settings.

Interventions and initiatives

Improving access to high quality, affordable rural otolaryngology care is a major challenge without a quick fix or single solution. There are a number of programs and strategies that are underway at a local and national level to help counter existing disparities. In addition, it is reasonable to use successes in other fields to project policies which may help to bridge the current gaps in otolaryngology. However, successful interventions require recognition of the problem and buy-in from all the relevant stakeholders including patients, families, providers, healthcare organizations, and government. Fig. 8.3 mapped some of the causes and subcauses for the relative inaccessibility of the rural otolaryngologist. Table 8.3 proposes a few potential solutions which may mitigate some of these barriers. This section will review interventions designed to improve rural physician recruitment and retention, supporting clinical resources, and limitations in travel, which currently limit access to high quality rural care in otolaryngology.

Otolaryngologist recruitment and retention to rural areas

Recruiting physicians to rural areas is a hot topic in the national media due to its impact on the healthcare system. The primary care physician shortage in rural areas is a major limitation to access to care and more commonly discussed, however specialist shortages are equally prevalent and meaningful. Healthcare groups should

Table 8.3 Solution analysis for rural otolaryngology care disparities.

Solution	Barrier(s) addressed
Increase rotations at rural centers during medical school and ENT residency training	Physician recruitment and retention, physician familiarity with rural care
Early recruitment of rural HS/college students	Physician recruitment and retention
Increase government support of critical access hospitals	Limited rural hospital resources, procedural capabilities, access to operating rooms
Rural–urban hospital partnerships	Limited rural hospital resources, travel limitations, lack of supporting clinicians and ancillary services
Rural loan forgiveness programs	Physician recruitment and retention, financial incentives for rural physicians
Telehealth expansion	Travel limitations, physician recruitment, hospital resources
Local/regional provider outreach; physician home visits	Travel limitations, medical mistrust, communication barriers, social stigma, privacy
Factor rurality and poverty into Medicare/Medicaid risk adjustment	Low provider reimbursement, financial incentives for rural physicians
Build supporting workforce	Lack of supporting clinicians and ancillary services

focus physician recruitment efforts toward the many desirable factors which are inherent to practice in a rural setting. Because rural health organizations are generally smaller, there are fewer bureaucratic layers and more direct surgeon access to administration and organizational policy. This allows for a very autonomous clinical practice with fewer administrative considerations or red tape and opportunities for customization. A solo private practice is much more prevalent for otolaryngologists in rural settings. Also, since real estate is generally less expensive and competitive, rural otolaryngologists may face fewer space constraints. In terms of clinical scope, practice in a rural setting is an opportunity for otolaryngologists to maintain an in-depth practice across the breadth of the field. Surgeons early in practice may refine clinical and procedural techniques without narrowing their expertise. In an era of increasing specialization, this has become increasingly challenging in competitive urban and suburban markets. Importantly, rural otolaryngologists may feel more freedom to provide individualized care with a focus on deepening interpersonal relationships with their patients rather than spending energy on navigating institutional protocols or treatment regimens. There is also a profound sense of duty by providing timely and important care to a greatly underserved population. Toman et al. recently surveyed otolaryngology residents and confirmed widespread interest in global health electives and humanitarian outreach.[97]

Despite the myriad benefits of a rural practice, a few major barriers continue to limit the flux of otolaryngologists into a rural setting. The most notable of these are geographic isolation, limited exposure during training, and economic considerations (see Fig. 8.3). Rural healthcare organizations looking to recruit physicians generally have somewhat limited control over geographic isolation, but a few offerings are available. Technological advancements continuously improve long distance connectivity. High-definition video conferencing and efficient air travel may help physicians to maintain a connection with friends and family. Rural employers may additionally mitigate the impact of geographic isolation by offering flexible schedules and practice options. Ample paid leave, part-time options, modified work weeks, and blocks for telehealth are among potential opportunities. Overall, tailoring the practice to individual preferences can improve physician satisfaction and aid both recruitment and retention.

Second, resident exposure to rural practice environments is critical to improving the rural otolaryngologist workforce. Unlike larger programs such as internal medicine, family medicine, or general surgery, the vast majority of otolaryngology residency programs are centered in urban academic centers, though some programs may encompass rural catchment areas. Experience with rural populations in training correlates with a future rural practice across multiple specialties.[95,98] In order to improve rural access to an otolaryngologist, it is imperative to ensure future otolaryngologists are adequately exposed to this patient population during training.[19] Otolaryngologists in general also have a desire to teach and train future generations, so the training partnership benefits not only resident physicians but also rural staff physicians and would likely improve rural physician retention. There is more than one effective structure to engaging residents with a role in rural health. As mentioned above, many residency programs with large academic affiliations encompass some rural populations in their catchment area; however, there is additional utility to experience to a formal rural practice setting. The chapter authors helped to design and implement a formal otolaryngology underserved care track with a significant rural health component at a large tertiary medical center in Chicago.[99] Interested residents travel with an attending from the home institution for regular clinic and surgical outreach at a nearby rural critical access hospital. Residents gain a diversity of clinical exposure, experience a different health system, and serve a population with very limited access to ear, nose, and throat care. The underserved care track requires prioritization from department leadership, but it is straightforward to implement, inexpensive, and does not interrupt existing clinical rotations. Resident interest and feedback have been very strong in the beginning years of this program. Specifics are noted in the cited publication.[99]

Next, economic considerations may drive otolaryngologists away from rural practice settings. The average medical school debt upon graduation is currently $200,000.[100] Physicians often owe much more than this amount upon completion of residency and fellowship due to additional undergraduate debt, compounding interest, and low incomes during graduate medical training. Loan forgiveness programs have become more available in recent years to help mitigate some of the immense financial burden. Government programs such as the federal Public Service Loan Forgiveness are in the early stages of implementation and reimburse individuals who seek employment in public servitude. Many rural hospitals qualify for reimbursement as part of their not-for-profit status. For-profit employers may also offer individual loan forgiveness programs which may be partial or complete and contingent upon employment for a set number of years. The National Health Service Corps (NHSC) offers loan forgiveness specifically for providers practicing in rural settings, although it is currently restricted to primary care and mental health providers. The most direct way to financially incentivize providers to practice in rural settings is with higher salaries. As mentioned above, however, reimbursements to rural physicians tend to be lower due to a less favorable payer mix and higher percentage of uninsured patients. Factoring rurality into risk adjustments for Medicare and Medicaid reimbursements could improve recruitment and retention of practices and providers.

Clinical resources to support the rural otolaryngologist

Another challenge for otolaryngologists in rural practice is integrating with supporting clinical services such as audiology, speech and language pathology, physical and occupational therapy, and rehabilitation services among others. Healthcare workforce shortages disproportionately impact rural areas. Healthcare organizations can mirror the recruitment efforts above to attract nonphysician clinicians. Some services may also be amenable to virtual conversion to allow rural patients access to otherwise niche services. For instance, facial retraining for patients with facial paralysis may be amenable to virtual consultations. Expanding virtual operations in audiology has also gained traction in the COVID era with the introduction of phone/tablet apps and other virtual services for patients with hearing loss. Rural otolaryngologists may be required to seek out virtual solutions for their patients who have difficulty accessing important supporting clinical services in rural settings.

Otolaryngology and distance

Travel is certainly one of the most substantial barriers to equity. Accessibility for rural patients is limited by both travel distance and infrastructure, but there are a number of emerging initiatives to help overcome this barrier. Of course, infrastructure improvements including expansion of low-cost public transportation services in rural settings would greatly facilitate travel particularly for rural patients requiring repeated services such as radiation oncology. Telemedicine has recently expanded in the setting of the coronavirus pandemic, and virtual otolaryngology care is an effective adjuvant to rural care. With the continued improvement of streaming technology and high-definition image sharing, virtual otolaryngology care is safe and effective. Seim et al. published a pilot cohort for a rural telemedicine clinic in 2018 that utilized in-person mid-level providers and virtual otolaryngologist consultation to delivery specialist care in a rural setting.[101] They confirmed 95% diagnostic agreement to in-person evaluation with equally high user satisfaction and without an increase in time for the encounters.[101] Mid-level providers can practice autonomously or semiautonomously depending on state and local regulations and help to expand a provider's reach. Visiting consultant clinics are another effective option. Otolaryngologists may establish recurring consultation dates with rural clinics in order to leverage the existing resources and maximize impact. Gruca et al. noted that almost half the otolaryngologists in Iowa participated in this type of outreach.[102] The chapter senior author (AAJ) also has a longstanding practice as a visiting rural consultant which integrates well with a large urban academic medical practice. Simply being present and available to see patients in rural communities allows for increased access to care. It also enables patients to receive treatment in a timely fashion, preventing further complications secondary to their illness. Surgeons visiting rural communities can help provide services to address basic needs, while patients who may require complex care can be referred to larger urban medical centers. Efficiency in patient evaluation and transfer may be improved via hospital partnerships. The "Endocrine Surgery" section above includes an example on sharing of ultrasound guided fine needle aspiration and pathology services between a large academic center and a very small rural critical access hospital and significant reductions in distance traveled for patients.[88] Suzanne Simard, a professor of forest ecology at the University of British Columbia, has shown in her extensive research how the interdependence of trees helps them thrive in their environment.[103] Trees essentially can communicate with each other in regard to their own well-being, with stronger trees able to share nutrients to help struggling neighbors. Just as Simard's research has shown that acts of sharing between trees help the forest thrive as one being, a symbiotic relationship between rural hospitals and larger medical centers is vital for the well-being of these respective institutions—and for the communities they serve.

Conclusions

There is a marked disparity in access to specialized otolaryngology services for patients living in rural areas of the US. Clearly defining disparities and recognizing opportunities for improvement are important first steps to bridging this gap. Some of the most studied areas of rural otolaryngology include hearing loss and head and neck cancer, while disparities in many other areas are experienced by many patients, but largely undescribed. Urban—rural classification systems are useful for research and mapping potential interventions. With a detailed knowledge of a broad anatomic region and many interventional capabilities, otolaryngologists are extremely well-suited to serving a rural population. A few strategies to expand rural access to otolaryngologists include: bolstering rural physician recruitment via flexible scheduling, favorable compensation, and loan repayment programs; developing a more extensive network of partnerships between rural hospitals and larger centers; and expanding otolaryngology rural training opportunities for residents and fellows. Overall, improving the access, quality, and cost of rural otolaryngology care is critical to improving the overall health of the US population.

References

1. U.S. Department of Health & Human Services. Social Determinants of Health | CDC. https://www.cdc.gov/socialdeterminants/index.htm. Accessed 29 September 2021.
2. Zahnd W, McLafferty S, Eberth J. Multilevel analysis in rural cancer control: a conceptual framework and methodological implications. *Prev Med.* 2019;129(105835): 139−148. https://doi.org/10.1016/j.ypmed.2019.105835.Multilevel.
3. Meit M, Knudson A, Gilbert T, et al. The 2014 Update of the Rural-Urban Chartbook. *Rural Heal Reform Policy Res Cent*; October 2014:44−45.
4. Womack LS, Rossen LM, Hirai AH, et al. Urban−rural infant mortality disparities by race and ethnicity and cause of death. *Am J Prev Med.* 2020;58(2):254−260. https:// doi.org/10.1016/j.amepre.2019.09.010.
5. Cosby AG, Maya McDoom-Echebiri M, James W, Khandekar H, Brown W, Hanna HL. Growth and persistence of place-based mortality in the United States: the rural mortality penalty. *Am J Publ Health.* 2019;109(1):155−162. https://doi.org/10.2105/AJPH.2018. 304787.
6. Centers for Disease Control and Prevention. *Rural Health*; 2019. https://www.cdc.gov/ chronicdisease/resources/publications/factsheets/rural-health.htm. Accessed October 19, 2021.
7. Jabbour J, Robey T, Cunningham MJ. Healthcare disparities in pediatric otolaryngology: a systematic review. *Laryngoscope.* 2018;128(7):1699−1713. https://doi.org/ 10.1002/lary.26995.
8. Boss EF, Smith DF, Ishman SL. Racial/ethnic and socioeconomic disparities in the diagnosis and treatment of sleep-disordered breathing in children. *Int J Pediatr Otorhinolaryngol.* 2011;75(3):299−307. https://doi.org/10.1016/j.ijporl.2010.11.006.
9. Keane E, Francis EC, Catháin EO, Rowley H. The role of race in thyroid cancer: systematic review. *J Laryngol Otol.* 2017;131(6):480−486. https://doi.org/10.1017/ S0022215117000688.
10. Lenze NR, Farquhar DR, Mazul AL, Masood MM, Zevallos JP. Racial disparities and human papillomavirus status in oropharyngeal cancer: a systematic review and meta-analysis. *Head Neck.* 2019;41(1):256−261. https://doi.org/10.1002/hed.25414.
11. Stein E, Lenze NR, Yarbrough WG, Hayes DN, Mazul A, Sheth S. Systematic review and meta-analysis of racial survival disparities among oropharyngeal cancer cases by HPV status. *Head Neck.* 2020;42(10):2985−3001. https://doi.org/10.1002/hed.26328.
12. Spielman DB, Liebowitz A, Kelebeyev S, et al. Race in rhinology clinical trials: a decade of disparity. *Laryngoscope.* 2021;131(8):1722−1728. https://doi.org/10.1002/ lary.29371.
13. Soler ZM, Mace JC, Litvack JR, Smith TL. Chronic rhinosinusitis, race, and ethnicity. *Am J Rhinol Allergy.* 2012;26(2):110−116. https://doi.org/10.2500/ajra.2012.26.3741.
14. James J, Tsvik AM, Chung SY, Usseglio J, Gudis DA, Overdevest JB. Association between social determinants of health and olfactory function: a scoping review. *Int Forum Allergy Rhinol.* March 2021:1−22. https://doi.org/10.1002/alr.22822.
15. Feit NZ, Wang Z, Demetres MR, Drenis S, Andreadis K, Rameau A. Healthcare disparities in laryngology: a scoping review. *Laryngoscope.* 2020:1−16. https://doi.org/ 10.1002/lary.29325.
16. Smith DF, Boss EF. Racial/Ethnic and socioeconomic disparities in the prevalence and treatment of otitis media in children in the United States. *Laryngoscope.* 2010;120(11): 2306−2312. https://doi.org/10.1002/lary.21090.

17. Barnett M, Hixon B, Okwiri N, et al. Factors involved in access and utilization of adult hearing healthcare: a systematic review. *Laryngoscope*. 2017;127(5):1187−1197. https://doi.org/10.1002/lary.26234.Factors.

18. Lovett B, Welschmeyer A, Johns JD, Mowry S, Hoa M. Health disparities in otology: a PRISMA-based systematic review. *Otolaryngol Head Neck Surg (United States)*. 2021. https://doi.org/10.1177/01945998211039490.

19. Urban MJ, Shimomura A, Shah S, Losenegger T, Westrick J, Jagasia AA. Rural otolaryngology care disparities: a scoping review. *Otolaryngol Head Neck Surg*. 2022;166(6):1219−1227. https://doi.org/10.1177/01945998211068822.

20. Emerson LP, Job A, Abraham V. A model for provision of ENT health care service at primary and secondary hospital level in a developing country. *Biomed Res Int*. 2013; 2013. https://doi.org/10.1155/2013/562643.

21. Singh A, Kumar S. A survey of ear, nose and throat disorders in rural India. *Indian J Otolaryngol Head Neck Surg*. 2010;62(2):121−124. https://doi.org/10.1007/s12070-010-0027-3.

22. United States Census Bureau. How does the U.S. Census Bureau define "Rural"? Rural America. https://mtgis-portal.geo.census.gov/arcgis/apps/MapSeries/index.html?appid=49cd4bc9c8eb444ab51218c1d5001ef6. Accessed 16 November 2021.

23. Ratcliffe M. *A Century of Delineating a Changing Landscape: The Census Bureau's Urban and Rural Classification, 1910 to 2010*; 2010. http://www2.census.gov/prod2/decennial/documents/00186079ch01.pdf.

24. Urban MJ, Wojcik C, Eggerstedt M, Jagasia AJ. Rural−urban disparities in otolaryngology: the state of Illinois. *Laryngoscope*. 2021;131(1):E70−E75. https://doi.org/10.1002/lary.28652.

25. Kiersz A. *The Most Average States in America - Business Insider*; 2014. https://www.businessinsider.com/the-most-average-states-in-america-2014-4. Accessed February 21, 2020.

26. Winters R, Pou A, Friedlander P. A "medical mission" at home: the needs of rural America in terms of otolaryngology care. *J Rural Health*. 2011;27(3):297−301. https://doi.org/10.1111/j.1748-0361.2010.00343.x.

27. Mackley HB, Teslova T, Camacho F, Short PF, Anderson RT. Does rurality influence treatment decisions in early stage laryngeal cancer? *J Rural Health*. 2014;30(4):406−411. https://doi.org/10.1111/jrh.12069.

28. Shah DR, Yang AD, Maverakis E, Martinez SR. Assessing rural-urban disparities in the use of sentinel lymph node biopsy for melanoma. *J Surg Res*. 2013;184(2):1157−1160. https://doi.org/10.1016/j.jss.2013.04.091.

29. Graboyes E, Cramer J, Balakrishnan K, et al. COVID-19 pandemic and health care disparities in head and neck cancer: scanning the horizon. *Head Neck*. 2020;42(7):1555−1559. https://doi.org/10.1002/hed.26345.COVID-19.

30. Rosemberg MAS, McCullagh MC, Nordstrom M. Farm and rural adolescents' perspective on hearing conservation: reports from a focus group study. *Noise Health*. 2015;17(76):134−140. https://doi.org/10.4103/1463-1741.155836.

31. Holt JJ, Broste SK, Hansen DA. Noise exposure in the rural setting. *Laryngoscope*. 1993;103:258−262.

32. Kramer M, Wood D. Noise-induced hearing loss in rural school children. *Scand Audiol*. 1982;11(4):279−280.

33. Hay-McCutcheon MJ, Hyams A, Yang X, et al. An exploration of the associations among hearing loss, physical health, and visual memory in adults from west central

Alabama. *J Speech Lang Hear Res.* 2017;60(8):2346−2359. https://doi.org/10.1044/2017_JSLHR-H-16-0369.

34. Karlovich RS, Wiley TL, Tweed T, Jensen DV. Hearing sensitivity in farmers. *Publ Health Rep.* 1988;103(1):61−71.

35. Ciletti L, Flamme GA. Prevalence of hearing impairment by gender and audiometric configuration: results from the National Health and Nutrition Examination Survey (1999−2004) and the Keokuk County Rural Health Study (1994−1998). *J Am Acad Audiol.* 2008;19(9):672−685. https://doi.org/10.3766/jaaa.19.9.3.

36. Flamme GA, Mudipalli VR, Reynolds SJ, et al. Prevalence of hearing impairment in a rural midwestern cohort: estimates from the Keokuk County Rural Health Study, 1994 to 1998. *Ear Hear.* 2005;26(3):350−360. https://doi.org/10.1097/00003446-200506000-00010.

37. Ives DG, Bonino P, Traven ND, Kuller LH. Characteristics and comorbidities of rural older adults with hearing impairment. *JAGS.* 1995;43:803−806.

38. Bush ML, Christian WJ, Bianchi K, Lester C, Schoenberg N. Targeting regional pediatric congenital hearing loss using a spatial scan statistic. *Ear Hear.* 2015;36(2):212−216. https://doi.org/10.1097/AUD.0000000000000101.

39. McCullagh MC, Yang JJ, Cohen MA. Community-based program to increase use of hearing conservation practices among farm and rural youth: a cluster randomized trial of effectiveness. *BMC Publ Health.* 2020;20(1):1−11. https://doi.org/10.1186/s12889-020-08972-3.

40. Marlenga B, Linneman JG, Pickett W, et al. Randomized trial of a hearing conservation intervention for rural students: long-term outcomes. *Pediatrics.* 2011;128(5). https://doi.org/10.1542/peds.2011-0770.

41. Powell W, Jacobs JA, Noble W, Bush ML, Snell-Rood C. Rural adult perspectives on impact of hearing loss and barriers to care. *J Community Health.* 2019;44(4):668−674. https://doi.org/10.1007/s10900-019-00656-3.

42. Shayman CS, Ha YM, Raz Y, Hullar TE. Geographic disparities in US veterans' access to cochlear implant care within the veterans health administration system. *JAMA Otolaryngol Head Neck Surg.* 2019;145(10):889−896. https://doi.org/10.1001/jamaoto.2019.1918.

43. Bush ML, Hardin B, Rayle C, Lester C, Studts CR, Shinn JB. Rural barriers to early diagnosis and treatment of infant hearing loss in Appalachia. *Otol Neurotol.* 2015;36(1):93−98. https://doi.org/10.1097/mao.0000000000000636.

44. Bush ML, Alexander D, Noblitt B, Lester C, Shinn JB. Pediatric hearing healthcare in Kentucky's Appalachian primary care setting. *J Community Health.* 2015;40(4):762−768. https://doi.org/10.1007/s10900-015-9997-0.

45. Chan S, Hixon B, Adkins M, Shinn J, Bush ML. Rurality and determinants of hearing healthcare in adult hearing aid recipients. *Laryngoscope.* 2017;127(10):2362−2367. https://doi.org/10.1016/j.physbeh.2017.03.040.

46. Bush ML, Bianchi K, Lester C, et al. Delays in diagnosis of congenital hearing loss in rural children. *J Pediatr.* 2014;164(2):393−397. https://doi.org/10.1016/j.jpeds.2013.09.047.

47. Bush ML, Osetinsky M, Shinn JB, et al. Assessment of Appalachian region pediatric hearing healthcare disparities and delays. *Laryngoscope.* 2014;124(7):1713−1717. https://doi.org/10.1002/lary.24588.

48. Bush M, Burton M, Loan A, Shinn JB. Timing discrepancies of early intervention hearing services in urban and rural cochlear implant recipients. *Otol Neurotol.* 2013;34(9):1−7. https://doi.org/10.1097/MAO.0b013e31829e83ad.

49. Hay-McCutcheon MJ, Yuk MC, Yang X. Accessibility to hearing healthcare in rural and urban populations of Alabama: perspectives and a preliminary roadmap for addressing inequalities. *J Community Health*. 2021;46(4):719–727. https://doi.org/10.1007/s10900-020-00943-4.

50. Cunningham M, Thomson V, McKiever E, Dickinson LM, Furniss A, Allison MA. Infant, maternal, and hospital factors' role in loss to follow-up after failed newborn hearing screening. *Acad Pediatr*. 2018;18(2):188–195. https://doi.org/10.1016/j.acap.2017.05.005.

51. Hixon B, Chan S, Adkins M, Shinn JB, Bush ML. Timing and impact of hearing healthcare in adult cochlear implant recipients: a rural-urban comparison. *Otol Neurotol*. 2016;37(9):1320–1324. https://doi.org/10.1097/MAO.0000000000001197.

52. Easterbrooks SR, Mordica JA. Teachers; ratings of functional communication in students with cochlear implants. *Am Ann Deaf*. 2000;145(1):54–59.

53. Ah-Tye C, Paradise JL, Colborn DK. Otorrhea in young children after tympanostomy-tube placement for persistent middle-ear effusion: prevalence, incidence, and duration. *Pediatrics*. 2021;107(6):1251–1258.

54. Crowson MG, Schulz KC, Tucci DL. Provider and patient drivers of ototopical antibiotic prescription variability. *Am J Otolaryngol Head Neck Med Surg*. 2015;36(6):814–819. https://doi.org/10.1016/j.amjoto.2015.07.001.

55. Kennedy KL, Connolly KM, Albert CL, Goldman JL, Cash ED, Severtson MA. Postoperative recurrent cholesteatoma in rural versus urban populations. *Otol Neurotol*. 2021;42(4):e459–e463. https://doi.org/10.1097/MAO.0000000000003003.

56. McEwen LN, Farjo R, Foxman B. Antibiotic prescribing for cystitis: how well does it match published guidelines? *Ann Epidemiol*. 2003;13(6):479–483. https://doi.org/10.1016/S1047-2797(03)00009-7.

57. Hashibe M, Kirchhoff AC, Kepka D, et al. Disparities in cancer survival and incidence by metropolitan versus rural residence in Utah. *Cancer Med*. 2018;7(4):1490–1497. https://doi.org/10.1002/cam4.1382.

58. Clarke JA, Despotis AM, Ramirez RJ, Zevallos JP, Mazul AL. Head and neck cancer survival disparities by race and rural–urban context. *Cancer Epidemiol Biomarkers Prev*. 2020;29(10):1955–1961. https://doi.org/10.1158/1055-9965.EPI-20-0376.

59. Papenberg BW, Allen JL, Markwell SM, et al. Disparate survival of late-stage male oropharyngeal cancer in Appalachia. *Sci Rep*. 2020;10(1):1–13. https://doi.org/10.1038/s41598-020-68380-w.

60. Pagedar NA, Davis AB, Sperry SM, Charlton ME, Lynch CF. Population analysis of socioeconomic status and otolaryngologist distribution on head and neck cancer outcomes. *Head Neck*. 2019;41(4):1046–1052. https://doi.org/10.1002/hed.25521. Population.

61. Harris JA, Hunter WP, Hanna GJ, Treister NS, Menon RS. Rural patients with oral squamous cell carcinoma experience better prognosis and long-term survival. *Oral Oncol*. 2020;111(July). https://doi.org/10.1016/j.oraloncology.2020.105037.

62. Ringstrom MJ, Christian J, Bush ML, Levy JE, Huang B, Gal TJ. Travel distance: impact on stage of presentation and treatment choices in head and neck cancer. *Am J Otolaryngol Head Neck Med Surg*. 2018;39(5):575–581. https://doi.org/10.1016/j.amjoto.2018.06.020.

63. White MG, Applewhite MK, Kaplan EL, Angelos P, Huo D, Grogan RH. A tale of two cancers: traveling to treat pancreatic and thyroid cancer. *J Am Coll Surg*. 2017;225(1):125–136.e6. https://doi.org/10.1016/j.jamcollsurg.2017.02.017.

64. Mukherjee A, Idigo AJ, Ye Y, et al. Geographical and racial disparities in head and neck cancer diagnosis in South-Eastern United States: using real-world electronic medical records data. *Heal Equity.* 2020;4(1):43−51. https://doi.org/10.1089/heq.2019.0092.

65. Logan HL, Guo Y, Emanuel AS, et al. Determinants of first-time cancer examinations in a rural community: a mechanism for behavior change. *Am J Publ Health.* 2015;105(7): 1424−1431. https://doi.org/10.2105/AJPH.2014.302516.

66. Pagedar NA, Kahl AR, Tasche KK, et al. Incidence trends for upper aerodigestive tract cancers in rural United States counties. *Head Neck.* 2020;41(8):2619−2624. https://doi.org/10.1002/hed.25736.Incidence.

67. Howren MB, Christensen AJ, Adamowicz JL, Seaman A, Wardyn S, Pagedar NA. Problem alcohol use among rural head and neck cancer patients at diagnosis: associations with health-related quality of life. *Psycho Oncol.* 2021;30(5):708−715. https://doi.org/10.1002/pon.5616.

68. Zuniga SA, Lango MN. Effect of rural and urban geography on larynx cancer incidence and survival. *Laryngoscope.* 2018;128(8):1874−1880. https://doi.org/10.1002/lary.27042.

69. Schreinemachers DM, Creason JP, Garry VF. Cancer mortality in agricultural regions of Minnesota. *Environ Health Perspect.* 1999;107(3):205−211. https://doi.org/10.1289/ehp.99107205.

70. Boakye EA, Johnston KJ, Moulin TA, et al. Factors associated with head and neck cancer hospitalization cost and length of stay-a national study. *Am J Clin Oncol Cancer Clin Trials.* 2019;42(2):172−178. https://doi.org/10.1097/COC.0000000000000487.

71. Allareddy V, Konety BR. Characteristics of patients and predictors of in-hospital mortality after hospitalization for head and neck cancers. *Cancer.* 2006;106(11): 2382−2388. https://doi.org/10.1002/cncr.21899.

72. Urban MJ, Shimomura A, Shah S, Losenegger T, Westrick J, Jagasia AA. Rural otolaryngology care disparities: a scoping review. *Otolaryngol Head Neck Surg.* 2022;166(6): 1219−1227. https://doi.org/10.1177/01945998211068822.

73. Ort S, Beus K, Isaacson J. Pediatric temporal bone fractures in a rural population. *Otolaryngol Head Neck Surg.* 2004;131(4):433−437. https://doi.org/10.1016/j.otohns.2004.04.006.

74. Yan F, Levy DA, Wen CC, et al. Rural barriers to surgical care for children with sleep-disordered breathing. *Otolaryngol Head Neck Surg (United States).* 2021. https://doi.org/10.1177/0194599821993383.

75. Cooper JN, Koppera S, Boss EF, Lind MN. Differences in tonsillectomy utilization by race/ethnicity, type of health insurance, and rurality. *Acad Pediatr.* 2021;21(6): 1031−1036. https://doi.org/10.1016/j.acap.2020.11.007.

76. McKee S, Yang A, Kidwai S, Govindaraj S, Shrivastava R, Iloreta A. The socioeconomic determinants for transsphenoidal pituitary surgery: a review of New York State from 1995 to 2015. *Int Forum Allergy Rhinol.* 2018;8(10):1145−1156. https://doi.org/10.1002/alr.22148.

77. Bhattacharyya N. Regional variation and factors associated with image guidance utilization during endoscopic sinus surgery in the ambulatory setting. *Ann Otol Rhinol Laryngol.* 2014;123(8):545−549. https://doi.org/10.1177/0003489414525344.

78. Thomas A, Smith K, Newberry C, et al. Operative time and cost variability for functional endoscopic sinus surgery. *Int Forum Allergy Rhinol.* 2019;9(1):23−29. https://doi.org/10.1002/alr.22198.Operative.

79. Hanley JP, Jackson E, Morrissey LA, et al. Geospatial and temporal analysis of thyroid cancer incidence in a rural population. *Thyroid.* 2015;25(7):812—822. https://doi.org/10.1089/thy.2015.0039.

80. McDow AD, Zahnd WE, Angelos P, Mellinger JD, Ganai S. Impact of rurality on national trends in thyroid cancer incidence and long-term survival. *J Rural Health.* 2020;36(3):326—333. https://doi.org/10.1111/jrh.12374.

81. Clarke C, Reynolds P, Oakley-Girvan I, et al. Indicators of microbial-rich environments and the development of papillary thyroid cancer in California Teachers Study. *Int J Cancer Epidemiol Detect Prev.* 2015;39:548—553.

82. Li N, Du XL, Reitzel LR, Xu L, Sturgis EM. Impact of enhanced detection on the increase in thyroid cancer incidence in the United States: review of incidence trends by socioeconomic status within the surveillance, epidemiology, and end results registry, 1980—2008. *Thyroid.* 2013;23(1):103—110. https://doi.org/10.1089/thy.2012.0392.

83. Al-Qurayshi Z, Hauch A, Srivastav S, Kandil E. Ethnic and economic disparities effect on management of hyperparathyroidism. *Am J Surg.* 2017;213(6):1134—1142. https://doi.org/10.1016/j.amjsurg.2016.07.008.

84. Biron VL, Bang H, Farwell DG, Bewley AF. National trends and factors associated with hospital costs following thyroid surgery. *Thyroid.* 2015;25(7):823—829. https://doi.org/10.1089/thy.2014.0495.

85. Richmond BK, Eads K, Flaherty S, Belcher M, Runyon D. Complications of thyroidectomy and parathyroidectomy in the rural community hospital setting. *Am Surg.* 2007;73(4):332—336. https://doi.org/10.1177/000313480707300404.

86. Haas S, Trujillo A, Kunstle J. Fine needle aspiration of thyroid nodules in a rural setting. *Am J Med.* 1993;94:357—361.

87. Guo A, Jenkinson S. Outcome of fine needle aspiration of thyroid nodules in the Bethesda system for reporting thyroid aspiration cytology: an institutional experience in a rural setting. *Thyroid.* 2014;24:A81—A82.

88. Le TQ, Sánchez Y, Misono AS, Saini S, Prabhakar AM. Improving access to image-guided procedures at an integrated rural critical access hospital: ultrasound-guided thyroid biopsy program. *Curr Probl Diagn Radiol.* 2017;46(6):419—422. https://doi.org/10.1067/j.cpradiol.2017.02.004.

89. Bonilha HS, Simpson AN, Ellis C, Mauldin P, Martin-Harris B, Simpson K. The one-year attributable cost of post-stroke dysphagia. *Dysphagia.* 2014;29(5):545—552. https://doi.org/10.1007/s00455-014-9543-8.

90. George BP, Kelly AG, Schneider EB, Holloway RG. Current practices in feeding tube placement for US acute ischemic stroke inpatients. *Neurology.* 2014;83(10):874—882. https://doi.org/10.1212/WNL.0000000000000764.

91. Cohen SM, Thomas S, Roy N, Kim J, Courey M. Frequency and factors associated with use of videolaryngostroboscopy in voice disorder assessment. *Laryngoscope.* 2014;124(9):2118—2124. https://doi.org/10.1002/lary.24688.

92. Roden KS, Tong W, Surrusco M, Shockley WW, Van Aalst JA, Hultman CS. Changing characteristics of facial fractures treated at a regional, level 1 trauma center, from 2005 to 2010: an assessment of patient demographics, referral patterns, etiology of injury, anatomic location, and clinical outcomes. *Ann Plast Surg.* 2012;68(5):461—466. https://doi.org/10.1097/SAP.0b013e31823b69dd.

93. Smith H, Peek-Asa C, Nesheim D, Nish A, Normandin P, Sahr S. Etiology, diagnosis, and characteristics of facial fracture at a midwestern level I trauma center. *J Trauma Nurs.* 2012;19(1):57—65. https://doi.org/10.1097/JTN.0b013e31823a4c0e.

94. Aaland MO, Smith K, Shuck JM, Weigelt J, Lucas C, Fischer J. Delayed diagnosis in a rural trauma center. *Surgery.* 1996;120(4):774—779. https://doi.org/10.1016/S0039-6060(96)80030-4.
95. Meaike JD, Cantwell S, Mills A, Singh K, Moran SL. Is rural plastic surgery feasible and important?: a survey and review of the literature. *Ann Plast Surg.* 2020;84(6): 626—631. https://doi.org/10.1097/SAP.0000000000002153.
96. Kezirian EJ, Maselli J, Vittinghoff E, Goldberg AN, Auerbach AD. Obstructive sleep apnea surgery practice patterns in the United States: 2000 to 2006. *Otolaryngol Head Neck Surg.* 2010;143(3):441—447. https://doi.org/10.1016/j.otohns.2010.05.009.
97. Toman J, Oussayef MB, Porterfield JZ. Going global: interest in global health among us otolaryngology residents. *Ann Glob Heal.* 2021;87(1):1—9. https://doi.org/10.5334/aogh.3283.
98. Bruksch-Meck K, Crouse B, Quinn G, McCart L, Traxler K. Graduate medical education initiatives to develop the physician workforce in rural Wisconsin. *Wis Med J.* 2018; 117(5):201—207. http://www.wisconsinmedicalsociety.org/_WMS/publications/wmj/pdf/117/5/201.pdf. Accessed September 20, 2019.
99. Urban MJ, Jagasia AA, Batra PS, Losavio P. Design and implementation of a global health and underserved care track in an otolaryngology residency. *OTO Open.* 2022; 6(1):1—5. https://doi.org/10.1177/2473974X221078857.
100. Calonia J. What's the average medical school debt in 2022? *Forbes.* 2022.
101. Seim NB, Philips RHW, Matrka LA, et al. Developing a synchronous otolaryngology telemedicine clinic: prospective study to assess fidelity and diagnostic concordance. *Laryngoscope.* 2018;128(5):1068—1074. https://doi.org/10.1002/lary.26929.
102. Gruca TS, Nam I, Tracy R. Reaching rural patients through otolaryngology visiting consultant clinics. *Otolaryngol Head Neck Surg.* 2014;151(6):895—898. https://doi.org/10.1177/0194599814553398.
103. Sam B, Chaloner T. *"Mother Tree" Ecologist Suzanne Simard Shares Secrets of Tree Communication: May 4, 2021 NPR*; 2021. https://www.npr.org/sections/health-shots/2021/05/04/993430007/trees-talk-to-each-other-mother-tree-ecologist-hears-lessons-for-people-too. Accessed September 19, 2022.

The impact of health literacy on patient care in otolaryngology

9

Uchechukwu C. Megwalu, Isaac A. Bernstein

Department of Otolaryngology—Head and Neck Surgery, Stanford University School of Medicine, Stanford, CA, United States

Introduction

Health literacy is the ability to access and understand information and services needed to make appropriate decisions regarding one's health.[1] It is a measure of an individual's ability to navigate the healthcare system. An estimated 90 million adults in the United States have inadequate health literacy.[2] Health literacy has been shown to impact outcomes in a number of medical conditions, including asthma, chronic obstructive pulmonary disease (COPD), diabetes, and hypertension.[3-9] Health literacy has also been shown to impact healthcare-seeking behavior. Patients with low health literacy are less likely to comply with colorectal, breast, and cervical cancer screening.[10-14]

Definition of health literacy

The Institute of Medicine (IOM) defines health literacy as "the degree to which individuals have the capacity to obtain, process, and understand basic health information needed to make appropriate health decisions."[1] Fundamental literacy is a core component of health literacy. In addition to the ability to read and write, fundamental literacy includes comprehension and reasoning abilities. The National Literacy Act of 1991 defines literacy as "an individual's ability to read, write, and speak in English, and compute and solve problems at levels of proficiency necessary to function on the job and in society, to achieve one's goals, and develop one's knowledge and potential."[15] Another component of health literacy is numeracy. This is the ability to perform quantitative computations using numbers that are embedded in printed materials.[2] This is exemplified by the ability to interpret nutritional labels and prescription drug instructions. In addition to fundamental literacy and numeracy, health literacy also includes skills such as the ability for self-advocacy, adequate background medical knowledge, health-related information seeking, and comprehension skills. These skills are critical for effectively navigating the current complex healthcare environment. A patient with functional health literacy should be

Healthcare Disparities in Otolaryngology. https://doi.org/10.1016/B978-0-443-10714-6.00013-4

151

proficient in tasks such as locating and assessing the accuracy of health information in the media, completing medical and financial forms, understanding prescription instructions, and comparing nutritional information of foods based on nutritional labels.

Epidemiology of low health literacy

An estimated 90 million adults in the United States have poor health literacy.[2] Several sociodemographic factors have been shown to be associated with inadequate health literacy. Health literacy is strongly associated with level of education. Low English proficiency and racial/ethnic minority status are also associated with increased risk of inadequate health literacy. The impact of age and gender on health literacy status is equivocal.

The 2003 National Assessment of Adult Literacy (NAAL) assessed approximately 19,000 adults in the United States and included a health literacy component.[2] The study found that lower level of education was associated with lower level of health literacy. They also found that younger age was associated with higher levels of health literacy. These finding are similar to the findings of subsequent studies in cancer patients and otolaryngology patients.[16,17] The NAAL study found that White and Asian/Pacific Islander adults had higher average health literacy than Black and American Indian/Alaska Native adults. In addition, Hispanic ethnicity was associated with low health literacy. Interestingly, adults who spoke only English before starting school had higher average health literacy than adults who spoke other languages alone or other languages and English. The study also found that women had average higher health literacy than men.

Health literacy and health outcomes

Health literacy has been shown to impact outcomes in a number of medical conditions. A recent retrospective cohort study examined the impact of health literacy on outcomes among patients admitted for heart failure.[18] Inadequate health literacy was associated with increased mortality, after adjusting for age, gender, race, insurance, highest level of education, hospital length of stay, and comorbid conditions. However, health literacy had no impact on 90-day rehospitalization and emergency department visits. Another retrospective cohort study by Peterson et al. examined the impact of health literacy on mortality and hospitalization among 1494 outpatients with heart failure.[19] Similarly, they found that inadequate health literacy was associated with increased mortality, but not hospitalization.

Among asthma patients, inadequate health literacy has been shown to be associated with poor medication adherence, poor asthma control, decreased asthma-related quality of life, and increased asthma-related hospitalizations and emergency department visits.[3–6] Federman et al. performed a prospective cohort study examining the impact of health literacy on asthma outcomes in 433 elderly patients.[3] They found that low health literacy was associated with having a predicted FEV <70% and with increased emergency department visits and hospitalization for asthma. However, health literacy was not associated with poor patient-reported asthma control or quality of life. Apter et al. performed a prospective cohort study examining the impact of health literacy on treatment compliance and asthma outcomes in 248 adult patients.[5] After controlling for age, sex, and race/ethnicity, inadequate health literacy was associated with poor asthma control and poor quality of life. Although inadequate health literacy was associated with poor adherence to inhaled steroids, this was not significant on multivariable analysis.

Inadequate health literacy is also associated with poor outcomes in diabetic patients. Schillinger et al. performed a cross-sectional study of 408 patients with diabetes.[8] After adjusting for sociodemographic characteristics, depressive symptoms, social support, treatment regimen, and years with diabetes, poor health literacy was associated with poor glycemic control and increased risk of developing retinopathy. The relationship between health literacy and blood pressure control in patients with hypertension is equivocal. Willens et al. performed a large cross-sectional study of 23,483 primary care clinic encounters in 10,644 patients with hypertension.[20] They found that higher health literacy was associated with higher systolic and diastolic blood pressures. Another cross-sectional study of 423 urban, primary care patients with hypertension and coronary disease also found that inadequate health literacy was associated with uncontrolled blood pressure ($\geq 140/90$ mmHg, $\geq 130/80$ mmHg for patients with diabetes), after adjusting for age, gender, race, employment, education, mental status, and self-reported adherence.[21]

Several studies suggest that the association between inadequate health literacy and poor outcomes may be partly mediated by poor understanding of medical information and erroneous illness and medication beliefs. Kale et al. found that COPD patients with inadequate health literacy were more likely to have beliefs about their illness and medication that are associated with poor adherence.[7] Similarly, another study on hypertensive and diabetic patients showed that patients with inadequate health literacy had poor knowledge of important information about their chronic disease.[9]

Health literacy has also been shown to impact cancer-related healthcare-seeking behavior. Patients with low health literacy are less likely to comply with colorectal, breast, and cervical cancer screening.[10–14] Sentell et al. performed a cross-sectional study of Chinese and White respondents in the 2007 California Health Interview Survey, examining the association between health literacy and compliance with US Preventive Service Task Force (USPSTF) guidelines for colorectal cancer screening.[10] They found that low health literacy and low English proficiency were associated with lower likelihood of compliance with colorectal screening guidelines. In another study, they examined the association between health literacy and compliance with USPSTF guidelines for cervical, colorectal, and breast cancer screening among Chinese Americans.[11] Low health literacy was associated with lower odds of meeting breast cancer screening guidelines, but not cervical cancer or colorectal cancer screening guidelines. Respondents with both low health literacy and low English proficiency were significantly less likely to have up-to-date colorectal and breast cancer screening. Another cross-sectional study of 722 Hispanic women in South Texas analyzed the impact of health literacy on mammography screening behavior and adherence.[12] The study revealed that 51% of survey respondents had inadequate or marginal health literacy. Inadequate health literacy was found to be strongly associated with lower rates of mammography screening.

Kobayashi et al. examined the association between health literacy and participation in colorectal cancer screening in England using data from the English Longitudinal Study of Ageing.[13] They found that 27% of participants had inadequate health literacy skills. Inadequate health literacy was associated with lower odds of participating in colorectal cancer screening, independent of other predictors of screening: age, sex, and personal wealth. Another study evaluating the association between health literacy and colorectal cancer screening among low-income patients also found that marginal and inadequate health literacy were associated with decreased likelihood of colorectal screening.[14] Furthermore, controlling for health literacy eliminated the association between educational attainment and colorectal cancer screening. This finding suggests that health literacy mediated the relationship between educational attainment and colorectal cancer screening.

Health literacy has also been shown to impact quality of life in cancer patients. Halverson et al. performed a cross-sectional study evaluating the impact of health literacy on health-related quality of life (HRQL) in 1841 adults in Wisconsin, diagnosed with lung, breast, colorectal, or prostate cancer 2–3 years prior.[22] They found that low health literacy was associated with low HRQL, after adjusting for cancer site, extent of disease, age, sex, race/ethnicity, education, income, and urban versus rural residence. Similarly, Song et al. investigated the association between health literacy and HRQL in men with prostate cancer.[23] The study included 1581 men with newly diagnosed clinically localized prostate cancer from the North Carolina–Louisiana Prostate Cancer Project. On univariable analysis, they found that lower health literacy was associated with both mental and physical well-being. However, after controlling for sociodemographic (age, race, marital status, income, and education) and illness-related factors (types of cancer treatment, tumor aggressiveness, and comorbidities), health literacy was only associated with the mental well-being.

Significance of health literacy for otolaryngology patients

Despite the well-documented impact of health literacy on health outcomes, health literacy is understudied in otolaryngology-head and neck surgery. Many of the available studies have focused on assessing the readability of patient education materials, instead of directly assessing health literacy in otolaryngology patients.[24,25] A few studies, however, have directly assessed health literacy. Beitler et al. assessed health literacy in eight patients, who had undergone total laryngectomy for laryngeal cancer, and found that three of the patients had inadequate health literacy.[26] In a larger study, Koay et al. examined health literacy in 60 patients with head and neck cancer (HNC) and 33 patients with lung cancer.[16] They found that 12% of the patients had limited health literacy. They also found that older age and lower education level were associated with inadequate health literacy. Megwalu et al. conducted the largest study to date assessing factors associated with inadequate health literacy among otolaryngology patients.[17] The study included 316 adult patients from a tertiary care otolaryngology clinic population. They found that 10% of the patients had inadequate health literacy. Similar to previous studies, they found an association between level of education and health literacy. Patients who had completed high school or less than high school education were more likely to have inadequate health literacy. Racial minority patients and patients who did not have English as their primary language were also more likely to have inadequate health literacy. Although univariable analysis suggested that age and Hispanic ethnicity were associated with health literacy, these factors were not found to be associated with health literacy on multivariable analysis. Gender was also not associated with health literacy. These findings differ from the NAAL study, which found that older age, Hispanic ethnicity, and male gender were associated with inadequate health literacy. Some of the differences in the findings between studies may be due to differences in the populations sampled and lack of multivariable analysis in the NAAL study.[2]

Health literacy may have a significant impact on healthcare-seeking behavior among otolaryngology patients. A recent single-institution cross-sectional study of 1295 patients undergoing audiometric testing found that patients with inadequate health literacy were more likely to present with more severe hearing loss than patients with adequate health literacy.[27] However, in a subset of patients identified as hearing aid candidates, health literacy was not associated with hearing aid adoption. These findings suggest that patients with low health literacy are more likely to seek care later in the course of their hearing loss, but are no less likely to obtain hearing aids compared with patients with adequate health literacy. It is likely that patients with inadequate health literacy present later because they are less likely to self-advocate for hearing assessment and experience more difficulty navigating the complex hearing healthcare system.

Health literacy also affects patient—clinician communication in otolaryngology. One study assessed factors associated with preferring remote versus in-person communication of fine needle aspiration biopsy results for patients in an otolaryngology clinic.[28] They found that, although approximately 70% of patients preferred remote notification of their biopsy results (either by telephone or via an online portal), patients with inadequate health literacy were more likely to prefer in-person notification. The study also found that patients who valued receiving a clear explanation of the results as the most important communication factor when receiving malignant biopsy results were more likely to prefer in-person notification. The preference for in-person communication by patients with low health literacy is probably due to concerns about misunderstanding results over the telephone or inability to interpret online results without the help of the healthcare provider.

It is critical for otolaryngologists to be aware of issues related to health literacy, given its significant impact on healthcare-seeking behavior, patient–clinician communication, and health outcomes. This is even more important in today's health-care environment with its emphasis on shared decision-making. Routine health literacy screening may be beneficial in otolaryngology practice, to identify and help patients who might require additional help in navigating the healthcare system. This may be particularly beneficial for patients with complex problems, such as HNC. A cross-sectional study of HNC patients in Ireland revealed that 47% of the patients had inadequate health literacy.[29] Furthermore, inadequate health literacy was associated with lower levels of self-management behaviors, lower functional well-being and HNC disease-specific quality of life, and higher levels of fear of recurrence. Another single-institution study from the United States also showed that inadequate health literacy was associated with lower social-emotional quality of life.[30] Management of HNC is complex and involves coordination of care across multiple disciplines, which increases the health literacy requirements for patients who have to assimilate new information and make complex decisions at times of physical and emotional stress.[31] Patients with HNC often need multiple diagnostic tests and evaluations by multiple providers prior to initiating treatment. Failure to comply with these pretreatment procedures may lead to treatment delay, which has been shown to adversely affect outcomes.[32–35] In addition, failure to comply with the treatment regimen, which may involve daily radiation treatments for 6–7 weeks, can lead to treatment breaks, which have also been shown to lead to poor locoregional control and survival.[36–38] Consequently, HNC patients with inadequate health literacy may be at risk for poor treatment compliance and outcomes due to difficulty in navigating the complex systems involved in their care. Health literacy screening, and provision of patient care navigators for those with inadequate health literacy, may help mitigate some of these issues.

The health literacy demands of the healthcare system

Patients with inadequate health literacy face many hurdles when navigating the healthcare system. These steps occur at multiple stages during the interaction with the healthcare system from scheduling the appointment to making decisions about the appropriate management plans. Take, for example, a patient who is seeing an otolaryngologist for a parotid mass. If this patient is not referred to a specific otolaryngologist, she would have to locate an appropriate provider, and determine whether they have the appropriate qualification and expertise to manage this condition. In addition to fundamental literacy, this would require adequate health-related information seeking and comprehension skills. After locating the appropriate provider, she would need to schedule an appointment. She might need to confirm with her health insurance company that the provider is in-network and that the services would be covered. She might have to determine the amounts of any possible co-pay or deductibles, which would require numeracy skills. If there is concern for potential malignancy or progression of disease, she may have to request that her appointment be expedited, which would require self-advocacy skills. Scheduling the appointment would require numeracy skills to coordinate between available appointment times and her schedule. Making it successfully to the appointment on would also require adequate numeracy and time management skills, accounting for factors such as traffic or altered public transportation schedules to ensure she makes it to her appointment on time. Locating the appropriate facility may require her to be able to interpret maps and directions that were provided during scheduling.

The clinical encounter also presents some health literacy challenges. In today's healthcare environment, patients are expected to engage with their healthcare providers in shared decision-making.[31,39] In our example, the clinician may discuss treatment options for the parotid mass, which may include parotidectomy or observation. Choosing the appropriate treatment requires the patient to have some basic medical knowledge, assimilate the new information that is provided by the clinician, rapidly perform a risk/benefit analysis of each treatment option, and convey her preferences to the clinician. If she decides to proceed with parotidectomy, informed consent is required.

The informed consent process is particularly challenging for patients with inadequate health literacy, given that consent is often provided after receiving a large amount of complex new information. In the case of our patient, if parotidectomy is recommended, the surgeon has the responsibility to provide the patient with basic details about the surgical procedure and inform the patient about the risks, benefits, and alternatives to the proposed operation. The patient, thus being "informed," can then decide whether to accept or refuse the operation. This process requires the patient to have some basic knowledge of human anatomy and the medical condition being treated. Furthermore, the process often includes discussions regarding probabilities such as the expected success rate, the risks of various complications, and recurrence rates. Consequently, patients need to employ numeracy skills in order to make an informed decision. Therefore, it is incumbent on the surgeon to ensure that the details of the proposed surgery are described very clearly without the use of medical jargon and that the patient has a clear understanding of what is to be expected from the procedure before providing consent. Finally, in addition to comprehension, the formal informed consent process usually requires the patient to sign the consent form. This poses a significant challenge for patients with low fundamental literacy, since most consent forms are written at a reading grade level much higher than recommended for patient materials.[40]

The practice of modern medicine also frequently involves the ordering of multiple diagnostic tests, especially when managing complex problems. Patients with inadequate health literacy may have difficulty coordinating the different tests that are ordered. Accessing and interpreting the test results can also be challenging for patients. The 2014 requirements of the Centers for Medicare & Medicaid Services (CMS) Electronic Health Record (EHR) Incentive Program led to the introduction of electronic medical record systems with patient portals.[41] Consequently, patients now have ready access to their test results and this often occurs before they have a chance to discuss the findings with their healthcare provider. Patients with inadequate health literacy may have difficulty interpreting these results and are more likely to prefer in-person notification due to concerns about misunderstanding the findings.[28] Therefore, it is important for clinicians to develop a clear plan for communication of test results based on patient preference.

The health literacy demands of patient education materials

The Agency for Healthcare Research and Quality recommends that patient education materials should be written at a reading level no greater than sixth grade.[42] Several studies assessing the readability of otolaryngology patient education materials have found that most of these are written at a higher reading grade level than recommended.

Kim et al. analyzed 128 patient education articles from three English-speaking otolaryngology societies and found that a grade 9 reading level or greater was required for comprehension.[43]

Wong et al. reviewed 502 pediatric otolaryngology-related articles from online patient health libraries from 16 institutions and found that 28.3% of articles were written at or below the reading ability of the average American adult.[44] Another study found that among 29 online patient education articles on vocal fold paralysis, readability ranged from grade 9 to 17 and understandability ranged from 29% to 82%.[45] In the management of HNC, the use of patient-reported outcome measures (PROMs) may support patient–physician communication and help assess patient satisfaction and outcomes.[46] However, a review of eight commonly used HNC PROMs found readabilities above the sixth grade reading level for each.[47] Similarly, Lee et al. studied eight PROMs for chronic rhinosinusitis, and three for skull base disease, and found that 100% and 67%, respectively, were above the recommended sixth grade reading level.[48] In the hearing healthcare literature, a systematic review of eight studies on readability of online hearing care information also consistently found readability levels above the recommended sixth grade reading level.[49]

It is important to address the fundamental literacy requirements of patient education materials by ensuring that materials are written at an appropriate reading grade level. However, other health literacy factors need to be considered. For the patient education material to be effective, it must be direct, concise, and easy to understand. A health literacy load analysis should be performed to examine the demands associated with interpreting and understanding the information presented. A health literacy load analysis involves structural and functional analysis of the text. The structural analysis includes analysis of the vocabulary, length, and complexity of phrases and sentences; the amount of repetition and reinforcement; and the coherence across sentence and paragraphs.[50,51] This goes beyond the standard readability tests and includes the assessment of appropriate font size, line spacing, and appropriate use of blank spaces and illustrations. The functional analysis involves identification of skills and knowledge that the consumer is assumed to already possess to understand the material. In addition to fundamental literacy (ability to read and write), this may include science literacy, civic literacy, and cultural literacy.

Health literacy measures

There are several validated measures of health literacy. Many of them are designed for research settings, are labor-intensive, and require a large amount of time to administer. However, a few of them are easy to apply in clinical practice and will be discussed in this section (Table 9.1).

The brief health literacy screen

The Brief Health Literacy Screen (BHLS) is a 3-item self-reported measure of health literacy.[52] It was developed to rapidly detect patients with inadequate health literacy, making it feasible to apply in clinical practice. The BHLS includes three questions:

1. "How confident are you filling out medical forms by yourself?"
2. "How often do you have someone help you read hospital materials?"
3. "How often do you have problems learning about your medical condition because of difficulty understanding written information?"

The response options for the first question are: "extremely," "quite a bit," "somewhat," "a little bit," or "not at all." The response options for the other two questions

Table 9.1 Validated health literacy measurement tools.

Health Literacy Tool	Method	Number of items	Notes
Brief Health Literacy Screen	Self-report	3	Assesses difficulty in filling out medical forms, reading hospital materials, and understanding written information about medical condition.
Newest Vital Sign	Test	6	Involves interpretation of the contents of an ice cream nutrition label.
Cancer Health Literacy Test (CHLT)	Test	CHLT-30: 30; CHLT-6: 6	Involves multiple-choice tests that specifically measure cancer-specific health literacy. Requires a computer algorithm to score.
Short Test of Functional Literacy in Adults	Test	40	Includes reading and numeracy assessments.
Rapid Estimate of Adult Literacy in Medicine	Test	66	Assigns a reading grade level. Does not assess numeracy or comprehension.

are: "all of the time," "most of the time," "some of the time," "a little of the time," or "none of the time." A response of "a little bit" or "not at all" for the first question is indicative of inadequate health literacy for that question. A response of "somewhat" or "some of the time" for the last two questions indicates inadequate health literacy for each of those questions. The main disadvantage of the BHLS is that it is a self-reported measure of health literacy and may be prone to reporting bias. On the other hand, it is easy to administer and can be easily incorporated into the physician's work-flow.

For research purposes, the response to each BHLS question is recorded on a 5 point Likert scale with the first question reverse-coded. The scores for the three questions are then summed to produce an overall BHLS score ranging between 3 and 15 points, with higher scores indicating higher health literacy.[20] A response of ≤ 3 on the Likert scale indicates inadequate health literacy for each question, while a summative BHLS score of ≤ 9 indicates overall inadequate health literacy.[53,54]

The newest vital sign

The Newest Vital Sign (NVS) is a quick health literacy that can be administered in 3 min. Health literacy assessment using the NVS involves the interpretation of the contents of an ice cream nutrition label (Fig. 9.1).[55] The nutrition label is accompanied by six questions. The first four questions require the subject to interpret and calculate caloric and nutritional contents from the label and apply them to daily life scenarios. The last two questions require the subject to use the ingredient information to answer questions related to patient allergies. Fewer than four correct answers are indicative of limited health literacy. The NVS is well suited for research applications due to its objective nature. However, it requires the patient to take a test and does not fit into the clinic work-flow as easily as the BHLS.

The Cancer Health Literacy Test

The Cancer Health Literacy Test (CHLT) is a validated health literacy measure, specifically designed to measure health literacy in cancer patients.[56] It consists of the longer Cancer Health Literacy Test-30 (CHLT-30) and the shorter Cancer Health Literacy Test-6 (CHLT-6). The CHLT-30 is a 30-item multiple choice test that can be completed in 10–15 min and measures cancer health literacy along a continuum. The test provides a score that is equal to the total number of correct responses and ranges from 0 to 30. The CHLT-6 is a 6-item multiple choice test that takes less than 2 min to administer. It is designed to quickly identify individuals with limited cancer health literacy. However, it requires the use of a computerized algorithm to score. The computerized test scoring yields the probability of belonging to the inadequate health literacy group and the probability of belonging to the adequate health literacy group. Using these probabilities, the CHLT-6 is able to designate patients as having adequate or inadequate cancer health literacy with a high degree of precision. The

Nutrition Facts

Serving Size	½ cup
Servings per container	4

Amount per serving		
Calories 250	Fat Cal	120

	%DV
Total Fat 13g	20%
Sat Fat 9g	40%
Cholesterol 28mg	12%
Sodium 55mg	2%
Total Carbohydrate 30g	12%
Dietary Fiber 2g	
Sugars 23g	
Protein 4g	8%

*Percentage Daily Values (DV) are based on a 2,000 calorie diet. Your daily values may be higher or lower depending on your calorie needs.

Ingredients: Cream, Skim Milk, Liquid Sugar, Water, Egg Yolks, Brown Sugar, Milkfat, Peanut Oil, Sugar, Butter, Salt, Carrageenan, Vanilla Extract.

FIGURE 9.1

The Newest Vital Sign ice cream nutritional label.

CHLT-30 was recently validated in Spanish-speaking patients.[57] The CHLT-6 has been validated only in English-speaking patients. Consequently, it can only be used in English-speaking patients.

Short Test of Functional Literacy in Adults

The Short Test of Functional Literacy in Adults (S-TOFHLA) is a 36-item reading and 4-item numeracy assessment.[58] There are two timed (7 min) clinically oriented reading passages that omit key words and phrases from sentences, and the study participant chooses among four options to correctly complete the sentence. The numeracy section assesses the patient's ability to read health information, such as that found on a prescription label, and interpret numerical information. Overall scores range from 0 to 100. The S-TOFHLA has been validated for use in both English and Spanish.[59]

Rapid Estimate of Adult Literacy in Medicine

The Rapid Estimate of Adult Literacy in Medicine (REALM) is a 66-item word recognition test designed to assess patients' reading skills.[60] It takes approximately 2–3 min to administer by trained personnel. A shortened version (REALM-SF) was created to facilitate literacy testing in clinical settings.[61] The REALM-SF contains a list of seven medical words from the original REALM. The subject is asked to read these words aloud. REALM-SF total score is defined as the number of words correctly pronounced and ranges from 0 to 7. A score of 0 indicates third grade reading level or below; 1–3 indicates fourth to sixth grade reading level; 4–6 indicates seventh to eighth grade reading level; and 7 indicates high school reading level. Unfortunately, REALM-SF, similar to other word recognition tests, does not assess writing, numeracy, or comprehension skills.

The Agency for Healthcare Research and Quality website has additional health literacy measures that may be useful for clinicians (http://www.ahrq.gov/professionals/quality-patient-safety/quality-resources/tools/literacy/index.html). To minimize interference with physician work-flow, and reduce the potential stigma attached to inadequate health literacy, health literacy assessment could be performed by a nurse or other nonphysician provider as part of the initial patient assessment or during assessment of vital signs. Consideration should be given to incorporating documentation of health literacy assessment into EHR systems. With the proliferation of EHR systems, this capability may already be present in some systems.

Conclusions

Inadequate health literacy is highly prevalent in the United States and is associated with poor health outcomes. Inadequate health literacy has also been shown to be associated with poor health-seeking behavior and poor treatment adherence and outcomes for a number of medical conditions. The healthcare system places significant burdens on patients with inadequate health literacy, due to complex processes involved in navigating the healthcare system. Health literacy is significantly understudied in the otolaryngology patient population. However, the few available studies show that inadequate health literacy is associated with poor health-seeking behavior and limitations in patient–clinician communication among otolaryngology patients. Consequently, it is critical for otolaryngologists to be aware of issues related to health literacy. Routine health literacy assessment in clinical practice may help identify patients that need additional assistance navigating the healthcare system. In addition, the use of clear and concise language when communicating with patients, and ensuring that patient education materials and patient documents are written at an appropriate grade reading level, may help mitigate the health literacy burden for patients during clinical encounters. Finally, there is a great need for future studies examining the impact of health literacy on access to care and treatment outcomes among otolaryngology patients, and the effectiveness of strategies aimed at improving access and outcomes for patients with inadequate health literacy.

References

1. Institute of Medicine. In: Nielsen-Bohlman L, Panzer AM, Kingdig DA, eds. *Health Literacy: A Prescription to End Confusion*. Washington, DC: National Academies Press; 2004.
2. Kutner M, Greenberg E, Jin Y, Paulsen C. *The Health Literacy of America's Adults: Results from the 2003 National Assessment of Adult Literacy (NCES 2006-483)*. Washington, DC: U.S. Department of Education, National Center for Education Statistics; 2006.
3. Federman AD, Wolf MS, Sofianou A, et al. Asthma outcomes are poor among older adults with low health literacy. *J Asthma Off J Assoc Care Asthma*. 2014;51(2):162−167. https://doi.org/10.3109/02770903.2013.852202.
4. Adams RJ, Appleton SL, Hill CL, Ruffin RE, Wilson DH. Inadequate health literacy is associated with increased asthma morbidity in a population sample. *J Allergy Clin Immunol*. 2009;124(3):601−603. https://doi.org/10.1016/j.jaci.2009.05.035.
5. Apter AJ, Wan F, Reisine S, et al. The association of health literacy with adherence and outcomes in moderate-severe asthma. *J Allergy Clin Immunol*. 2013;132(2):321−327. https://doi.org/10.1016/j.jaci.2013.02.014.
6. Mancuso CA, Rincon M. Impact of health literacy on longitudinal asthma outcomes. *J Gen Intern Med*. 2006;21(8):813−817. https://doi.org/10.1111/j.1525-1497.2006.00528.x.
7. Kale MS, Federman AD, Krauskopf K, et al. The association of health literacy with illlness and medication beliefs among patients with chronic obstructive pulmonary disease. *PLoS One*. 2015;10(4):e0123937. https://doi.org/10.1371/journal.pone.0123937.
8. Schillinger D, Grumbach K, Piette J, et al. Association of health literacy with diabetes outcomes. *JAMA*. 2002;288(4):475−482.
9. Williams MV, Baker DW, Parker RM, Nurss JR. Relationship of functional health literacy to patients' knowledge of their chronic disease. A study of patients with hypertension and diabetes. *Arch Intern Med*. 1998;158(2):166−172.
10. Sentell T, Braun KL, Davis J, Davis T. Colorectal cancer screening: low health literacy and limited English proficiency among Asians and Whites in California. *J Health Commun*. 2013;18(Suppl 1):242−255. https://doi.org/10.1080/10810730.2013.825669.
11. Sentell TL, Tsoh JY, Davis T, Davis J, Braun KL. Low health literacy and cancer screening among Chinese Americans in California: a cross-sectional analysis. *BMJ Open*. 2015;5(1):e006104. https://doi.org/10.1136/bmjopen-2014-006104.
12. Pagán JA, Brown CJ, Asch DA, Armstrong K, Bastida E, Guerra C. Health literacy and breast cancer screening among Mexican American women in South Texas. *J Cancer Educ Off J Am Assoc Cancer Educ*. 2012;27(1):132−137. https://doi.org/10.1007/s13187-011-0239-6.
13. Kobayashi LC, Wardle J, von Wagner C. Limited health literacy is a barrier to colorectal cancer screening in England: evidence from the English Longitudinal Study of Ageing. *Prev Med*. 2014;61:100−105. https://doi.org/10.1016/j.ypmed.2013.11.012.
14. Ojinnaka CO, Bolin JN, McClellan DA, Helduser JW, Nash P, Ory MG. The role of health literacy and communication habits on previous colorectal cancer screening among low-income and uninsured patients. *Prev Med Rep*. 2015;2:158−163. https://doi.org/10.1016/j.pmedr.2015.02.009.
15. US Congress. *National Literacy Act of 1991 (1991 - H.R. 751)*. GovTrack.us; 1991. https://www.govtrack.us/congress/bills/102/hr751. Accessed October 21, 2016.
16. Koay K, Schofield P, Gough K, et al. Suboptimal health literacy in patients with lung cancer or head and neck cancer. *Support Care Cancer*. 2013;21(8):2237−2245. https://doi.org/10.1007/s00520-013-1780-0.

17. Megwalu UC, Lee JY. Health literacy assessment in an otolaryngology clinic population. *Otolaryngol Head Neck Surg.* August 23, 2016. https://doi.org/10.1177/019459981 6664331.

18. McNaughton CD, Cawthon C, Kripalani S, Liu D, Storrow AB, Roumie CL. Health literacy and mortality: a cohort study of patients hospitalized for acute heart failure. *J Am Heart Assoc.* 2015;4(5):e001799. https://doi.org/10.1161/JAHA.115.001799.

19. Peterson PN, Shetterly SM, Clarke CL, et al. Health literacy and outcomes among patients with heart failure. *JAMA.* 2011;305(16):1695–1701. https://doi.org/10.1001/jama.2011.512.

20. Willens DE, Kripalani S, Schildcrout JS, et al. Association of brief health literacy screening and blood pressure in primary care. *J Health Commun.* 2013;18(sup1):129–142. https://doi.org/10.1080/10810730.2013.825663.

21. McNaughton CD, Jacobson TA, Kripalani S. Low literacy is associated with uncontrolled blood pressure in primary care patients with hypertension and heart disease. *Patient Educ Counsel.* 2014;96(2):165–170. https://doi.org/10.1016/j.pec.2014.05.007.

22. Halverson JL, Martinez-Donate AP, Palta M, et al. Health literacy and health-related quality of life among a population-based sample of cancer patients. *J Health Commun.* 2015;20(11):1320–1329. https://doi.org/10.1080/10810730.2015.1018638.

23. Song L, Mishel M, Bensen JT, et al. How does health literacy affect quality of life among men with newly diagnosed clinically localized prostate cancer? Findings from the North Carolina-Louisiana Prostate Cancer Project (PCaP). *Cancer.* 2012;118(15):3842–3851. https://doi.org/10.1002/cncr.26713.

24. Hansberry DR, Agarwal N, Shah R, et al. Analysis of the readability of patient education materials from surgical subspecialties. *Laryngoscope.* 2014;124(2):405–412. https://doi.org/10.1002/lary.24261.

25. Alamoudi U, Hong P. Readability and quality assessment of websites related to microtia and aural atresia. *Int J Pediatr Otorhinolaryngol.* 2015;79(2):151–156. https://doi.org/10.1016/j.ijporl.2014.11.027.

26. Beitler JJ, Chen AY, Jacobson K, Owens A, Edwards M, Johnstone PAS. Health literacy and health care in an inner-city, total laryngectomy population. *Am J Otolaryngol.* 2010;31(1):29–31. https://doi.org/10.1016/j.amjoto.2008.09.011.

27. Tran ED, Vaisbuch Y, Qian ZJ, Fitzgerald MB, Megwalu UC. Health literacy and hearing healthcare use. *Laryngoscope.* December 11, 2020. https://doi.org/10.1002/lary.29313.

28. Saraswathula A, Lee JY, Megwalu UC. Patient preferences regarding the communication of biopsy results in the general otolaryngology clinic. *Am J Otolaryngol.* 2019;40(1):83–88. https://doi.org/10.1016/j.amjoto.2018.10.002.

29. Clarke N, Dunne S, Coffey L, et al. Health literacy impacts self-management, quality of life and fear of recurrence in head and neck cancer survivors. *J Cancer Surviv Res Pract.* 2021;15(6):855–865. https://doi.org/10.1007/s11764-020-00978-5.

30. Nilsen ML, Moskovitz J, Lyu L, et al. Health literacy: impact on quality of life in head and neck cancer survivors. *Laryngoscope.* 2020;130(10):2354–2359. https://doi.org/10.1002/lary.28360.

31. Katz SJ, Belkora J, Elwyn G. Shared decision making for treatment of cancer: challenges and opportunities. *J Oncol Pract.* 2014;10(3):206–208. https://doi.org/10.1200/JOP.2014.001434.

32. Kowalski LP, Carvalho AL. Influence of time delay and clinical upstaging in the prognosis of head and neck cancer. *Oral Oncol.* 2001;37(1):94–98. https://doi.org/10.1016/S1368-8375(00)00066-X.

33. Murphy CT, Galloway TJ, Handorf EA, et al. Survival impact of increasing time to treatment initiation for patients with head and neck cancer in the United States. *J Clin Oncol.* 2016;34(2):169–178. https://doi.org/10.1200/JCO.2015.61.5906.

34. Jensen AR, Nellemann HM, Overgaard J. Tumor progression in waiting time for radiotherapy in head and neck cancer. *Radiother Oncol.* 2007;84(1):5–10. https://doi.org/10.1016/j.radonc.2007.04.001.

35. Sharma S, Bekelman J, Lin A, et al. Clinical impact of prolonged diagnosis to treatment interval (DTI) among patients with oropharyngeal squamous cell carcinoma. *Oral Oncol.* 2016;56:17–24. https://doi.org/10.1016/j.oraloncology.2016.02.010.

36. Pajak TF, Laramore GE, Marcial VA, et al. Elapsed treatment days—a critical item for radiotherapy quality control review in head and neck trials: RTOG report. *Int J Radiat Oncol.* 1991;20(1):13–20. https://doi.org/10.1016/0360-3016(91)90132-N.

37. Ferreira BC, Sá-Couto P, Lopes MC, Khouri L. Compliance to radiation therapy of head and neck cancer patients and impact on treatment outcome. *Clin Transl Oncol Off Publ Fed Span Oncol Soc Natl Cancer Inst Mex.* October 12, 2015. https://doi.org/10.1007/s12094-015-1417-5.

38. Patel UA, Patadia MO, Holloway N, Rosen F. Poor radiotherapy compliance predicts persistent regional disease in advanced head/neck cancer. *Laryngoscope.* 2009;119(3):528–533. https://doi.org/10.1002/lary.20072.

39. Charles C, Gafni A, Whelan T. Decision-making in the physician-patient encounter: revisiting the shared treatment decision-making model. *Soc Sci Med.* 1999;49(5):651–661. https://doi.org/10.1016/s0277-9536(99)00145-8.

40. Hopper KD, TenHave TR, Tully DA, Hall TE. The readability of currently used surgical/procedure consent forms in the United States. *Surgery.* 1998;123(5):496–503. https://doi.org/10.1067/msy.1998.87236.

41. Tieu L, Schillinger D, Sarkar U, et al. Online patient websites for electronic health record access among vulnerable populations: portals to nowhere? *J Am Med Inform Assoc JAMIA.* 2017;24(e1):e47–e54. https://doi.org/10.1093/jamia/ocw098.

42. Agency for Healthcare Research and Quality. The AHRQ Health Literacy Universal Precautions Toolkit, In: Assess, select, and create easy-to-understand materials: tool #11. 2nd ed. Accessed 11 May 2022. https://www.ahrq.gov/health-literacy/improve/precautions/tool11.html.

43. Kim JH, Grose E, Philteos J, et al. Readability of the American, Canadian, and British otolaryngology—head and neck surgery societies' patient materials. *Otolaryngol Neck Surg.* 2022;166(5):862–868. https://doi.org/10.1177/01945998211033254.

44. Wong K, Levi JR. Readability of pediatric otolaryngology information by children's hospitals and academic institutions. *Laryngoscope.* 2017;127(4):E138–E144. https://doi.org/10.1002/lary.26359.

45. Balakrishnan V, Chandy Z, Hseih A, Bui TL, Verma SP. Readability and understandability of online vocal cord paralysis materials. *Otolaryngol Neck Surg.* 2016;154(3):460–464. https://doi.org/10.1177/0194599815626146.

46. Marshall S, Haywood K, Fitzpatrick R. Impact of patient-reported outcome measures on routine practice: a structured review. *J Eval Clin Pract.* 2006;12(5):559–568. https://doi.org/10.1111/j.1365-2753.2006.00650.x.

47. Lee SE, Farzal Z, Ebert Jr CS, Zanation AM. Readability of patient-reported outcome measures for head and neck oncology. *Laryngoscope.* 2020;130(12):2839–2842. https://doi.org/10.1002/lary.28555.

48. Lee SE, Farzal Z, Kimple AJ, et al. Readability of patient-reported outcome measures for chronic rhinosinusitis and skull base diseases. *Laryngoscope*. 2020;130(10):2305–2310. https://doi.org/10.1002/lary.28330.

49. Ariane L-L, Thorén ES. Readability of internet information on hearing: systematic literature review. *Am J Audiol*. 2015;24(3):284–288. https://doi.org/10.1044/2015_AJA-14-0091.

50. Zarcadoolas C. The simplicity complex: exploring simplified health messages in a complex world. *Health Promot Int*. 2011;26(3):338–350. https://doi.org/10.1093/heapro/daq075.

51. Czaja SJ, Zarcadoolas C, Vaughon WL, Lee CC, Rockoff ML, Levy J. The usability of electronic personal health record systems for an underserved adult population. *Hum Factors*. 2015;57(3):491–506. https://doi.org/10.1177/0018720814549238.

52. Chew LD, Bradley KA, Boyko EJ. Brief questions to identify patients with inadequate health literacy. *Fam Med*. 2004;36(8):588–594.

53. Chew LD, Griffin JM, Partin MR, et al. Validation of screening questions for limited health literacy in a large VA outpatient population. *J Gen Intern Med*. 2008;23(5):561–566. https://doi.org/10.1007/s11606-008-0520-5.

54. Wallace LS, Cassada DC, Rogers ES, et al. Can screening items identify surgery patients at risk of limited health literacy? *J Surg Res*. 2007;140(2):208–213. https://doi.org/10.1016/j.jss.2007.01.029.

55. Weiss BD, Mays MZ, Martz W, et al. Quick assessment of literacy in primary care: the Newest Vital Sign. *Ann Fam Med*. 2005;3(6):514–522. https://doi.org/10.1370/afm.405.

56. Dumenci L, Matsuyama R, Riddle DL, et al. Measurement of cancer health literacy and identification of patients with limited cancer health literacy. *J Health Commun*. 2014;19(sup2):205–224. https://doi.org/10.1080/10810730.2014.943377.

57. Echeverri M, Anderson D, Nápoles AM. Cancer health literacy test-30-Spanish (CHLT-30-DKspa), a new Spanish-Language version of the cancer health literacy test (CHLT-30) for Spanish-Speaking Latinos. *J Health Commun*. 2016;21(Suppl 1):69–78. https://doi.org/10.1080/10810730.2015.1131777.

58. Nurss JR, Parker RM, Williams MV, Baker DW. *TOFHLA. Test of Functional Health Literacy in Adults*. Snow Camp: Peppercorn Books and Press; 2003.

59. Baker DW, Williams MV, Parker RM, Gazmararian JA, Nurss J. Development of a brief test to measure functional health literacy. *Patient Educ Counsel*. 1999;38(1):33–42.

60. Davis TC, Long SW, Jackson RH, et al. Rapid estimate of adult literacy in medicine: a shortened screening instrument. *Fam Med*. 1993;25(6):391–395.

61. Arozullah AM, Yarnold PR, Bennett CL, et al. Development and validation of a short-form, rapid estimate of adult literacy in medicine. *Med Care*. 2007;45(11):1026–1033. https://doi.org/10.1097/MLR.0b013e3180616c1b.

Healthcare disparities in laryngology and speech language pathology

10

Grace M. Wandell[1], Anaïs Rameau[2]

[1]*Department of Otolaryngology—Head and Neck Surgery, University of Washington School of Medicine, Seattle, WA, United States;* [2]*Sean Parker Institute for Voice, Weill Cornell Medicine, New York, NY, United States*

Introduction

The field of laryngology includes fellowship-trained otolaryngologists and speech pathologists specializing in the care of adult patients with voice, swallowing, and upper airway disorders. Speech therapy (ST) is an integral part of treatment in many upper airway disorders for which a patient visits a laryngologist.[1,2] Although these issues affect many individuals, examining disparities in laryngology is understudied.[3] While still in its early stages overall, attention to this topic is growing, with an increasing number of publications in this subspecialty.[1,4] This chapter is grounded in an analysis of the primary literature to describe current research in health disparities as it relates to laryngeal cancer, voice, airway, swallowing, and general laryngology care in North America. In addition, we summarize barriers in access to gender-affirming voice care for transgender and nonbinary (TNB) individuals. Finally, we examine how innovations in telehealth and technology have the potential to improve access to this subspecialty, though implementation of these modalities must be examined for bias that may potentially reinforce disparities.

General laryngology disparities

Some of the current literature examining disparities in laryngology focuses on patient factors affecting access to outpatient laryngology clinics. For instance, in an analysis of >7000 tertiary laryngological visits at the Medical College of Wisconsin, patients were more likely older, female, and insured.[5] Analysis of the referred and treated population at one laryngology clinic at an academic medical center in the South revealed an overrepresentation of White as compared to Black patients.[6]

In general, laryngology is a field reliant on technology, concentrated in urban centers, tending to provide services to people with insurance. Equity in care access remains limited by the concentration of laryngologists in urban areas.[7] Further, the field's emphasis on technological advancement can impede the equitable provision of care and services to patients. This challenge is highlighted in national variations in video laryngostroboscopy (VLS) billing. VLS is used in approximately 6% of otolaryngology outpatient visits; however, studies suggest its use is concentrated in urban centers.[8,9] A recent study analyzing CMS claims found that VLS provision varies widely across the United States (US), being most utilized in the Mid-Atlantic region and least utilized in the contiguous western mountain states (Fig. 10.1). Using Pearson correlation, VLS density was associated with a greater density of Medicare enrollees ($r = 0.26$, $P < .001$), population density ($r = 0.14$, $P = .01$), median household income ($r = 0.19$, $P < .001$), concentration of otolaryngologists

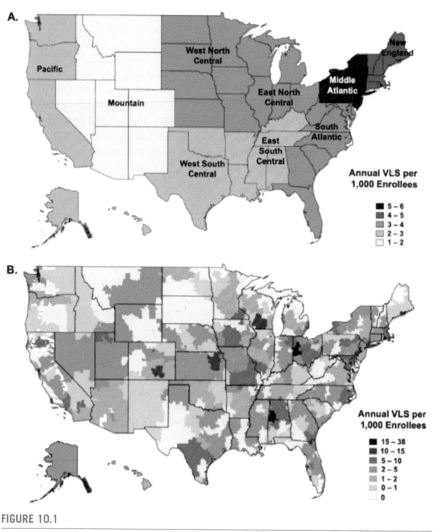

FIGURE 10.1

(A) Map of annual VLS per 1000 medical enrollees by US census division and (B) by HRR.

$(r = 0.016, = < 0.001)$, and other medical specialists $(r = 0.23, P < .001)$.[9] This study highlights the clustering of evaluation and referral of upper airway diseases in urban and tertiary centers.

Although limited geographic access to laryngology and ST services is prevalent, some studies suggest it may not always impact ST initiation and attendance. In a study of barriers to voice therapy (VT) at Boston University among >400 patients, distance from the hospital did not significantly impact VT attendance.[2] In a cross-sectional study among 95 patients in Wisconsin, the distance of the clinic did not significantly impact initiation of VT.[10] Further larger studies are needed to examine this relationship.

Laryngeal cancer care disparities

Laryngeal squamous cell carcinoma (LSCC) represents 1.2%−2.4% of new cancers diagnosed each year.[11−13] LSCC care is one of the best studied areas when examining healthcare disparities in laryngology.[4,14] In understanding disparities in LSCC care, patient factors, barriers to access, and differences in the quality of available care may be considered.[14]

Disparities in LSCC incidence, diagnosis, and treatment by race and ethnicity have been examined extensively.[15] Stage of presentation is a major factor influencing prognosis in LSCC, especially as it relates to race and ethnicity.[16] In a Surveillance, Epidemiology, and End Results (SEER) database study from Chen et al. (2021), disease presentation, treatment patterns, and survival metrics were analyzed in 14,506 patients with LSCC by race.[17] Overall, Black patients were more likely to present with LSCC at a younger age and a higher stage in this study and others, and their mortality was higher.[17,18] The authors concluded that stage is one of the greatest predictors of cancer-specific mortality (CSM). It should be noted, however, that although Black patients had higher CSM on univariate analysis, controlling for year of age, geography, marital status, education, subsite, stage, nodal metastasis, and treatment on multivariable analysis, Black race did not significantly affect CSM.[17] The finding that Black patients present at a later stage of disease has also been reported by others.[15,19] Additionally, in other national analyses, Black patients have been shown to have lower overall survival in advanced laryngeal cancer.[20] These findings highlight an opportunity to focus on earlier diagnosis of LSCC in Black communities.

Delays and differences in LSCC treatment by race and ethnicity are widespread. In a recent National Cancer Database (NCDB) analysis by Shaikh et al. (2022), patients in ethnic minorities demonstrated a longer diagnosis to treatment interval.[21] Treatment options in LSCC, including surgery, radiation, and chemotherapy, have long-term, impactful consequences on morbidity, lifestyle, and financial concerns.[14,22] Racial disparities in treatment modalities have also been highlighted. Studies of advanced laryngeal cancer suggest that Black patients are less likely to undergo larynx-preserving treatment modalities compared to other ethnic groups.[18,23] An earlier SEER analysis, published by Hou et al. (2012), found that Black patients were less likely to receive larynx-preservation treatment in multivariate analysis (OR 0.78, 95% CI 0.63−0.96).[23] A different SEER analysis from 1998 to 2010 demonstrated that Black patients were more likely than White patients to undergo total laryngectomy (TL) for early stage tumors (T1-T2), for which the procedure is rarely indicated.[18] The reasons for these differences are unknown, but important to consider given the huge physical and psychosocial sequelae involved after undergoing TL.

Studies of the Veteran's Administration (VA), an equal-access system, provide insight on the source of these disparities. In one Texas VA, no significant differences in treatment choice, recurrence-specific survival, or overall survival in early glottic cancer were found in a racially balanced cohort.[24] In a large SEER analysis examining and comparing VA care, Black patients had a similar stage at diagnosis and survival compared to others.[19] These studies suggest that racial differences in outcomes at other locations are more likely due to factors related to cancer diagnosis and care access, rather than biological predispositions.[24] Therefore, improving equal access to care is a strategy to decrease racial disparities in LSCC.[19]

Insurance status, which may also be related to race and ethnicity, is a major factor in laryngeal cancer outcomes and treatment.[4,15,16] Comparing LSCC to other and head and neck cancers, patients with LSCC are the most uninsured. Predictors of being uninsured include living in states that did not expand the Affordable Care Act and identifying as a Black or Hispanic individual.[25] Insurance status in itself correlates with diagnosis of Stage IV laryngeal cancer.[15] In Mehta et al.'s NCDB study examining demographic and insurance effects on relative survival (RS) in LSCC,[15] the difference or the ratio of the survival compared to a population's expected survival, uninsured and Medicaid patients had five-year RS estimates of 0.59 (95% CI 0.5−0.61) and 0.50 (95% CI 0.48−0.52), respectively. In multivariate modeling, having private insurance reduced the risk of mortality by 26% in comparison to being uninsured.[15] In a different NCDB study, Medicaid insurance was associated with delays in most intervals, including diagnosis to treatment and surgery to radiation initiation, as well as radiation and total treatment duration.[26] Similarly, in Chen and Halpern's (2007) NCDB analysis,[20] being uninsured or having Medicaid, Medicare, or government health insurance increased the risk of mortality in advanced stage laryngeal cancer as compared to private insurance (HR 1.29−1.57, $P < .001$). Conversely, in Chen et al.'s (2021) SEER study, a lack of insurance influenced overall mortality (OM) in univariate analysis, but not in multivariate analysis or when analyzing CSM.[17]

In addition to race and health insurance, geography influences diagnosis and treatment outcomes in LSCC.[14,21,27−29] The greater prevalence of smoking in rural communities likely raises rates of LSCC.[14] On top of this, lower socioeconomic status and worse access to health care result in delays in both diagnosis and treatment in rural communities.[30] Though most laryngeal cancers are diagnosed within cities, Zuniga et al. analyzed SEER data and found that patients living in rural areas have a higher incidence rate of laryngeal cancer compared to urban areas (5.3 vs.

2.8 per 100,000 person years).[29] Interestingly, they did not see a significant association between rural location and stage of diagnosis.[29] Conversely, Morse et al. found using the NCDB that travel distance significantly predicted stage of presentation; traveling >50 miles for care was associated with 1.5 higher odds (95% CI 1.36–165) of presenting with T4 disease and 2.52 higher odds (95% CI 2.28–2.79) of undergoing TL.[31] In Shaikh et al.'s NCDB paper, living >30 miles from the treatment facility predicted a prolonged diagnosis to treatment interval (OR 1.4, 95% CI 1.3–1.4).[21] Patients living in rural areas are less likely to undergo radiation[3,29] and more likely to receive TL.[29] Adjusting for socioeconomic factors, patients living in rural areas may be less likely to undergo primary radiation for early laryngeal cancer (OR 0.74, 95% CI 0.58–0.95).[27] To address these disparities, future efforts should focus on education on LSCC screening via primary care providers (PCPs) and improving access to cancer care services.[29]

Disparities in voice care

Voice disorders affect a substantial proportion of the US population and yearly healthcare costs, with approximately 18 million Americans reporting a voice disorder per year amounting to $178–294 million in direct healthcare costs.[32–34] The annual incidence of a voice disorder among US adults is estimated to be 6%–8%.[35] As it relates to examining disparities, access to voice care is the second most frequently studied disparity in laryngology and speech language pathology (SLP).[1] Examining these disparities is important because delayed diagnosis and treatment of voice disorders contributes to inequity and higher healthcare costs.[35]

Gender differences in dysphonia care and reporting are frequently studied.[4,35] Women and older adults compromise the greatest utilizers of voice care.[5,36] In Bertelsen et al.'s analysis of National Health Interview Survey (NHIS), men were less likely than women to report a voice disorder (OR 0.70, 95% CI 0.057–0.86).[36] Hur et al. corroborated this result analyzing a national health survey (OR for reporting a voice disorder men-women: 0.63, $P < .01$).[35] Nevertheless, men are more likely to be referred to an otolaryngologist for a voice complaint by a PCP.[37]

A commonly described disparity in VT is often observed by gender. Besides reporting more voice disorders, women are more likely to be referred to SLP[38] and frequently reported to attend VT more than men.[10,39,40] However, gender did not impact ST attendance in some publications.[2,41,42] Additionally, women may have slightly higher rates of VT dropout.[42] In a systematic review on upper airway-related ST disparities, gender significantly impacted voice therapy attendance in four out of nine studies.[1] In Bertelsen et al.'s NHIS study, men were also less likely to seek treatment for a voice disorder compared to women (36% vs. 64%, OR 0.7 [95% CI 0.6–0.9]).[36]

Studies on racial and ethnic inequities in dysphonia prevalence and access to care are varied. Hur et al.[35] found in a national health survey, while controlling for other socioeconomic variables, that Black, Hispanic, and other minority individuals were less likely to report a voice disorder. Racial minorities often delayed presenting with a voice complaint due to transportation issues, while Hispanic patients struggled with making appointments over the phone.[35] However, another large population-based study found that race was unassociated with likelihood of reporting a voice disorder in older adults.[36] Conversely, in a cross-sectional, retrospective, single-institution study performed at the Medical College of Wisconsin, Black patients presented with dysphonia to their clinic with a greater relative prevalence compared to others.[5]

There are a few studies examining the impact of race and ethnicity on specific laryngeal disorders associated with dysphonia. Varelas et al. examined differences in laryngopharyngeal reflux (LPR) symptom indices by demographics among 170 patients. Using the Reflux Symptom Index (RSI), risk factors for reporting a higher RSI included Black race or Latinx ethnicity and Medicaid insurance. Controlling for insurance type eliminated the observed racial disparity.[43]

Laryngeal dystonia (LD) is a less common voice disorder which significantly influences quality of life and requires frequent, chronic visits to the laryngologist for treatment with regular Botox injections.[44] One single institution study in Canada assessed socioeconomic status in their LD population and found that most patients receiving botox treatment were Caucasian, educated, English-speaking, and employed.[44] Though the majority of patients receiving treatment for LD are frequently White individuals,[44,45] ethnicity was not associated with outcomes in one single institution study.[45] These studies provide evidence that greater outreach to non-White communities is needed.

Studies vary with regards to the impact of race and ethnicity on VT attendance or adherence, when controlling for other variables.[2,39–41,44] Lim et al. (2021)[2] published a single-center retrospective study analyzing VT attendance among 422 patients. In multivariate analysis including language, race, and ethnicity, none of these factors significantly impacted the probability of VT attendance.[2] In a prospective, multicenter survey study of 172 patients, Misono et al.[46] found that identifying with Black or White race did not affect the likelihood of attending VT, while being "other" race did. Hapner et al.[41] investigated the impact of demographic variables on VT dropout and found no association with race, though importantly, 23% of their 147-patient cohort lacked complete information on this variable.[41] In one tertiary academic practice in Miami, Latinx patients who were recommended VT for vocal fold nodules were less adherent: 57% of Hispanic patients were adherent compared to 78% of non-Hispanic patients ($P = .025$).[47] A recent systematic review on ST disparities noted that a lack of racial diversity and representation in some these studies is a barrier to the validity of these varied results.[1]

Interplaying with race and ethnicity, the impact of language on VT participation is pertinent, given the importance of communication in forming a therapeutic relationship. In Lim et al.'s study in Boston, non-English language or interpreter use did not impact VT attendance.[2] These results differ from other studies. Huwyler et al.[40] analyzed compliance with ST referrals among >7000 patients within the Kaiser Permanente system in Northern California. Though their proportion of non-English speaking patients was small ($\sim$2%), 63% of them completed ST referrals compared to 74% of English speakers ($P = .0011$). In this study, speaking a non-English primary language was associated with 1.56 (95% CI 1.11-1-2.18) higher odds of VT noncompliance in multivariate analysis.[40]

Insurance status appears to be the major factor modifying dysphonia evaluation and VT initiation and attendance. Individuals with public insurance may be more likely report a voice disorder and are also more likely to delay evaluation due long wait times of clinic availability.[35] In Lim et al.'s study,[2] only insurance status significantly impacted VT attendance in multivariate analysis. Patients with private versus public insurance were 2.35 times more likely to attend (95% CI 1.18–4.71).[2] Analyzing factors facilitating voice therapy attendance among 170 patients at different sites, Misono et al. (2016) identified insurance and co-pay as a significant factors.[39] Again, in a single-center retrospective review from Atlanta, lack of insurance was identified as a barrier to VT initiation.[42]

There are some regional differences in voice and ST care, though studies vary on this subject. Patients living in urban areas are more likely to be referred to otolaryngology by PCPs for a voice disorder and evaluated by an SLP.[38] Travel distance to attend VT appointments may influence patients' likelihood of attendance.[39] Patients living in the North Central and Western US are more likely to be referred from primary care to otolaryngology for a voice disorder than patients living in the South.[37] Living in the Midwest has been associated with increased odds of reporting a voice disorder compared to those living in the Northeast.[35] Additionally, patients in the Western US are more likely to report a voice disorder and be referred to SLP.[36,38]

Disparities in airway, tracheostomy, and laryngotracheal stenosis care

Laryngotracheal stenosis (LTS) is a fixed extrapulmonary narrowing in the airway, which may be due to inflammatory, traumatic, or iatrogenic causes. Despite the commonality of procedures associated with iatrogenic LTS, namely intubation and tracheostomy, literature examining disparities in airway disorders are understudied.[4] Some research suggests certain populations are more at risk for iatrogenic LTS. In a retrospective study at Boston Medical Center, rates of etiologies of LTS were examined by ethnicity among 132 patients. Black patients were overrepresented in the iatrogenic cohort and had 4.2 greater odds of presenting with LTS secondary to an iatrogenic cause as compared to White patients (95% CI 2.2–11, $P < .001$).[48]

Nevertheless, a recent single-institution study found no difference in age, race, or sex when examining laryngeal pathology precluding tracheostomy decannulation.[49] Posterior glottic stenosis (PGS) is a serious complication of intubation related to abnormal wound healing of the posterior commissure. In a smaller case control study of risk factors for PGS among three tertiary care centers, age, race, and sex did not significantly affect the incidence of PGS.[50] Length of intubation significantly correlated with PGS incidence.[50]

Idiopathic inflammatory subglottic stenosis primarily affects Caucasian females.[48,51] The North American Airway Collaborative prospectively recruited a cohort of individuals diagnosed with idiopathic subglottic stenosis and examined how sociodemographic factors influence treatment outcomes. Among 810 patients, who were mostly Caucasian (97%), there was no association between income or education on time to diagnosis or need for recurrent surgical intervention.[52]

When examining outcomes in LTS, tracheostomy may be considered treatment failure. In a case control study of patients undergoing treatment for LTS at one tertiary hospital, sociodemographic factors impacting outcomes were examined. In this population, public insurance was associated with tracheostomy dependence in univariate and multivariate analyses. Race, sex, and education did not significantly influence the probability of tracheostomy dependence.[51]

Disparities in tracheostomy practices and outcomes

Though there are few studies looking at disparities in practice and outcomes of tracheostomy, this is an important topic that deserves more scholarship. Many studies looking at tracheostomy outcomes discuss the benefits to the patient and hospital system of early tracheotomy (ET) versus late tracheotomy (LT). ET is frequently defined as <7−10 days since intubation, but ranges from 3 to 10 days.[53,54] On the systems level, ET has been associated with shorter ICU and hospital stays.[55,56] LT has been associated with greater tracheostomy-related deaths.[57]

Considering these factors, it is important to consider the likelihood of ET versus LT for different groups. In one retrospective study of 1640 patients in New York state, there were no differences in timing of tracheostomy placement based on age, ethnicity, and income. However, the authors found that more men (30%) had ET (defined as 3−7 days postintubation) compared to women (28%; $P = .05$).[58] Another smaller, single-institution study found no difference in ET disparities by race or sex.[57] Shaw et al. (2015) examined disparities in tracheostomy timing in 49,191 patients at 185 different academic medical centers. In their multivariate analysis, women (OR 0.84, 95% CI 0.81−0.87), Black patients (OR 0.85, 95% CI 0.81−90), Hispanic patients (0.85, 95% CI 0.78−0.92), and Medicaid-insured or uninsured (OR 0.95, 95% CI 0.89−0.99) were less likely to undergo ET.[59] Black, Hispanic, and Medicaid-insured patients had longer hospital stays when tracheotomy is performed and were less likely to receive ET in another study.[60] Hispanic patients with tracheostomy have been shown to have a higher 30-day mortality rate, despite having a lower rate of co-morbidity compared to other ethnic groups.[61] Given these associations, and mounting evidence that ET improves outcomes, providers will need to pay attention to and investigate the factors driving these disparities among vulnerable populations.

Disparities in dysphagia care

Disparities in dysphagia care are among the least studied in laryngology, although there is a richer literature in gastroenterology and speech pathology.[4] Swallowing problems are common in the elderly, but they frequently do not access appropriate treatment.[62] Myotomy and diverticulectomy are commonly performed for dysphagia associated with cricopharyngeal pathology. One study using the Nationwide Claims Database reported on demographic factors influencing morbidity following surgery for hypopharyngeal and esophageal diverticula. On multivariate analysis, accounting for several variables including co-morbidities, Black patients had higher odds of morbidity as compared to White patients following treatment (OR 2.29, 95% CI 1.02–5.17).[63] Racial disparities in aspiration pneumonia incidence have also been described. In an older study of Medicare inpatient bills, Black men were at the highest risk of developing aspiration pneumonia.[64]

Disparities in care following cerebrovascular accident (CVA) are the best described and studied in relation to healthcare disparities in dysphagia. Asian patients have been reported to have a greater risk of developing dysphagia following stroke.[65,66] However, other studies have found no association between race, ethnicity, sex, or insurance with rates of dysphagia following CVA.[67]

There is variability in feeding tube placement practices following stroke, and race has been implicated as an associated disparity.[4,65,68,69] Patients who are Asian or Black had higher odds of feeding tube placement (OR 1.62 and 1.42, respectively).[4,69] In a different study, Black and Hispanic patients had significantly greater likelihood as well, with adjusted odds ratios (AORs) of 1.34 (95% 1.25–1.42) and 1.39 (95% Ci 1.27–1.53), respectively.[70] In a different study, feeding tube placement correlated more with lower socioeconomic status, though patients in this category were more likely to be a minority race.[68]

There are access issues impacting dysphagia diagnosis and treatment following CVA. Insurance may also impact the likelihood of feeding tube placement following stroke. In a large insurance claims database study, having private insurance compared to Medicare or Medicaid was associated with reduced risk of feeding tube placement (AOR 0.90; 95% CI 0.83–0.98).[70] Geographic disparities for dysphagia swallow therapy also exist, as the southern US is the area with the highest concentration of CVA and also the least therapists.[71] US governmental healthcare payors, such as Medicare, may be limiting some therapy due to caps placed on SLP services, which may be less problematic when patients are privately insured.[71]

Gender-affirming voice care

Voice-gender incongruence is important to the psychosocial health and quality of life of many individuals who are TNB individuals.[72–74] Therefore, gender-affirming voice care and voice surgery are integral facets of gender-affirming care (GAC). The primary method of teaching TNB individuals to habituate their voice is through voice care with SLP. Behavioral treatments are designed to educate clients on strategies to alter voice fundamental and formant frequencies. Voice care is associated with significant improvements in both quality of life and gender perception.[75]

Unlike individuals assigned female at birth who want to present more masculine and can use hormonal therapy to lower their voice, hormone therapy does not affect the pitch of those wishing to present more feminine. When voice therapy is insufficient, an elevated vocal pitch sometimes necessitates surgical intervention by increasing tension, shortening length, or reducing the mass of the vocal folds.[74] Feminization laryngoplasty has been shown to heighten mean speaking fundamental frequency, lowest fundamental frequency, and improved self-perception among trans females.[76] Nevertheless, a recent meta-analysis of surgical techniques to feminize the voice concluded that studies in this field are limited by low power and short length of follow-up.[74]

There is a need for studies on access to VT services for gender-affirming voice care.[1] Kennedy et al.[72] surveyed the impact of voice-gender incongruence among the TNB population and found that it is high (88%), and that specifically, individuals seeking a more masculine voice may perceive greater barriers to care. Expense and a lack of nearby qualified professionals are the two most commonly cited reasons for not seeking voice care. Other reasons include fear of judgment or harassment by providers, and lack of time to invest in therapy sessions or travel. TNB people also reported that a major obstacle to seeking treatment for voice-gender incongruence is financial difficulties.[72]

Expanding on the impact of cost on GAC, there are significant differences in access to care for TNB individuals based on geographic and insurance factors, though more studies are needed. Insurance coverage for GAC has improved in recent years; however, there are significant variations across states and insurers for coverage for gender-affirming surgery (GAS). Some states, mostly located in the Northeast and West, prohibit transgender exclusions.[77] Among Medicaid state policies, only 30 states have policies regarding GAS and 18 states mandated its coverage.[78] Devore et al. (2020)[79] examined insurance policies for coverage of gender-affirming voice care. Only four of the 149 examined companies provided favorable policies; 75.8% of insurance companies provided no coverage and 13.4% had unclear policies. A figure delineating coverage status of different interventions is displayed in Fig. 10.2. They concluded that coverage for voice care, whether behavioral or surgical, is scarce.[79] Thyroid chondroplasty, which can feminize the appearance of the larynx, is offered in 30.4% of insurance policies in states that prohibit transgender exclusions and 7.7% of states that do have such prohibitions.[77] A lack of robust studies demonstrating the positive impact of gender-affirming voice care may be limiting insurer coverage of these therapies,[79] thus this is a major area for future investigation in laryngology and voice-related SLP.

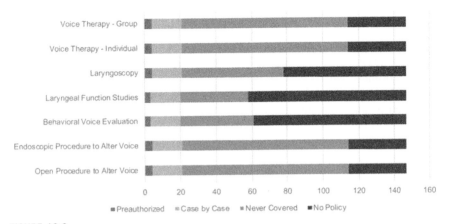

FIGURE 10.2

Distributions of laryngeal interventions by coverage status.[79]

The promise of telemedicine

A hopeful solution to some of the difficulties with geographic access in the field is telemedicine. Telepractice refers to the delivery of diagnostic and therapeutic interventions using telecommunication services with a distance between the patient and clinician.[80] Prior the COVID-19 pandemic, many advocated for the use of telemedicine to provide services in medically underserved areas. Following the World Health Organization's declaration of the COVID-19 pandemic in March 2020, laryngologists and voice and swallowing-focused SLPs adopted telepractice more broadly. Following the height of the pandemic, the Centers for Medicare and Medicaid Services (CMS) allowed for continuation of voice therapy under this model, promoting long-term adoption of telehealth. Successful remote treatment of dysphonia-related muscle tension, Parkinson's disease, and vocal fold nodules has been reported.[80] CMS did not initially cover evaluation and therapy for swallowing disorders on a telemedicine platform, but coverage has since been expanded to include swallow therapy.[81]

Growth of telepractice in otolaryngology has lagged behind other specialty fields in part due to its reliance on office laryngoscopy for clinical diagnosis.[80,82] Additional barriers to implementation of telepractice are inadequate internet and computer equipment for teleconferencing, limited digital literacy, potential language barriers, and differences in insurance coverage.[80,83] Further, it is also unknown whether CMS will continue to support SLP telepractice long term.[80] As insurance status and income affected telehealth utilization given disparities in technology access,[84] it will be important to examine and consider how vulnerable populations may benefit from the growth of telehealth or whether it has the potential to widen existing disparities in laryngology.

Representation of voice diversity in technology and media

Voice is a ubiquitous, noninvasive, and informative biomarker,[85,86] and voice assistants are embedded in many homes and cell phones currently.[87] Machine learning (ML) algorithms and artificial intelligence (AI) are poised to become integral in health care and hopefully in laryngology.[88] Current evaluation of persistent dysphonia requires limited specialist resources and expensive equipment to endoscopically examine the larynx.[89] There is excitement that ML could improve dysphonia triage based on voice recordings, via earlier diagnosis and facilitating appropriate or urgent specialist referral.[86,90–93] There are numerous studies using ML for the detection of dysphonia and identification of specific pathology.[90]

As AI applications using voice analysis and speech develop, it will become increasingly critical that the populations used to develop these algorithms are representative of our diverse communities. As further innovation develops in voice analysis and speech assistance, new research and technology should adhere to reporting standards which require a description of the patient cohort characteristics on which the technology was developed and tested on, including descriptions of cohort age, sex, gender, race, and ethnicity.[94] Voice and speech present with unique privacy issues, which also need to be considered in the development of these technologies. The Open Voice Network has created a white paper examining these specific issues with regard to ML applications in voice.[95]

Another challenge is the representation of a diversity of voices, including ones associated with pathology in medias and technology. Voice-activated technologies like Google Home, Amazon's Alexa, or Apple's Siri are very useful for individuals with physical mobility limitations. Yet, they may not be able to recognize impaired voices or speech patterns that the same individuals with physical disabilities may also suffer from, making their successful use limited in those who might benefit the most from their technology. A Google research endeavor, Project Euphonia, is attempting to bridge this divide by training a speech recognition model on a population with dysarthria.[87]

Diversity among laryngologists and speech language pathologists

A diverse and inclusive workforce is important in building a professional culture focused on reducing health disparities within their field. A study published in Laryngoscope in 2022 characterized representation in the field of academic laryngology. This study reported that 77% were Caucasian, followed by 16% Asian, 4% African American, and 1% Latinx individuals. Of the 47 full professors, 83% were Caucasian and 92% were male. Examining the impact of diverse leadership in the field, they reported that 90% of American Laryngological Association and 75% of American Broncho-Esophagological Association past presidents have been male. The authors concluded that the field lags behind other surgical subspecialties in its representation of ethnic and gender diversity.[96] Examining some of the reasons for differences in academic rank, laryngology follows similar patterns to the overall otolaryngology field, with men having significantly higher h-indices, greater number of citations, and coauthorship.[97]

Improving diversity in the field of communication sciences is also needed. The field of SLP was ranked among the top five "whitest" jobs in the country, and 92.2% of members in the American Speech-Language-Hearing Association are White.[98]

Conclusion

Examining health disparities in the fields of laryngology and SLP is in its infancy, though publications in this area are increasing. Better studied areas in the field include disparities in LSCC and factors influencing VT attendance. The field can improve in this area by improved reporting on race and ethnicity in published research.[1] Although there are some studies examining differences in tracheostomy and LTS disparities, given the frequency of the procedure and rising numbers of LTS following the COVID pandemic, more studies are needed in this area. There is literature examining mostly racial disparities in dysphagia care following CVA; however, more investigation is needed examining other topics in the field, especially performed from the laryngologist or speech therapist's perspective. Laryngologists and speech language pathologists are uniquely poised to serve the nonbinary community. There is a paucity of literature regarding the efficacy and patient satisfaction associated with gender-affirming voice care, which is likely needed to improve insurance policy coverage of GAC. Voice healthcare professionals can contribute to our understanding of the impact of voice-based new technologies on existing disparities, and they could advocate for greater representation of disabled voices and speech patterns in media and technology. Finally, improving diversity in the fields of laryngology and SLP is needed to address an ever-diversifying patient population.

References

1. Morton ME, Easter S, Brown M, Sandage MJ. Potential risks for healthcare disparities among individuals with voice and upper airway disorders: a systematic review. *J Voice*. 2021. https://doi.org/10.1016/j.jvoice.2021.11.003.
2. Lim KWR, Zambare W, Rubin BR, Tracy LF. Barriers to voice therapy attendance in a language-diverse population. *Laryngoscope*. 2021;131(8):1835–1839. https://doi.org/10.1002/lary.29149.
3. Urban MJ, Shimomura A, Shah S, Losenegger T, Westrick J, Jagasia AA. Rural otolaryngology care disparities: a scoping review. *Otolaryngol Head Neck Surg*. 2022. https://doi.org/10.1177/01945998211068822.

4. Feit NZ, Wang Z, Demetres MR, Drenis S, Andreadis K, Rameau A. Healthcare disparities in laryngology: a scoping review. *Laryngoscope.* 2022;132(2):375−390. https://doi.org/10.1002/lary.29325.

5. White SW, Bock JM, Blumin JH, et al. Analysis of socioeconomic factors in laryngology clinic utilization for treatment of dysphonia. *Laryngoscope Investig Otolaryngol.* 2022;7(1):202−209. https://doi.org/10.1002/lio2.715.

6. Madden LL, Hernandez BO, Russell GB, Wright SC, Kiell EP. The demographics of patients presenting for laryngological care at an academic medical center. *Laryngoscope.* 2022;132(3):626−632. https://doi.org/10.1002/lary.29831.

7. Urban MJ, Wojcik C, Eggerstedt M, Jagasia AJ. Rural−urban disparities in otolaryngology: the state of Illinois. *Laryngoscope.* 2021;131(1):E70−E75. https://doi.org/10.1002/lary.28652.

8. Cohen SM, Thomas S, Roy N, Kim J, Courey M. Frequency and factors associated with use of videolaryngostroboscopy in voice disorder assessment. *Laryngoscope.* 2014;124(9):2118−2124. https://doi.org/10.1002/lary.24688.

9. Davis RJ, Exilus S, Best S, Willink A, Akst LM. The geographic distribution of videolaryngostroboscopy in the United States. *J Voice.* 2021. https://doi.org/10.1016/j.jvoice.2021.05.002.

10. Pasternak K, Diaz J, Thibeault SL. Predictors of voice therapy initiation: a cross-sectional cohort study. *J Voice.* 2022;36(2):194−202. https://doi.org/10.1016/j.jvoice.2020.05.003.

11. Ferlay J, Shin HR, Bray F, Forman D, Mathers C, Parkin DM. Estimates of worldwide burden of cancer in 2008: GLOBOCAN 2008. *Int J Cancer.* 2010;127(12):2893−2917. https://doi.org/10.1002/ijc.25516.

12. Parkin DM, Bray F, Ferlay J, Pisani P. *Global cancer statistics, 2002.* 2002. https://doi.org/10.3322/caac.21262.

13. Reiter R, Hoffman TK, Pickhard A, Brosch S. Hoarseness - causes and treatments. *Med Monatsschr Pharm.* 2016;39(10):429−435. https://doi.org/10.3238/arztebl.2015.0329.

14. Cox SR, Daniel CL. Racial and ethnic disparities in laryngeal cancer care. *J Racial Ethn Heal Disparities.* 2022;9(3):800−811. https://doi.org/10.1007/s40615-021-01018-3.

15. Mehta V, Shi Z, Mills GM, Nathan CAO, Shi R. Effect of payer status on relative survival of patients with laryngeal cancer. *Anticancer Res.* 2016;36(1):327−333.

16. Chen AY, Schrag NM, Halpern M, Stewart A, Ward EM. Health insurance and stage at diagnosis of laryngeal cancer: does insurance type predict stage at diagnosis? *Arch Otolaryngol Head Neck Surg.* 2007;133(8):784−790. https://doi.org/10.1001/archotol.133.8.784.

17. Chen S, Dee EC, Muralidhar V, Nguyen PL, Amin MR, Givi B. Disparities in mortality from larynx cancer: implications for reducing racial differences. *Laryngoscope.* 2021;131(4):E1147−E1155. https://doi.org/10.1002/lary.29046.

18. Shin JY, Truong MT. Racial disparities in laryngeal cancer treatment and outcome: a population-based analysis of 24,069 patients. *Laryngoscope.* 2015;125(7):1667−1674. https://doi.org/10.1002/lary.25212.

19. Voora RS, Kotha NV, Kumar A, et al. Association of race and health care system with disease stage and survival in veterans with larynx cancer. *Cancer.* 2021;127(15):2705−2713. https://doi.org/10.1002/cncr.33557.

20. Chen AY, Halpern M. Factors predictive of survival in advanced laryngeal cancer. *Arch Otolaryngol Head Neck Surg.* 2007;133(12):1270−1276. https://doi.org/10.1001/archotol.133.12.1270.

21. Shaikh N, Morrow V, Stokes C, et al. Factors associated with a prolonged diagnosis-to-treatment interval in laryngeal squamous cell carcinoma. *Otolaryngol Neck Surg*. 2022, 019459982210901. https://doi.org/10.1177/01945998221090115.

22. Cox SR, Theurer JA, Spaulding SJ, Doyle PC. The multidimensional impact of total laryngectomy on women. *J Commun Disord*. 2015;56:59–75. https://doi.org/10.1016/j.jcomdis.2015.06.008.

23. Hou WH, Daly ME, Lee NY, Farwell DG, Luu Q, Chen AM. Racial disparities in the use of voice preservation therapy for locally advanced laryngeal cancer. *Arch Otolaryngol Head Neck Surg*. 2012;138(7):644–649. https://doi.org/10.1001/archoto.2012.1021.

24. Fullmer TM, Shi J, Skinner HD, et al. Early glottic cancer in a veteran population: impact of race on management and outcomes. *Laryngoscope*. 2020;130(7):1733–1739. https://doi.org/10.1002/lary.28262.

25. Babu A, Wassef DW, Sangal NR, Goldrich D, Baredes S, Park RCW. The Affordable Care Act: implications for underserved populations with head & neck cancer. *Am J Otolaryngol Head Neck Med Surg*. 2020;41(4). https://doi.org/10.1016/j.amjoto.2020.102464.

26. Morse E, Fujiwara RJT, Judson B. Treatment delays in laryngeal squamous cell carcinoma: a national cancer database analysis. *Laryngoscope*. 2018. https://doi.org/10.1002/lary.27247.

27. Mackley HB, Teslova T, Camacho F, Short PF, Anderson RT. Does rurality influence treatment decisions in early stage laryngeal cancer? *J Rural Health*. 2014;30(4):406–411. https://doi.org/10.1111/jrh.12069.

28. Clarke JA, Despotis AM, Ramirez RJ, Zevallos JP, Mazul AL. Head and neck cancer survival disparities by race and rural–urban context. *Cancer Epidemiol Biomarkers Prev*. 2020;29(10):1955–1961. https://doi.org/10.1158/1055-9965.EPI-20-0376.

29. Zuniga SA, Lango MN. Effect of rural and urban geography on larynx cancer incidence and survival. *Laryngoscope*. 2017. https://doi.org/10.1002/lary.27042.

30. Zuniga MG, Turner JH. Treatment outcomes in acute invasive fungal rhinosinusitis. *Curr Opin Otolaryngol Head Neck Surg*. 2014;22(3):242–248. https://doi.org/10.1097/MOO.0000000000000048.

31. Morse E, Lohia S, Dooley LM, Gupta P, Roman BR. Travel distance is associated with stage at presentation and laryngectomy rates among patients with laryngeal cancer. *J Surg Oncol*. 2021;124(8):1272–1283. https://doi.org/10.1002/jso.26643.

32. Cohen SM, Kim J, Roy N, Asche C, Courey M. Prevalence and causes of dysphonia in a large treatment-seeking population. *Laryngoscope*. 2012;122:343–348.

33. Cohen SM, Kim J, Roy N, Asche C, Courey M. Direct health care costs of laryngeal diseases and disorders. *Laryngoscope*. 2012. https://doi.org/10.1002/lary.23189.

34. Bhattacharyya N. The prevalence of voice problems among adults in the United States. *Laryngoscope*. 2014;124(10):2359–2362. https://doi.org/10.1002/lary.24740.

35. Hur K, Zhou S, Bertelsen C, Johns MM. Health disparities among adults with voice problems in the United States. *Laryngoscope*. 2018;128(4):915–920. https://doi.org/10.1002/lary.26947.

36. Bertelsen C, Zhou S, Hapner ER, Johns MM. Sociodemographic characteristics and treatment response among aging adults with voice disorders in the United States. *JAMA Otolaryngol Head Neck Surg*. 2018;144(8):719–726. https://doi.org/10.1001/jamaoto.2018.0980.

37. Cohen S, Kim J, Roy N, Courey M. Factors influencing referral of patients with voice disorders from primary care to otolaryngology. *Laryngoscope*. 2014;124(1):1−7. https://doi.org/10.1002/lary.24280.Factors.

38. Cohen SM, Dinan MA, Kim J, Roy N. Otolaryngology utilization of speech-language pathology services for voice disorders. *Laryngoscope*. 2016;126(4):906−912. https://doi.org/10.1002/lary.25574.

39. Misono S, Marmor S, Roy N, Mau T, Cohen SM. Factors influencing likelihood of voice therapy attendance. *Otolaryngol Head Neck Surg*. 2017;156(3):518−524. https://doi.org/10.1177/0194599816679941.

40. Huwyler C, Merchant M, Jiang N. Disparities in speech therapy for voice disorders between English- and non-English-speaking patients. *Laryngoscope*. 2021;131(7): E2298−E2302. https://doi.org/10.1002/lary.29429.

41. Hapner E, Portone-Maira C, Johns MM. A study of voice therapy dropout. *J Voice*. 2009; 23(3):337−340. https://doi.org/10.1016/j.jvoice.2007.10.009.

42. Portone C, Johns MM, Hapner ER. A review of patient adherence to the recommendation for voice therapy. *J Voice*. 2008;22(2):192−196. https://doi.org/10.1016/j.jvoice.2006.09.009.

43. Varelas EA, Houser TK, Husain IA. Laryngopharyngeal reflux: effect of race and insurance status on symptomology. *Ann Otol Rhinol Laryngol*. 2022. https://doi.org/10.1177/00034894221100025.

44. Valenzuela D, Singer J, Lee T, Hu A. The impact of socioeconomic status on voice outcomes in patients with spasmodic dysphonia treated with botulinum toxin injections. *Ann Otol Rhinol Laryngol*. 2019;128(4):316−322. https://doi.org/10.1177/0003489418823013.

45. O'Connell Ferster AP, Sataloff RT, Shewokis PA, Hu A. Socioeconomic variables of patients with spasmodic dysphonia: a preliminary study. *J Voice*. 2018;32(4):479−483. https://doi.org/10.1016/j.jvoice.2017.07.015.

46. Misono S, Marmor S, Roy N, Mau T, Cohen SM. *Multi-institutional Study of Voice Disorders and Voice Therapy Referral: Report from the CHEER Network*. 2016. https://doi.org/10.1177/0194599816639244.

47. Rosow DE, Diaz J, Pan DR, Lloyd AT. Hispanic ethnicity as a predictor of voice therapy adherence. *J Voice*. 2021;35(2):329.e1−329.e5. https://doi.org/10.1016/j.jvoice.2019.09.011.

48. Plocienniczak M, Sambhu KM, Tracy L, Noordzij JP. Impact of socioeconomic demographics and race on laryngotracheal stenosis etiology and outcomes. *Laryngoscope*. 2022:1−6. https://doi.org/10.1002/lary.30321.

49. Meenan K, Bhatnagar K, Guardiani E. Intubation-related laryngeal pathology precluding tracheostomy decannulation: incidence and associated risk factors. *Ann Otol Rhinol Laryngol*. 2021;130(9):1078−1084. https://doi.org/10.1177/0003489421995285.

50. Hillel AT, Karatayli-Ozgurosoy S, Samad I, et al. Predictors of posterior glottic stenosis: a multi-institutional case-control study. *Ann Otol Rhinol Laryngol*. 2016;125(3):257−263. https://doi.org/10.1177/0003489415608867.

51. Dang S, Shinn JR, Campbell BR, Garrett G, Wootten C, Gelbard A. The impact of social determinants of health on laryngotracheal stenosis development and outcomes. *Laryngoscope*. 2020;130(4):1000−1006. https://doi.org/10.1002/lary.28208.

52. Lee J, Huang L-C, Berry LD, et al. Association of social determinants of health with time to diagnosis and treatment outcomes in idiopathic subglottic stenosis. *Ann Otol Rhinol Laryngol*. 2021;130(10):1116−1124. https://doi.org/10.1177/0003489421995283.Association.

53. Halum SL, Ting JY, Plowman EK, et al. A multi-institutional analysis of tracheotomy complications. *Laryngoscope*. 2012;122(1):38−45. https://doi.org/10.1002/lary.22364.

54. Koch T, Hecker B, Hecker A, et al. Early tracheostomy decreases ventilation time but has no impact on mortality of intensive care patients: a randomized study. *Langenbeck Arch Surg*. 2012;397(6):1001−1008. https://doi.org/10.1007/s00423-011-0873-9.

55. Altman KW, Ha TAN, Dorai VK, Mankidy BJ, Zhu H. Tracheotomy timing and outcomes in the critically ill: complexity and opportunities for progress. *Laryngoscope*. 2021;131(2):282−287. https://doi.org/10.1002/lary.28657.

56. Chorath K, Hoang A, Rajasekaran K, Moreira A. Association of early vs late tracheostomy placement with pneumonia and ventilator days in critically ill patients: a meta-analysis. *JAMA Otolaryngol Head Neck Surg*. 2021;78229:1−10. https://doi.org/10.1001/jamaoto.2021.0025.

57. Park C, Bahethi R, Yang A, Gray M, Wong K, Courey M. Effect of patient demographics and tracheostomy timing and technique on patient survival. *Laryngoscope*. 2020:10−12. https://doi.org/10.1002/lary.29000.

58. Gillis A, Pfaff A, Ata A, Giammarino A, Stain S, Tafen M. Are there variations in timing to tracheostomy in a tertiary academic medical center? *Am J Surg*. 2020;219(4):566−570. https://doi.org/10.1016/j.amjsurg.2020.01.035.

59. Shaw JJ, Santry HP. Who gets early tracheostomy? evidence of unequal treatment at 185 academic medical centers. *Chest*. 2015;148(5):1242−1250. https://doi.org/10.1378/chest.15-0576.

60. Yang A, Gray ML, McKee S, et al. Percutaneous versus surgical tracheostomy: timing, outcomes, and charges. *Laryngoscope*. 2018;128(12):2844−2851. https://doi.org/10.1002/lary.27334.

61. Bahethi R, Park C, Yang A, et al. Influence of insurance status and demographic factors on outcomes following tracheostomy. *Laryngoscope*. 2021;131(7):1463−1467. https://doi.org/10.1002/lary.28967.

62. Turley R, Cohen S. Impact of voice and swallowing problems in the elderly. *Otolaryngol Head Neck Surg*. 2009;140(1):33−36. https://doi.org/10.1016/j.otohns.2008.10.010.

63. Onwugbufor MT, Obirieze AC, Ortega G, Allen D, Cornwell EE, Fullum TM. Surgical management of esophageal diverticulum: a review of the Nationwide Inpatient Sample database. *J Surg Res*. 2013;184(1):120−125. https://doi.org/10.1016/j.jss.2013.05.036.

64. Baine WB, Yu W, Summe JP. Epidemiologic trends in the hospitalization of elderly Medicare patients for pneumonia, 1991−1998. *Am J Public Health*. 2001;91(7):1121−1123. https://doi.org/10.2105/AJPH.91.7.1121.

65. Bussell SA, Gonzlez-Fernndez M. Racial disparities in the development of dysphagia after stroke: further evidence from the Medicare database. *Arch Phys Med Rehabil*. 2011;92(5):737−742. https://doi.org/10.1016/j.apmr.2010.12.005.

66. Gonzalez-Fernandez M, Kuhlemeier KV, Palmer JB. Racial disparities in the development of dysphagia after stroke: analysis of the California (MIRCal) and New York (SPARCS) inpatient databases. *Arch Phys Med Rehabil*. 2008;89(7):1358−1365. https://doi.org/10.1016/j.apmr.2008.02.016.

67. Bonilha HS, Simpson AN, Ellis C, Mauldin P, Martin-Harris B, Simpson K. The one-year attributable cost of post-stroke dysphagia. *Dysphagia*. 2014;29(5):545−552. https://doi.org/10.1007/s00455-014-9543-8.

68. Garcia RM, Prabhakaran S, Richards CT, Naidech AM, Maas MB. Race, socioeconomic status, and gastrostomy after spontaneous intracerebral hemorrhage. *J Stroke Cerebrovasc Dis*. 2020;29(2). https://doi.org/10.1016/j.jstrokecerebrovasdis.2019.104567.

69. Faigle R, Cooper LA, Gottesman RF. Race differences in gastrostomy tube placement after stroke in majority-white, minority-serving, and racially integrated US hospitals. *Dysphagia*. 2018;33(5):636–644. https://doi.org/10.1007/s00455-018-9882-y.

70. George BP, Kelly AG, Schneider EB, Holloway RG. Current practices in feeding tube placement for US acute ischemic stroke inpatients. *Neurology*. 2014;83(10):874–882. https://doi.org/10.1212/WNL.0000000000000764.

71. González-Fernández M, Huckabee ML, Doeltgen SH, Inamoto Y, Kagaya H, Saitoh E. Dysphagia rehabilitation: similarities and differences in three areas of the World. *Curr Phys Med Rehabil Reports*. 2013;1(4):296–306. https://doi.org/10.1007/s40141-013-0035-9.

72. Kennedy E, Thibeault SL. Voice-gender incongruence and voice health information – seeking behaviors in the transgender community. *Am J Speech-Lang Pathol*. 2020; 29(August):1563–1573.

73. Awe AM, Burkbauer L, Pascarella L. Surgical implications of LGBTQ+ health disparities: a review. *Am Surg*. 2022. https://doi.org/10.1177/00031348221096577.

74. Song TE, Jiang N. Transgender phonosurgery: a systematic review and meta-analysis. *Otolaryngol Head Neck Surg*. 2017;156(5):803–808. https://doi.org/10.1177/0194599817697050.

75. Chadwick KA, Coleman R, Andreadis K, Pitti M, Rameau A. Outcomes of gender-affirming voice and communication modification for transgender individuals. *Laryngoscope*. 2022;132(8):1615–1621. https://doi.org/10.1002/lary.29946.

76. Nuyen BA, Qian ZJ, Campbell RD, Erickson-DiRenzo E, Thomas J, Sung CK. Feminization laryngoplasty: 17-year review on long-term outcomes, safety, and technique. *Otolaryngol Head Neck Surg*. 2022;167(1):112–117. https://doi.org/10.1177/0194599821036870.

77. Almazan AN, Benson TA, Boskey ER, Ganor O. Associations between transgender exclusion prohibitions and insurance coverage of gender-affirming surgery. *LGBT Health*. 2020;7(5):254–263. https://doi.org/10.1089/lgbt.2019.0212.

78. Gorbea E, Gidumal S, Kozato A, Pang JH, Safer JD, Rosenberg J. Insurance coverage of facial gender affirmation surgery: a review of Medicaid and commercial insurance. *Otolaryngol Head Neck Surg*. 2021;165(6):791–797. https://doi.org/10.1177/0194599821997734.

79. DeVore EK, Gadkaree SK, Richburg K, et al. Coverage for gender-affirming voice surgery and therapy for transgender individuals. *Laryngoscope*. 2021;131(3):E896–E902. https://doi.org/10.1002/lary.28986.

80. Becker DR, Gillespie AI. In the zoom where it happened: telepractice and the voice clinic in 2020. *Semin Speech Lang*. 2021;42(1):64–72. https://doi.org/10.1055/s-0040-1722750.

81. American Speech-Language-Hearing Association. Providing Telehealth Services Under Medicare During the COVID-19 Pandemic. https://www.asha.org/practice/reimbursement/medicare/providing-telehealth-services-under-medicare-during-the-covid-19-pandemic/#Covered. Accessed October 9, 2022.

82. McCool RR, Davies L. Where does telemedicine fit into otolaryngology? An assessment of telemedicine eligibility among otolaryngology diagnoses. *Otolaryngol Head Neck Surg*. 2018;158(4):641–644. https://doi.org/10.1177/0194599818757724.

83. Ramirez AV, Ojeaga M, Espinoza V, Hensler B, Honrubia V. Telemedicine in minority and socioeconomically disadvantaged communities amidst COVID-19 pandemic. *Otolaryngol Head Neck Surg*. 2021;164(1):91–92. https://doi.org/10.1177/01945998 20947667.

84. Darrat I, Tam S, Boulis M, Williams AM. Socioeconomic disparities in patient use of telehealth during the coronavirus disease 2019 surge. *JAMA Otolaryngol Head Neck Surg*. 2021;147(3):287–295. https://doi.org/10.1001/jamaoto.2020.5161.

85. Fagherazzi G, Fischer A, Ismael M, Despotovic V. Voice for health: the use of vocal biomarkers from research to clinical practice. *Digit Biomark*. 2021:78–88. https://doi.org/10.1159/000515346.

86. Bensoussan Y, Vanstrum EB, Johns MM, Rameau A. Artificial intelligence and laryngeal cancer: from screening to prognosis: a state of the art review. *Otolaryngol Head Neck Surg*. 2022. https://doi.org/10.1177/01945998221110839.

87. Holloway C, Barbareschi G. Future disability interactions. In: Carroll JM, ed. *Disability Interactions. Synthesis Lectures on Human-Centered Informatics*. Cham: Springer; 2022: 1–23. https://doi.org/10.1007/978-3-031-03759-7_7.

88. Topol E. Digital medicine: empowering both patients and clinicians. *Lancet*. 2016; 388(10046):740–741. https://doi.org/10.1016/S0140-6736(16)31355-1.

89. Powell ME, Cancio MR, Young D, et al. Decoding phonation with artificial intelligence (DEP AI): proof of concept. *Laryngoscope*. 2019;4(June):328–334.

90. Hegde S, Shetty S, Rai S, Dodderi T. A survey on machine learning approaches for automatic detection of voice disorders. *J Voice*. 2018;33(6):947e.11–947.e33.

91. Gelzinis A, Verikas A, Bacauskiene M. Automated speech analysis applied to laryngeal disease categorization. *Comput Methods Progr Biomed*. 2008;91(1):36–47. https://doi.org/10.1016/j.cmpb.2008.01.008.

92. Alhussein M, Muhammad G. Voice pathology detection using deep learning on mobile healthcare framework. *IEEE Access*. 2018;6:41034–41041.

93. Obermeyer Z, Emanuel EJ. Predicting the future - big data, machine learning, and clinical medicine. *N Engl J Med*. 2016;375(13):1212–1216. https://doi.org/10.1056/NEJMp1606181.Predicting.

94. Crowson MG, Rameau A. Standardizing machine learning manuscript reporting in otolaryngology-head & neck surgery. *Laryngoscope*. 2022;132(September): 1598–1700. https://doi.org/10.1002/lary.30264.

95. Ethical Guidelines for Voice Experiences. https://openvoicenetwork.org/documents/ovn_ethical_guidlines_voice_experiences.pdf.

96. Kollu T, Giutashvili T, Uppal P, Ruffner R, Mortensen M. Diversity in academic laryngology: an evaluation of academic advancement and research productivity. *Laryngoscope*. 2022;132(6):1245–1250. https://doi.org/10.1002/lary.29918.

97. Okafor S, Tibbetts K, Shah G, Tillman B, Agan A, Halderman AA. Is the gender gap closing in otolaryngology subspecialties? An analysis of research productivity. *Laryngoscope*. 2020;130(5):1144–1150. https://doi.org/10.1002/lary.28189.

98. Ellis C, Kendall D. Time to act: confronting systemic racism in communication sciences and disorders academic training programs. *Am J Speech Lang Pathol*. 2021;30(5): 1916–1924. https://doi.org/10.1044/2021_AJSLP-20-00369.

Social determinants of health and demographic disparities in rhinology

11

Michael Ghiam, David A. Gudis

Department of Otolaryngology—Head and Neck Surgery, Columbia University Irving Medical Center, New York-Presbyterian Hospital, New York, NY, United States

Introduction

In recent years, research across numerous medical specialties and healthcare disciplines has demonstrated the impact of demographic disparities and social determinants of health (SDH) on patients. Rhinology is the subspecialty of otolaryngology focusing on sinonasal and skull base disorders. Demographic disparities and SDH have been shown to affect several dimensions of rhinology care and research, including patient presentation, management, outcomes, and clinical trial enrollment. This chapter aims to summarize the current literature surrounding disparities in rhinology including rhinosinusitis, sinonasal malignancies, olfactory dysfunction (OD), and clinical research.

Adult chronic rhinosinusitis

Chronic rhinosinusitis (CRS) represents a heterogenous set of disorders affecting the paranasal sinuses and nasal cavities, historically categorized by the presence of polyps as CRS with nasal polyposis (CRSwNP) and CRS without nasal polyposis (CRSsNP). Recent research has focused on subtyping CRS into more specific phenotypes and endotyping CRS into specific cellular and molecular etiologies.[1] CRS is a common condition, associated with reduced quality of life (QOL) and both indirect and direct financial costs.[2–4]

To improve delivery of care for chronic conditions such as CRS, healthcare providers and healthcare systems must understand how SDH influence the presentation, management, and outcomes of such disorders. Clinicians must understand how disparities related to sociodemographic and socioeconomic factors, access and utilization of care, and practice patterns interact to affect disease presentation, severity, and patient healthcare outcomes.[5]

Broadly speaking, rhinosinusitis is a disease characterized by inflammation of the nasal cavity and paranasal sinuses. The clinical definition of CRS (with or without nasal polyps) in adults is:[5]

Healthcare Disparities in Otolaryngology. https://doi.org/10.1016/B978-0-443-10714-6.00007-9

- The presence of *two* or more symptoms for ≥ 12 weeks, *one* of which should be either nasal blockage, obstruction, congestion, or nasal discharge
  - $\pm$ facial pain/pressure
  - $\pm$ reduction or loss of smell
- Objective evidence of inflammation, which could include:
  - Endoscopic signs of:
    - Nasal polyps and/or
    - Mucopurulent discharge
  - And/or CT changes

The prevalence of CRS is reported to range from 10% to 15%.[6] However, capturing the true prevalence of CRS has been challenging as many population studies are based on surveys of subjective symptoms. The diagnosis of CRS is based on a combination of both subjective symptoms and objective findings as discussed above. Furthermore, a growing body of evidence has demonstrated CRS represents a heterogenous set of disease with different cellular and molecular etiologies such as allergic fungal rhinosinusitis (AFRS), aspirin-exacerbated respiratory disease (AERD), and pediatric CRS. Secondary causes of CRS further add to the diversity of disease which include autoimmune disease (e.g., granulomatosis with polyangiitis and eosinophilic granulomatosis with polyangiitis), primary mucociliary disorders (e.g., cystic fibrosis and primary ciliary dyskinesia), and immunodeficiency.[1,7,8] Historically categorized by phenotypic presence or absence of polyps, recent literature has focused on subtyping CRS based on cellular and molecular etiologies (Type 2 Inflammation vs. non-Type 2 Inflammation).[5]

An increasing body of evidence has demonstrated that SDH, including race, ethnicity, socioeconomic status (SES), education level, nutrition, and several other factors impact health outcomes for various chronic diseases. Recent literature has begun to demonstrate how SDH and geographic variation affect the prevalence of CRS and its subtypes and contribute to the pathogenesis, natural history, and outcomes.[9–14] Large knowledge gaps regarding how these complex factors affect CRS patients persist. Understanding these disparities may help improve access to care, improve health outcomes, and better inform enrollment of populations in CRS studies.

Demographic and regional differences

The overall prevalence of symptom-based CRS in the population has been reported to range from 5.5% to 28%.[15–18] While prevalence of CRS has shown variability across countries, several studies on United States populations have also demonstrated both demographic and regional variations in the prevalence of CRS and its subtypes.[10,11]

Studies reporting on the incidence of CRS in the general US population have shown that CRS patient demographics may not mirror the demographics of the US population as a whole. One systematic review of national databases by Ma et al. explored the demographic characteristics of CRS and its subtypes by geographic region in the United States. The authors found the CRS population in the US is distinct from the overall US population, with CRS patients more likely to be older and of White race and less likely to be Black, Asian, or other minority races or ethnicities.[11] Additionally, when stratified by the various CRS subtypes, the authors found that male sex was more predominant in CRSwNP patients, whereas female sex was more prevalent in CRSsNP patients. Interestingly, while nearly all subtypes of CRS have a higher proportion of White patients, Black patients were overrepresented in AFRS and AERD subtypes (both Type 2 CRS endotypes).[11]

Geographic variations were also identified, with AFRS more prevalent in the South, affecting a significantly higher proportion of Black patients compared to other regions in the United States.[11,19] A retrospective cohort study of patients with CRS in Chicago also demonstrated African Americans with medically refractory CRS to have higher prevalence of nasal polyposis and AERD and have increased disease severity based on Lund—Mackay CT imaging scores than White patients with CRS.[20] These findings suggest that CRS subtypes may affect distinct patient subpopulations reflecting distinct socioeconomic and demographic risk factors that alter disease processes.[11] In particular, Type-2 CRS endotypes such as AFRS appear to disproportionally affect Black patients and patients in Southern US.

Differences in ethnic prevalence may also be associated with demographic regionalization. The study by Ma et al. found that the South had a significantly higher proportion of Black patients compared to other regions (20% vs. 5.7%—13.4%) and the highest frequency of Black patients with CRS (17.8% vs. 2.1%—4.2%). Furthermore, the West had the highest prevalence of Asian (12% vs. 3.9%—7.4%) and Hispanic (30.2% vs. 8.1%—18.3%) populations as well as the highest prevalence of Asian (4.5% vs. 0.4%—1.3%) and Hispanic (12.3% vs. 0.8%—3%) patients with CRS.[11]

Additional studies are needed to elucidate demographic disparities in CRS, as most of the studies examined patients who were receiving care for CRS and thus may capture patients with more bothersome disease. Furthermore, the use of survey data may overestimate the prevalence of CRS as it is limited to subjective symptoms rather than both objective and subjective criteria. Understanding the demographic and regional differences of CRS can help reduce healthcare disparities and guide development of representative populations in CRS research.

Disease severity and presentation

The cardinal symptoms in CRS are nasal obstruction, nasal discharge, alterations in sense of smell, and facial pain/pressure. In patients with CRS, the clinical course is highly variable—some patients may only be bothered by mild intermittent nasal obstruction while others may have severe and persistent symptoms.[21] Furthermore, various subtypes of CRS may predispose patients to recalcitrant disease.[22,23] CRS is associated with adverse effects on overall QOL, and it imposes both direct and indirect financial burden in the United States.[4,24] The severity of CRS can be measured along several axes using a variety of validated outcome metrics based on subjective and objective symptoms.[25,26]

Extensive literature for other chronic diseases has demonstrated that sociodemographic factors are associated with disease severity and presentation. One mechanism by which such disparities occur is the impact of SES on access to care. Studies investigating such disparities in symptomatology and presentation in CRS patients have been limited, and results have been mixed.

Some studies have failed to show an association between SDH and disease severity at presentation. Bergmark et al. prospectively investigated presenting CRS symptomatology using the 22-Item Sino-Nasal Outcome Test (SNOT-22) at a single Northeastern tertiary care rhinology practice. The authors found that patients with CRS had similar metrics on SNOT-22 scores and prepresentation medical management regardless of various SDH such as race, ethnicity, education, income, and insurance status.[9] However, the results of this study are limited by the study population. Patients were recruited from a single tertiary care center and were disproportionately White, highly educated, and with a lower proportion of uninsured patients than the general US population.

Studies incorporating minority populations to reflect national demographics more accurately have shown disparities in CRS presentation and severity across various socioeconomic levels and demographic cohorts. These studies have generally shown that patients of minority racial and/or ethnic groups and patients with lower income may have more severe CRS symptoms on presentation.[10,27,28] In a retrospective cohort analysis of US database registries, Soler et al. demonstrated disparities in baseline preoperative QOL scores as measured by the Rhinosinusitis Disability Index (RSDI) across different racial and ethnic groups. Hispanic and Black patients had significantly worse preoperative QOL scores as determined by the total RSDI particularly on the physical and emotional subscales.[10] In a similar study, Shen et al. evaluated baseline QOL scores (SNOT-22) in preoperative patients planning to undergo endoscopic sinus surgery (ESS). In this study that included 30% non-White minority individuals, the authors found that non-White patients (difference in means: 8.3, 96% CI: 1, 15) and lower income patients (difference in means: 8.5, 95% CI: 2, 14) had more severe baseline symptoms compared to White and higher income patients, respectively. On adjusted multivariate regression, the authors found that low-income status was persistently associated with worse baseline severity ($\beta = 7.7$; 95% CI: 1.1, 14).[27]

In a study by Levine et al., investigators measured both subjective disease burden using SNOT-22 and objective disease severity using the Lund Kennedy Endoscopy (LKE) score in patients with medically refractory CRS. Their study cohort included 40% Hispanic individuals from a South Florida tertiary care center. The authors found that the Hispanic patients presented with worse subjective preoperative disease burden as well as worse objective CRS disease severity compared to the non-Hispanic cohort.[28]

Kuhar et al. sought to correlate histopathological variables in CRS patients undergoing ESS with clinical features by race and insurance status. Tissue specimens from surgical patients were examined for various histopathologic variables and retrospectively compared to clinical variables such as demographics, insurance, and preoperative symptoms. Their findings demonstrated that Black race and Medicaid insurance status were associated with worse SNOT-22 scores compared with non-Black CRS patients, suggesting more severe preoperative symptoms. Furthermore, Black patients had more severe disease based on histopathological findings, including higher levels of tissue eosinophilia. However, after controlling for insurance status, Black race was no longer associated with increased SNOT-22 scores nor tissue eosinophilia. When comparing insurance status, Medicaid was associated with worse SNOT-22 scores as well as more severe histopathological variables such as increased polypoid disease, subepithelial edema, hyperplastic/papillary changes, fibrosis, and eosinophilia.[29] Their findings suggest that the most prevailing factor influencing CRS disease severity is insurance status, which served as a marker for access to care. These disparities are associated with longstanding and inadequately controlled CRS consistent with lack of access to care and delayed treatment.[29]

While studies on presenting disease severity in CRS are limited and mixed, study cohorts that more closely reflect the broader US population have shown an association between demographic minorities and lower SES with worse disease severity. Future studies that more accurately represent the general and regional US demographic and socioeconomic variability are needed to better understand how SDH affect disease presentation. Reducing obstacles to care and improving access may help to mitigate disparities.

Utilization and access of care

Improving access to care is an important step in improving outcomes in patients with CRS. A clear understanding of how SDH such as race, insurance status, education, and income impact access to care is needed to reduce healthcare disparities. While studies in healthcare utilization and access are limited in CRS patients, several studies have identified associations between SDH and utilization of tertiary care.[10]

In a national survey study by Soler et al., the authors found that Hispanic and Black patients were most likely to delay medical care due to cost-related concerns and less likely to see a medical specialist or undergo surgery. In the same study, the authors found that these two minority groups had the highest rate of being uninsured. Twenty-four percent of Hispanic and 18% of African American respondents were uninsured compared to 11% of White and 11% of Asian respondents with CRS.[10] These findings highlight the disparities in utilization and access to care seen in minority and uninsured populations.

Higher utilization of tertiary care rhinology services has been associated with higher SES, insurance status, and education level, which may reflect easier access to care.[12,13] In a retrospective review of CRS patients at a single tertiary care hospital, Samuelson et al. found higher utilization of rhinology services in patients from zip codes with higher income, lower minority populations, higher rates of private insurance, and higher rates of college education. However, on adjusted analysis, only college education was independently associated with increased utilization. The authors concluded that economically advantaged patients have greater access to care, particularly with access to a specialist. Furthermore, patients who are insured and have higher education tend to have better health literacy and thus are more likely to have their chronic medical conditions addressed.[12] However, it is possible that the study was underpowered to identify other SDH in the adjusted analysis. In a similar study from a Midwest tertiary care center, Poetker et al. also found higher utilization of tertiary rhinology services in patients with higher income, higher education, and White race. Although private insurance alone was not independently associated with rhinology utilization, the authors felt that this was due to the low rate of uninsured patients in their region.[13] These two studies further corroborate disparities in healthcare utilization that may result from access to care due to SDH.

While the previous two studies solely looked at utilization at a single tertiary care center, other studies have analyzed disparities in utilization between public and private hospital systems. Such studies have demonstrated that demographic minority patients and Medicaid/uninsured patients are more likely to utilize public hospital systems.[30] Duerson et al. retrospectively reviewed patient demographics in CRS patients who underwent ESS at a public versus private hospital. The authors found that patients at public hospitals were significantly more likely to be non-White (73% vs. 25%, $P > .0001$) and to have Medicaid or no insurance (86% vs. $4.0\% < P < .001$). Furthermore, public hospital patients had longer wait times for surgery and were more likely to be lost to follow up.[30] These findings represent the relative decrease of healthcare utilization in minority and low SES populations and the potential for treatment delays and inadequate disease control.

Similarly, in a study by Levine et al. evaluating disparities in Hispanic patients from South Florida, the authors found that Hispanic patients had lower education and income compared to non-Hispanic patients. Interestingly, there was no difference in insurance status. The study also determined Hispanic patients were less likely to see an otolaryngologist prior to initial consultation and had greater symptom duration compared to non-Hispanic patients. It was postulated that these disparities were attributed to Hispanic patients' preference for Spanish speaking providers, lower income, and lower education levels.[28] This study underscores the intricate interplay of sociodemographic factors and healthcare utilization.

Treatment

The socioeconomic variables that influence disease burden and access to care may also influence treatment patterns. Several studies have shown that insurance status, race, and ethnicity can impact treatment patterns and outcomes in CRS patients.[10,30,31]

A study by Duerson et al. evaluated disparities in patients with CRS undergoing ESS in private versus public hospitals. Patients in the public hospital represented low SES (86% with Medicaid or no insurance vs. 4%, $P < .001$) and minority populations (73% non-White vs. 25% White, $P < .001$). Patients treated at the public hospital were less likely to be seen by an allergist (16% vs. 55%, $P < .001$) and thus less likely to be diagnosed and treated for allergic rhinitis (30% vs. 65%, $P < .001$). They also had longer delays to surgery (68 vs. 45 days, $P < .001$) and were less likely to receive postoperative antibiotics (43% vs. 24%, $P = .0021$). Patients seen at public hospitals were also more likely to be lost to follow up (26% vs. 16%, $P = .0310$).[30] These findings represent decreased access to physicians and specialists which may limit disease control.

Other studies have also shown lower rates of ESS in minority groups. In a study based on the National Health Interview Survey, Soler et al. found that minority individuals accounted for only 18% of ESS patients in the United States, compared with national population census estimates of 35%.[10] Within this study, 19% of White patients underwent surgery compared to 13% of African American, 12% of Hispanic, and 9% of Asian patients. A second study by Woodard et al. corroborated the aforementioned findings. Minority groups across the United States were found to undergo ESS less frequently. Over a five-year period from 2009–13, surgery rates for Black patients were 47%–56% lower than for White patients. Similarly, Hispanic patients underwent ESS 33%–62% less than non-Hispanic individuals.[31]

Understanding disparities in practice patterns in CRS patients is important to help close the gap in healthcare delivery. Timely assessment and treatment are paramount in helping control disease burden and improving delivery of care. Delays in treatment not only affect patients' QOL, but also may have downstream clinical and financial impacts such as increasing the risk for comorbid asthma and reducing societal productivity due to absenteeism, respectively.

Outcomes

While disease presentation and burden have been shown to be influenced by SDH, data on outcomes suggest surgery may mitigate disparities and improve outcomes across all races and ethnicities.

In a retrospective cohort analysis of US database registries by Soler et al., the authors found significant improvement from baseline QOL scores as measured by the RSDI and Chronic Sinusitis Survey (CSS) across all races and ethnicities. While Hispanic and Black patients had significantly lower baseline RSDI scores, postoperative RSDI and CSS scores increased significantly and were statistically similar across all groups ($P < .001$).[10] Similar findings have been corroborated in other studies. Shen et al. retrospectively compared QOL scores (SNOT-22) in patients before and after ESS. The authors found non-White patients to have significantly worse baseline symptoms (SNOT-22, 52 vs. 44, $P = .021$) compared to White patients. However, non-White patients showed larger benefit (41% vs. 37%, $P = .015$) and fewer CRS symptoms following ESS (SNOT-22, 24 vs. 29, p 0.035).[27] Their findings suggest minority patients may be more sensitive to QOL changes following surgery. Lastly, Levine et al. also found Hispanic patients to have worse preoperative disease burden compared to non-Hispanic patients.

However, postoperative SNOT-22 scores were clinically and statistically similar between both groups with Hispanic individuals having a larger improvement. These studies suggest that disparities in baseline CRS symptoms may resolve with surgery across all races and ethnicities.

Gender-specific differences have been reported in surgical outcomes following ESS. Sharma et al. evaluated predictors of complications following ESS and found women to have a significantly lower risk of complications than men (OR = 0.61, 95% CI 0.37–0.99, $P = .046$). Women were found to have lower rate of reoperation (4.4% vs. 1.8%, $P < .001$) and deep venous thromboses (0.6% vs. 0.0%, $P = .005$) compared to men.[32] These findings suggest there may be gender-based differences in complications following ESS which may be confounded by chronic conditions more prevalent in men such as hypertension. Additional studies are needed to identify such risk factors.

Pediatric rhinology

Within pediatric otolaryngology, disparities related to insurance status, access to care, race, SES, and education have been demonstrated to affect the treatment and outcome of several conditions including otitis media, sleep disordered breathing, and rhinosinusitis.[33] Data are limited to explore specifically how such disparities impact rhinologic disorders. With respect to acute rhinosinusitis, prior studies have identified that children with Medicaid or without insurance utilize emergency departments more frequently and are more likely to develop intracranial complications compared to privately insured children.[34,35]

Pediatric patients with CRS differ by race and SES from general pediatric otolaryngology patients seen at academic centers. Children with CRS are more likely to be male (63% vs. 52%, $P = .018$), of White race (77% vs. 47%, $P < .0001$), and less likely to be uninsured (14% vs. 44%, $P < .0001$). Overall, 79% of pediatric CRS patients are treated medically, while 21% are treated with surgery. Subsequent analysis has not shown differences in practice management by race or insurance status. However, privately insured pediatric patients are more likely to have had an allergy referral. Further studies are needed to better understand disparities in rhinologic pediatric patients.[36]

Sinonasal malignancies

Demographic and socioeconomic disparities impact the presentation, treatment, and outcomes for many cancers. Current literature on head and neck cancers (HNCs) have demonstrated disparities related to both race, ethnicity, and socioeconomic factors on cancer prognosis.[33] However, due to the complexity and heterogenous nature of HNCs, elucidating the effect of each of these risk factors on prognosis is elusive. The etiology of survival differences is likely multifactorial and influenced by patient demographics, socioeconomic factors, patient risk factors, and tumor biology.[37] Racial minorities such as Black Americans have been shown to have higher incidence of HNCs, greater tumor burden at presentation, and increased mortality for HNCs.[37−40] However, minorities are often uninsured or Medicaid patients. Barriers to care due to low SES can confound the magnitude of other SDH on prognosis.

Within HNC, sinonasal malignancies represent a subset of vastly heterogenous tumors that affect the paranasal sinuses. Histological subtypes include tumors of epithelial, mesenchymal, lymphoproliferative, and neuroendocrine origin.[41] Studies investigating the impact of SDH on sinus cancer outcomes are therefore understandably limited. However, the current literature available on disparities in sinonasal tumors highlights the complex interactions of both demographic and socioeconomic factors in influencing treatment outcomes.[33,42−45]

Recent studies have demonstrated roles for both socioeconomic and racial/ethnic factors in disparities related to presentation, survival, and treatment patterns in sinonasal tumors.[42,43,45] In a cross-sectional analysis by Sharma et al., authors evaluated the impact of SES on sinonasal cancer disease-specific survival (DSS) and conditional disease-specific survival (CDSS). While DSS measures the percentage who have survived from cancer at a specific time point, CDSS is the probability that a patient will live an additional 5 years given that the patient has already survived t years since diagnosis. The authors stratified the cohort into three socioeconomic tiers. After controlling for patient-specific factors including race, authors found patients in the lowest SES tertile exhibited worse mortality with a 15%−20% increased risk of death (HR 1.22; 95% CI 1.07−1.39). However, after controlling for treatment and pathology, disparities between SES tertiles were no longer statistically significant. These findings suggest treatment and tumor biology may mitigate survival differences based on SES. The study also found that patients in the lowest SES tertile were more often diagnosed at a later stage (OR 1.52; 95% CI 1.12−2.06), and for patients with regional and distant metastatic disease, the middle and lowest tertile SES were less likely to receive multimodal therapy than those in the highest SES tertile.[42] These findings suggest that those in the lowest SES may lack equal access to medical care and other healthcare resources or are receiving disparate treatment. Care for patients with sinonasal malignancies often requires multidisciplinary and highly specialized care including tertiary care rhinology services, medical oncology, radiation oncology, and others. Lastly, the authors showed that CDSS for all stages converged over time, suggesting that establishment of care and posttreatment surveillance may mitigate differences in SES following diagnosis.[42]

A second study by Sharma et al. demonstrated that race and ethnicity also impact sinonasal malignancy outcomes.[43] After controlling for demographic factors including income, authors found that Black patients (HR 1.29; 95% CI 1.13−1.45) and American Indian/Alaskan Native patients (HR 1.94; 95% CI 1.37−2.74) exhibited increased mortality compared to White patients. Black patients also had worse CDSS for regional and distant staged cancers compared to other races, and American Indian/Alaskan Native patients had worse CDSS for cancers of all stages. The authors also demonstrated racial disparities related to disease presentation and treatment patterns. Hispanic patients were more likely to present with advanced disease, and Indian/Alaskan Native patients were less likely than White patients to receive surgical therapy.[43]

A study by Irace et al. further elucidates the impact of SDH on sinonasal malignancies. Study investigators examined the impact of Medicaid expansion on rhinologic malignancies including sinonasal and nasopharyngeal tumors. In comparing cohorts before and after Medicaid expansion from the Affordable Care Act in 2014, investigators found that patients in states without the expansion of Medicaid were more likely to be diagnosed with advanced stage cancer. Uninsured status was associated with advanced stage disease at diagnosis and significantly increased risk of disease-specific death. Racial disparities were also identified in minority populations. Black and Asian/Pacific Islander race were associated with advanced stage of disease at diagnosis.[45] Advanced stage disease is often a proxy to reduced healthcare access and treatment delays. Minority patients often represent low SES populations with higher rates of uninsured/Medicaid insurance. These findings suggest that advanced stage disease is not only associated with increased mortality but also disproportionately affects racial minorities.[45]

While these studies included a heterogenous set of sinonasal tumors, a third study by Sharma et al. investigated the association of demographic and socioeconomic factors with outcomes in patients with esthesioneuroblastoma. The authors found that both race, ethnicity, and SES impact various oncologic outcomes in this tumor subset. After controlling for confounders, authors found patients in the lowest SES tertile experienced 70% worse DSS (HR 1.70, 95% CI 1.05−2.75) and were 85% more likely to present with advanced stage cancer (OR 1.84, 95% CI 1.06−3.30) at diagnosis when compared to the highest SES tertile. While racial/ethnic disparities were not associated with DSS, racial disparities did impact treatment patterns. Black patients were 60% less likely to receive multimodal therapy (OR 0.44, 95% CI 0.24−0.84) compared to White patients.[44] These findings suggest that SES mitigates outcomes, but racial disparities remain in treatment patterns in patients with esthesioneuroblastoma. In conjunction with the aforementioned articles, this study demonstrates how disparities can vary across different tumor subtype, further corroborating the complex interplay of social determinants of health and tumor biology.

Olfactory dysfunction

While OD may be the most common form of sensory impairment, the prevalence of OD varies markedly in the literature.[46] These variations are due to differences in definitions of impairment, sample demographics, and assessment of techniques used. OD can be characterized as hyposmia or anosmia, as well as parosmia and phantosmia.[47] Subjective olfactory outcome measures include the SNOT-22, RSDI, and the Questionnaire of Olfactory Disorders. Objective measures include the University of Pennsylvania Smell Identification Test (UPSIT), San Diego Odor Identification Test

(SDOIT), Olfactory Function Field Exam (OFFE), Pocket Smell and Taste Test (PSTT), and Sniffin' Sticks Test.[48] Studies using subjective measures tend to underestimate prevalence of OD. Furthermore, the prevalence of OD increases with age, making comparisons between studies difficult in dissimilar sample demographics.[49]

Common etiologies of OD include aging, sinonasal inflammatory disease such as CRS, postinfectious olfactory loss, traumatic brain injury, and occupational exposures.[47] While the association of OD has been linked to poor QOL including depression, the associations of SDH and OD are not well described in the literature. The published literature suggests that OD is more prevalent in patients with lower SES, minority racial/ethnic status, and certain environmental/occupational exposures, while the associations with education and other patient risk factors remain indeterminate.[50]

The cumulative body of literature on the role of SES in OD suggests an association between OD and lower SES. Several studies have demonstrated low SES is associated with objective OD as measured by the PSTT as well as self-reported phantosmia and general smell alterations.[51,52] Interestingly, prospective studies suggest the effect of low SES in developing OD is gradual, with significant decline noted after 10 years.[53,54]

Studies have also demonstrated the association between occupational/environmental exposures and OD, particularly to heavy metals, pesticides, and herbicides.[53] Exposure to heavy metals such as lead and manganese has been associated with objective OD.[55–57] Farmers with "high risk" exposures to pesticides, as well as those exposed to ambient air pollution were at increased risk of OD.[58] The underlying pathophysiology is not well understood but may involve damage to the olfactory epithelium or central olfactory processing systems.

Associations between subjective and objective OD have been identified in minority patients including Black and Hispanic patients.[50,51,54,59] Whether these findings represent true biological predispositions or are confounded by the higher prevalence of blue collar/industry jobs and neurogenerative disease in minority groups has yet to be determined by prospective studies.

The associations between education and OD remain mixed. Studies have shown both a significant association between decreased years of education and OD, as well as no association.[50] Interestingly, higher education has been shown to associate with odor identification, but not olfactory threshold, which may be linked to the association of OD and cognition seen in older patients and those with neurodegenerative disease.[60–63] Furthermore, studies examining the association of education and OD may be limited by the various psychophysical tests available along with cultural/lingual barriers.

Several studies have linked alcohol dependence to OD; however, the overall evidence in the literature remains mixed. Studies linking mild to moderate alcohol use to OD have been inconclusive, with some even suggesting a possible protective effect.[50,64] Heavy drinking has been found to be associated with OD which may be due to alterations in the orbitofrontal cortex and limbic systems from alcohol dependence.[65] Several studies demonstrated a dose-dependent, negative effect of smoking on olfactory function.[66,67] The pathophysiology of smoking-related OD may be related to direct inflammation of olfactory epithelium to irritants. Studies have also shown that current smokers are more likely to have OD than nonsmokers and former smokers suggesting the possibility of reversal.[68] However, other studies have demonstrated contradictory findings, suggesting protective effects of smoking on OD caused by the memory-enhancing effects of nicotine.[69,70]

Disparities in clinical research

Racial and ethnic disparities seen in rhinologic diseases are interconnected with disparities in the clinical research sector. Clinical trials are conducted in sample populations with the goal of generalizing findings to the remaining population. However, the disparities that affect prevalence, disease burden, healthcare utilization, treatments, and outcomes can similarly affect the quality and accuracy of clinical research. For example, disparities that portend to healthcare utilization can lead to unrepresentative cohorts which may lead to results that do not represent the broader population. Misrepresentative study populations may also fail to capture treatment failures or adverse events.[71–73]

A recent systemic review and population analysis of prospective CRS trials in the United States found the racial/ethnic composition of study cohorts to differ significantly from the general US population. The review included 83 studies between 2010 and 2020 comprising nearly 12,000 patients. The authors found the racial composition of the study population to significantly underrepresent Black, Asian, Pacific Island, and American Indian minorities. With regard to ethnicity, the composite study populations included 1.6% Hispanic patients, compared to 18% within the general US population ($P < .0001$). On further regional subanalysis, all minorities were underrepresented in the Northeast and West. However, in the South and Midwest, enrollment of Black patients mirrored the US census data, while other demographic minorities remained underrepresented.[71]

In an effort to reduce disparities in medical research, the US National Institute of Health (NIH) introduced the Revitalization Act of 1993. This act required NIH-funded clinical trials to improve representation of women and minority groups. These mandates have since expanded to be more inclusive of other underrepresented demographic cohorts. Despite these federal regulations, sociodemographic disparities persist in rhinologic research populations.

Speilman et al. compared pooled data from 18 prospective clinical trials for CRSwNP to the national US census and found significant racial, ethnic, and gender disparities. Of the studies exclusive to the United States, the pooled study population significantly underrepresented women, as well as Asian, American Indian, and Hispanic patients ($P < .005$). Subanalyses of individual medication cohorts demonstrated similar disparities. Women were significantly underrepresented in dupilumab, mepolizumab, and omalizumab trials. With regard to race and ethnicity, all minority patients were significantly underrepresented in mepolizumab and oma-lizumab trials, while Black patients were significantly underrepresented in dupilu-mab trials. In studies evaluating intranasal corticosteroids, disparities were less severe, although gender and racial/ethnic disparities were still present.[72]

Liebowitz et al. analyzed demographic disparities of clinical trials in new drug applications (NDAs) and biologic license applications (BLAs) approved by the Food and Drug Administrations for allergic rhinitis and found demographic dis-parities in study cohorts compared to the US population. White patients were overrepresented in most NDAs, while Black, Asian, and Native American patients were underrepresented in most studies. Ethnic disparities were also found, as His-panic individuals were similarly underrepresented in NDA studies. Authors also compared cohort demographics before and after implementation of the Demo-graphic Rule in 1998; they found an improvement in representation of race but not ethnicity.[74]

While these mandates have yet to narrow the gap in rhinology-related trials, Mehta et al. have shown that federal mandates have improved demographic report-ing in rhinitis clinical trials. Patient demographics from trials conducted from 2001 to 2009 were compared to trials from 2010 to 2020. The authors found that racial disparities significantly improved between the two time periods, with improved rep-resentation of Black and Asian subjects. Similarly, adherence to racial and ethnic de-mographic reporting increased significantly from 45% to 77% ($P < .001$) and 6% to 51% ($P < .001$), respectively. However, women continued to be overrepresented in rhinitis trials.[73] This disparity may be attributed to women's increased likelihood to visit healthcare providers or to experience greater disease severity.

While federal mandates have helped reduce disparities in rhinitis clinical trials, disparities are still present in CRS research. Identifying disparities and barriers to minority participation in research is essential in improving the generalizability of study results. Continued disparities may be related to (1) access to tertiary care and clinical trials, (2) SES factors that limit participation, (3) patients' beliefs and willingness to participate, (4) cultural and language barriers, and (5) recruitment. In order to conduct the most reliable and accurate studies generalizable to the gen-eral population, enrollment of representative study populations is paramount in clin-ical research.

Conclusion

Social determinants of health play an important role in the care of rhinology patients. Understanding how SDH affect the epidemiology, disease burden, treatment, and outcomes of patients is an important step in mitigating disparities between demo-graphic cohorts. The rhinology research community can improve recruitment of representative study populations in order to develop more accurate and generalizable findings to subsequently improve patient care.

References

1. Tomassen P, Vandeplas G, Van Zele T, et al. Inflammatory endotypes of chronic rhinosinusitis based on cluster analysis of biomarkers. *J Allergy Clin Immunol*. May 2016; 137(5):1449−1456 e4. https://doi.org/10.1016/j.jaci.2015.12.1324.
2. Gliklich RE, Metson R. The health impact of chronic sinusitis in patients seeking otolaryngologic care. *Otolaryngol Head Neck Surg*. July 1995;113(1):104−109. https://doi.org/10.1016/s0194-5998(95)70152-4.
3. Wahid NW, Smith R, Clark A, Salam M, Philpott CM. The socioeconomic cost of chronic rhinosinusitis study. *Rhinology*. April 1, 2020;58(2):112−125. https://doi.org/10.4193/Rhin19.424.
4. Lourijsen ES, Fokkens WJ, Reitsma S. Direct and indirect costs of adult patients with chronic rhinosinusitis with nasal polyps. *Rhinology*. June 1, 2020;58(3):213−217. https://doi.org/10.4193/Rhin19.468.
5. Fokkens WJ, Lund VJ, Hopkins C, et al. European position paper on rhinosinusitis and nasal polyps 2020. *Rhinology*. February 20, 2020;58(Suppl S29):1−464. https://doi.org/10.4193/Rhin20.600.
6. Halawi AM, Smith SS, Chandra RK. Chronic rhinosinusitis: epidemiology and cost. *Allergy Asthma Proc*. July-August 2013;34(4):328−334. https://doi.org/10.2500/aap.2013.34.3675.
7. Cho SH, Hamilos DL, Han DH, Laidlaw TM. Phenotypes of chronic rhinosinusitis. *J Allergy Clin Immunol Pract*. May 2020;8(5):1505−1511. https://doi.org/10.1016/j.jaip.2019.12.021.
8. Bailey LN, Garcia JAP, Grayson JW. Chronic rhinosinusitis: phenotypes and endotypes. *Curr Opin Allergy Clin Immunol*. February 1, 2021;21(1):24−29. https://doi.org/10.1097/ACI.0000000000000702.
9. Bergmark RW, Hoehle LP, Chyou D, et al. Association of socioeconomic status, race and insurance status with chronic rhinosinusitis patient-reported outcome measures. *Otolaryngol Head Neck Surg*. March 2018;158(3):571−579. https://doi.org/10.1177/0194599817745269.
10. Soler ZM, Mace JC, Litvack JR, Smith TL. Chronic rhinosinusitis, race, and ethnicity. *Am J Rhinol Allergy*. March-April 2012;26(2):110−116. https://doi.org/10.2500/ajra.2012.26.3741.
11. Ma C, Mehta NK, Nguyen SA, Gudis DA, Miglani A, Schlosser RJ. Demographic variation in chronic rhinosinusitis by subtype and region: a systematic review. *Am J Rhinol Allergy*. May 2022;36(3):367−377. https://doi.org/10.1177/19458924211056294.
12. Samuelson MB, Chandra RK, Turner JH, Russell PT, Francis DO. The relationship between social determinants of health and utilization of tertiary rhinology care. *Am J Rhinol Allergy*. November 1, 2017;31(6):376−381. https://doi.org/10.2500/ajra.2017.31.4476.
13. Poetker DM, Friedland DR, Adams JA, Tong L, Osinski K, Luo J. Socioeconomic determinants of tertiary rhinology care utilization. *OTO Open*. April-June 2021;5(2): 2473974X211009830. https://doi.org/10.1177/2473974X211009830.
14. Beswick DM, Mace JC, Soler ZM, et al. Socioeconomic status impacts postoperative productivity loss and health utility changes in refractory chronic rhinosinusitis. *Int Forum Allergy Rhinol*. September 2019;9(9):1000−1009. https://doi.org/10.1002/alr.22374.
15. Hastan D, Fokkens WJ, Bachert C, et al. Chronic rhinosinusitis in Europe–an underestimated disease. A GA(2)LEN study. *Allergy*. September 2011;66(9):1216−1223. https://doi.org/10.1111/j.1398-9995.2011.02646.x.

16. Hirsch AG, Stewart WF, Sundaresan AS, et al. Nasal and sinus symptoms and chronic rhinosinusitis in a population-based sample. *Allergy.* February 2017;72(2):274−281. https://doi.org/10.1111/all.13042.

17. Pilan RR, Pinna FR, Bezerra TF, et al. Prevalence of chronic rhinosinusitis in Sao Paulo. *Rhinology.* June 2012;50(2):129−138. https://doi.org/10.4193/Rhino11.256.

18. Shi JB, Fu QL, Zhang H, et al. Epidemiology of chronic rhinosinusitis: results from a cross-sectional survey in seven Chinese cities. *Allergy.* May 2015;70(5):533−539. https://doi.org/10.1111/all.12577.

19. Smith WM, Davidson TM, Murphy C. Regional variations in chronic rhinosinusitis, 2003−2006. *Otolaryngol Head Neck Surg.* September 2009;141(3):347−352. https://doi.org/10.1016/j.otohns.2009.05.021.

20. Mahdavinia M, Benhammuda M, Codispoti CD, et al. African American patients with chronic rhinosinusitis have a distinct phenotype of polyposis associated with increased asthma hospitalization. *J Allergy Clin Immunol Pract.* July-August 2016;4(4): 658−664 e1. https://doi.org/10.1016/j.jaip.2015.11.031.

21. Bachert C, Marple B, Schlosser RJ, et al. Adult chronic rhinosinusitis. *Nat Rev Dis Prim.* October 29, 2020;6(1):86. https://doi.org/10.1038/s41572-020-00218-1.

22. Woodbury K, Ferguson BJ. Recalcitrant chronic rhinosinusitis: investigation and management. *Curr Opin Otolaryngol Head Neck Surg.* February 2011;19(1):1−5. https://doi.org/10.1097/MOO.0b013e3283420e92.

23. Kong IG, Kim DW. Pathogenesis of recalcitrant chronic rhinosinusitis: the emerging role of innate immune cells. *Immune Netw.* April 2018;18(2):e6. https://doi.org/10.4110/in.2018.18.e6.

24. Rudmik L, Smith TL. Quality of life in patients with chronic rhinosinusitis. *Curr Allergy Asthma Rep.* June 2011;11(3):247−252. https://doi.org/10.1007/s11882-010-0175-2.

25. Ting F, Hopkins C. Outcome measures in chronic rhinosinusitis. *Curr Otorhinolaryngol Rep.* 2018;6(3):271−275. https://doi.org/10.1007/s40136-018-0215-3.

26. Rudmik L, Hopkins C, Peters A, Smith TL, Schlosser RJ, Soler ZM. Patient-reported outcome measures for adult chronic rhinosinusitis: a systematic review and quality assessment. *J Allergy Clin Immunol.* December 2015;136(6):1532−1540 e2. https://doi.org/10.1016/j.jaci.2015.10.012.

27. Shen SA, Jafari A, Qualliotine JR, DeConde AS. Socioeconomic and demographic determinants of postoperative outcome after endoscopic sinus surgery. *Laryngoscope.* February 2020;130(2):297−302. https://doi.org/10.1002/lary.28036.

28. Levine CG, Casiano RR, Lee DJ, Mantero A, Liu XZ, Palacio AM. Chronic rhinosinusitis disease disparity in the south Florida hispanic population. *Laryngoscope.* December 2021;131(12):2659−2665. https://doi.org/10.1002/lary.29664.

29. Kuhar HN, Ganti A, Eggerstedt M, et al. The impact of race and insurance status on baseline histopathology profile in patients with chronic rhinosinusitis. *Int Forum Allergy Rhinol.* June 2019;9(6):665−673. https://doi.org/10.1002/alr.22295.

30. Duerson W, Lafer M, Ahmed O, et al. Health care disparities in patients undergoing endoscopic sinus surgery for chronic rhinosinusitis: differences in disease presentation and access to care. *Ann Otol Rhinol Laryngol.* July 2019;128(7):608−613. https://doi.org/10.1177/0003489419834947.

31. Woodard T, Sindwani R, Halderman AA, Holy CE, Gurrola 2nd J. Variation in delivery of sinus surgery in the Medicaid population across ethnicities. *Otolaryngol Head Neck Surg.* May 2016;154(5):944−950. https://doi.org/10.1177/0194599816628460.

32. Sharma RK, Dodhia S, Golub JS, Overdevest JB, Gudis DA. Gender as a predictor of complications in endoscopic sinus surgery. *Ann Otol Rhinol Laryngol.* August 2021; 130(8):892–898. https://doi.org/10.1177/0003489420987418.

33. Russo DP, Tham T, Bardash Y, Kraus D. The effect of race in head and neck cancer: a meta-analysis controlling for socioeconomic status. *Am J Otolaryngol.* November-December 2020;41(6):102624. https://doi.org/10.1016/j.amjoto.2020.102624.

34. Bergmark RW, Ishman SL, Scangas GA, Cunningham MJ, Sedaghat AR. Socioeconomic determinants of overnight and weekend emergency department use for acute rhinosinusitis. *Laryngoscope.* November 2015;125(11):2441–2446. https://doi.org/10.1002/lary.25390.

35. Sedaghat AR, Wilke CO, Cunningham MJ, Ishman SL. Socioeconomic disparities in the presentation of acute bacterial sinusitis complications in children. *Laryngoscope.* July 2014;124(7):1700–1706. https://doi.org/10.1002/lary.24492.

36. Smith DF, Ishman SL, Tunkel DE, Boss EF. Chronic rhinosinusitis in children: race and socioeconomic status. *Otolaryngol Head Neck Surg.* October 2013;149(4):639–644. https://doi.org/10.1177/0194599813498206.

37. Goodwin WJ, Thomas GR, Parker DF, et al. Unequal burden of head and neck cancer in the United States. *Head Neck.* March 2008;30(3):358–371. https://doi.org/10.1002/hed.20710.

38. Swango PA. Cancers of the oral cavity and pharynx in the United States: an epidemiologic overview. *J Public Health Dent.* Fall 1996;56(6):309–318. https://doi.org/10.1111/j.1752-7325.1996.tb02458.x.

39. Horner MJ, Ries LAG, Krapcho M, et al. *SEER Cancer Statistics Review, 1975.* National Cancer Institute; 2006.

40. Molina MA, Cheung MC, Perez EA, et al. African American and poor patients have a dramatically worse prognosis for head and neck cancer: an examination of 20,915 patients. *Cancer.* November 15, 2008;113(10):2797–2806. https://doi.org/10.1002/cncr.23889.

41. Bracigliano A, Tatangelo F, Perri F, et al. Malignant sinonasal tumors: update on histological and clinical management. *Curr Oncol.* July 1, 2021;28(4):2420–2438. https://doi.org/10.3390/curroncol28040222.

42. Sharma RK, Del Signore A, Govindaraj S, Iloreta A, Overdevest JB, Gudis DA. Impact of socioeconomic status on paranasal sinus cancer disease-specific and conditional survival. *Otolaryngol Head Neck Surg.* June 2022;166(6):1070–1077. https://doi.org/10.1177/01945998211028161.

43. Sharma RK, Schlosser RJ, Beswick DM, et al. Racial and ethnic disparities in paranasal sinus malignancies. *Int Forum Allergy Rhinol.* November 2021;11(11):1557–1569. https://doi.org/10.1002/alr.22816.

44. Sharma RK, Irace AL, Overdevest JB, Turner JH, Patel ZM, Gudis DA. Association of race, ethnicity, and socioeconomic status with esthesioneuroblastoma presentation, treatment, and survival. *OTO Open.* January-March 2022;6(1):2473974X221075210. https://doi.org/10.1177/2473974X221075210.

45. Irace AL, Sharma RK, Smith TL, Stewart MG, Gudis DA. Impact of Medicaid expansion on rhinologic cancer presentation, treatment, and outcomes. *Laryngoscope.* February 11, 2022. https://doi.org/10.1002/lary.30049.

46. Yang J, Pinto JM. The epidemiology of olfactory disorders. *Curr Otorhinolaryngol Rep.* May 2016;4(2):130–141. https://doi.org/10.1007/s40136-016-0120-6.

47. Schafer L, Schriever VA, Croy I. Human olfactory dysfunction: causes and consequences. *Cell Tissue Res*. January 2021;383(1):569−579. https://doi.org/10.1007/s00441-020-03381-9.

48. Hummel T, Whitcroft KL, Andrews P, et al. Position paper on olfactory dysfunction. *Rhinol Suppl*. March 2017;54(26):1−30. https://doi.org/10.4193/Rhino16.248.

49. Schlosser RJ, Desiato VM, Storck KA, et al. A community-based study on the prevalence of olfactory dysfunction. *Am J Rhinol Allergy*. September 2020;34(5):661−670. https://doi.org/10.1177/1945892420922771.

50. James J, Tsvik AM, Chung SY, Usseglio J, Gudis DA, Overdevest JB. Association between social determinants of health and olfactory function: a scoping review. *Int Forum Allergy Rhinol*. October 2021;11(10):1472−1493. https://doi.org/10.1002/alr.22822.

51. Noel J, Habib AR, Thamboo A, Patel ZM. Variables associated with olfactory disorders in adults: a U.S. population-based analysis. *World J Otorhinolaryngol Head Neck Surg*. March 2017;3(1):9−16. https://doi.org/10.1016/j.wjorl.2017.02.005.

52. Schlosser RJ, Storck KA, Rudmik L, et al. Association of olfactory dysfunction in chronic rhinosinusitis with economic productivity and medication usage. *Int Forum Allergy Rhinol*. January 2017;7(1):50−55. https://doi.org/10.1002/alr.21841.

53. Schubert CR, Cruickshanks KJ, Nondahl DM, Klein BE, Klein R, Fischer ME. Association of exercise with lower long-term risk of olfactory impairment in older adults. *JAMA Otolaryngol Head Neck Surg*. October 2013;139(10):1061−1066. https://doi.org/10.1001/jamaoto.2013.4759.

54. Pinto JM, Schumm LP, Wroblewski KE, Kern DW, McClintock MK. Racial disparities in olfactory loss among older adults in the United States. *J Gerontol A Biol Sci Med Sci*. March 2014;69(3):323−329. https://doi.org/10.1093/gerona/glt063.

55. Grashow R, Sparrow D, Hu H, Weisskopf MG. Cumulative lead exposure is associated with reduced olfactory recognition performance in elderly men: the Normative Aging Study. *Neurotoxicology*. July 2015;49:158−164. https://doi.org/10.1016/j.neuro.2015.06.006.

56. Casjens S, Pesch B, van Thriel C, et al. Associations between blood lead, olfaction and fine-motor skills in elderly men: results from the Heinz Nixdorf Recall Study. *Neurotoxicology*. September 2018;68:66−72. https://doi.org/10.1016/j.neuro.2018.06.013.

57. Casjens S, Pesch B, Robens S, et al. Associations between former exposure to manganese and olfaction in an elderly population: results from the Heinz Nixdorf Recall Study. *Neurotoxicology*. January 2017;58:58−65. https://doi.org/10.1016/j.neuro.2016.11.005.

58. Ajmani GS, Suh HH, Pinto JM. Effects of ambient air pollution exposure on olfaction: a review. *Environ Health Perspect*. November 2016;124(11):1683−1693. https://doi.org/10.1289/EHP136.

59. Dong J, Pinto JM, Guo X, et al. The prevalence of anosmia and associated factors among U.S. Black and White older adults. *J Gerontol A Biol Sci Med Sci*. August 1, 2017;72(8):1080−1086. https://doi.org/10.1093/gerona/glx081.

60. Bainbridge KE, Byrd-Clark D, Leopold D. Factors associated with phantom odor perception among US adults: findings from the national health and nutrition examination survey. *JAMA Otolaryngol Head Neck Surg*. September 1, 2018;144(9):807−814. https://doi.org/10.1001/jamaoto.2018.1446.

61. Seo HS, Jeon KJ, Hummel T, Min BC. Influences of olfactory impairment on depression, cognitive performance, and quality of life in Korean elderly. *Eur Arch Otorhinolaryngol*. November 2009;266(11):1739−1745. https://doi.org/10.1007/s00405-009-1001-0.

62. Orhan KS, Karabulut B, Keles N, Deger K. Evaluation of factors concerning the olfaction using the Sniffin' Sticks test. *Otolaryngol Head Neck Surg*. February 2012;146(2):240−246. https://doi.org/10.1177/0194599811425019.

63. Richardson JT, Zucco GM. Cognition and olfaction: a review. *Psychol Bull*. May 1989;105(3):352−360. https://doi.org/10.1037/0033-2909.105.3.352.

64. Hoffman HJ, Rawal S, Li CM, Duffy VB. New chemosensory component in the U.S. National Health and Nutrition Examination Survey (NHANES): first-year results for measured olfactory dysfunction. *Rev Endocr Metab Disord*. June 2016;17(2):221−240. https://doi.org/10.1007/s11154-016-9364-1.

65. Maurage P, Rombaux P, de Timary P. Olfaction in alcohol-dependence: a neglected yet promising research field. *Front Psychol*. 2013;4:1007. https://doi.org/10.3389/fpsyg.2013.01007.

66. Vennemann MM, Hummel T, Berger K. The association between smoking and smell and taste impairment in the general population. *J Neurol*. August 2008;255(8):1121−1126. https://doi.org/10.1007/s00415-008-0807-9.

67. Katotomichelakis M, Balatsouras D, Tripsianis G, et al. The effect of smoking on the olfactory function. *Rhinology*. December 2007;45(4):273−280.

68. Ajmani GS, Suh HH, Wroblewski KE, Pinto JM. Smoking and olfactory dysfunction: a systematic literature review and meta-analysis. *Laryngoscope*. August 2017;127(8):1753−1761. https://doi.org/10.1002/lary.26558.

69. Mullol J, Alobid I, Marino-Sanchez F, et al. Furthering the understanding of olfaction, prevalence of loss of smell and risk factors: a population-based survey (OLFACAT study). *BMJ Open*. 2012;2(6). https://doi.org/10.1136/bmjopen-2012-001256.

70. Rushforth SL, Allison C, Wonnacott S, Shoaib M. Subtype-selective nicotinic agonists enhance olfactory working memory in normal rats: a novel use of the odour span task. *Neurosci Lett*. March 3, 2010;471(2):114−118. https://doi.org/10.1016/j.neulet.2010.01.022.

71. Spielman DB, Liebowitz A, Kelebeyev S, et al. Race in rhinology clinical trials: a decade of disparity. *Laryngoscope*. August 2021;131(8):1722−1728. https://doi.org/10.1002/lary.29371.

72. Spielman DB, Schlosser RJ, Liebowitz A, et al. Do federal regulations affect gender, racial, and ethnic disparities in chronic rhinosinusitis research? *Otolaryngol Head Neck Surg*. June 2022;166(6):1211−1218. https://doi.org/10.1177/01945998211021011.

73. Mehta NK, Ma C, Miglani A, Gudis DA, Nguyen SA, Schlosser RJ. Impact of federal mandates on demographic reporting in rhinitis clinical trials. *Int Forum Allergy Rhinol*. January 2022;12(1):116−119. https://doi.org/10.1002/alr.22876.

74. Liebowitz A, Spielman DB, Schlosser RJ, Stewart MG, Gudis DA. Demographic disparities in the federal drug approval process for allergic rhinitis medications. *Laryngoscope*. April 8, 2022. https://doi.org/10.1002/lary.30129.

Hearing health disparities: applying social epidemiologic principles and new approaches

12

Kelly A. Malcolm[1], Carrie L. Nieman[1,2]

[1]*Cochlear Center for Hearing & Public Health, Johns Hopkins Bloomberg School of Public Health, Baltimore, MD, United States;* [2]*Department of Otolaryngology—Head and Neck Surgery, Johns Hopkins School of Medicine, Baltimore, MD, United States*

Introduction

An estimated 1.5 billion people have some degree of hearing loss, making hearing loss a global public health priority.[1] In the United States (US), there are an estimated 38.2 million individuals over the age of 12 years with bilateral hearing loss.[2] Older adults are disproportionately affected, where two thirds of adults 70 years and older have a clinically significant hearing loss.[2] Age-related hearing loss is the most common etiology of hearing loss at a population level and occurs secondary to degradation of cochlear inner and outer hair cells, with disruption of the mechanotransduction process, along with dysfunction of the stria vascularis and degradation of the auditory nerve.[3] Currently, these changes are irreversible and often progressive. As the aging population continues to grow in the US and globally, hearing loss will remain a highly prevalent chronic condition in the geriatric population.

Untreated hearing loss can have substantial effects on individuals across the life course, as well as their families, communities, and society. Hearing loss early in life, particularly if identification and treatment are delayed, can lead to poor speech and language outcomes, as well as poor educational and employment outcomes.[4,5] For older adults, hearing loss has been independently associated with increased loneliness, social isolation, depression, healthcare spending, and risk of accelerated cognitive decline and incident dementia, as well as reduced satisfaction with healthcare overall.[6–9] Management of hearing loss, most frequently through hearing aid use, has been shown to reduce some negative effects of untreated hearing loss, including communication function, as well as mental health and social outcomes.[10]

Despite the high prevalence of hearing loss and its potential negative implications across the life span, many Americans lack access to hearing care. This chapter will discuss disparities in hearing health care through a social epidemiological lens and provide examples of novel approaches to address these disparities for individuals who have routinely gone without care.

Healthcare Disparities in Otolaryngology. https://doi.org/10.1016/B978-0-443-10714-6.00012-2

Application of social epidemiological principles to hearing care

Epidemiology is the study of the distribution of disease or health phenomena in a population, which includes understanding prevalence as well as determining related risk factors and health outcomes.[11] Traditionally, epidemiology employs a biologic model of disease and does not always capture additional influences, such as an individual's social context, which may affect disease processes. Social epidemiology, as a branch of epidemiology, seeks to capture social factors and mechanisms associated with the risk of disease and health outcomes from a societal, community, and individual level, alongside biological explanations of disease.[12,13] This is especially important as groups of individuals may be affected by disease or health phenomena differently depending on their social environment.

Everyone's sociodemographic context is a unique set of factors relating to the environment in which they live and work, their social interactions and status in communities and societies, their access to education and health care, and their economic stability, among others.[14] Differences in these social factors between populations influence health and have been associated with large variations in health outcomes.[15,16] Defined as the social determinants of health (SDOH) by the World Health Organization (WHO), "the circumstances in which people are born, grow, live, work, and age,"[14] these social conditions create complex associations with disease at a population level. Social epidemiology applies theory-driven frameworks to understand and capture the influence of SDOH on populations, which can help explain the differential distribution of disease across populations.[12–14] These differences in health outcomes due to social factors, such as geospatial access to care and socioeconomic position (SEP), are known as disparities.[17] Disparities differ from inequities in that inequities are at a systemic level, are avoidable, and often seen as unjust.[17] Social epidemiology considers both disparities and inequities in mechanisms impacting health of various populations.

The complexity of the relationship between SDOH and health outcomes relates to the numerous interactions and pathways between social factors and disease and can inform where and how to target interventions to address disparities (Fig. 12.1). Some pathways are considered upstream, in that social and structural factors can affect individuals at a community and societal level and lead to increased risk of disease.[18] Upstream factors include policies, laws, the built environment, poverty, racism, group norms, and social networks that affect health.[18] For example, addressing policies that disrupt structural barriers to hearing care, such as reforming state-level Medicaid coverage of hearing aids and associated services for adults, is a way to address disparities through a focus on upstream factors. Downstream factors, on the other hand, are social factors that influence the individual and interpersonal levels.[18] For example, the use of telemedicine or care models that partner with community health workers (CHWs) to deliver hearing health care are ways to address downstream factors related to access to quality hearing care in low resource settings.

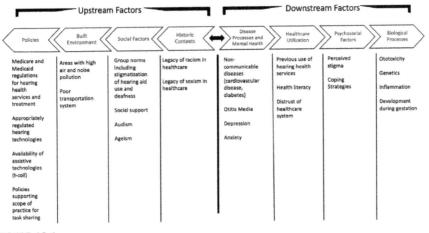

Upstream Factors				Downstream Factors			
Policies	Built Environment	Social Factors	Historic Contexts	Disease Processes and Mental Health	Healthcare Utilization	Psychosocial Factors	Biological Processes
Medicare and Medicaid regulations for hearing health services and treatment	Areas with high air and noise pollution	Group norms including stigmatization of hearing aid use and deafness	Legacy of racism in healthcare	Non-communicable diseases (cardiovascular disease, diabetes)	Previous use of hearing health services	Perceived stigma	Ototoxicity
	Poor transportation system		Legacy of sexism in healthcare		Health literacy	Coping Strategies	Genetics
Appropriately regulated hearing technologies		Social support		Otitis Media	Distrust of healthcare system		Inflammation
Availability of assistive technologies (t-coil)		Audism		Depression			Development during gestation
		Ageism		Anxiety			
Policies supporting scope of practice for task sharing							

FIGURE 12.1

Representative list of upstream and downstream factors that may affect hearing health.

Both upstream and downstream social factors are important to consider when delivering hearing health care to a population, particularly in terms of identifying where and how to intervene to improve hearing health at a population level.

Fundamental to social epidemiology is the ability to measure complex concepts, namely SDOH. For hearing health specifically, social determinants, such as race, place, and SEP, can affect an individual's hearing health from an individual to a societal level.[18] While measurements for race, place, and SEP attempt to capture various social factors that can influence an individual's health, limitations exist as these proxies do not always capture the full scope of social factors affecting health for every individual.[18] Regardless, a more detailed examination of these concepts can be helpful in understanding a social epidemiological approach to identifying and, ultimately, addressing hearing health disparities.

Race

Disparities in hearing health by race have been primarily explored at the individual level, with a reliance on self-reported race and ethnicity as the primary measure of race.[19] Importantly, when discussing race, caution must be taken to ensure race is not portrayed as a biologic difference or a direct cause of differences in health.[20] Race is a social construct and not a biological one.[20] Though racism and segregation can affect the health of the individual, the social construct of race does not affect directly.[20] Race is often used as a proxy for underlying factors, for instance, in terms of hearing loss, race has been used as a proxy for skin pigmentation, where the prevalence of age-related hearing loss has been associated with variations in skin pigmentation.[19,21,22] Care should be taken when interpreting such findings as they do not support biologic race-based differences, but rather differences in skin pigmentation which can be distinct from an individual's self-identified race.

Place

At the community level, the place in which an individual is geographically located can influence hearing health, especially when considering access to hearing health care. Persons living in areas with increased air and noise pollution are at greater risk for hearing loss, and individuals living in these areas are often of low SEP and identify as a racial or ethnic minority.[23] Considering geospatial data by state can lead to hearing interventions targeted toward the needs of different communities.

Socioeconomic position

Lastly, SEP reflects an individual's access to various opportunities and resources, both material and social. The term socioeconomic status (SES) commonly used throughout the literature differs from SEP in that only an individual's class and status in society are considered. SEP is more broadly defined and includes several aspects from a systemic and societal level to an individual and biologic level.[18] This includes access to education, employment, money, social status in society, and even time and happiness. Measuring SEP in hearing health-related research and practice can vary and, when considering a life course approach, often depends on age (Fig. 12.2).[18] For example, measuring SEP in children should reflect an emphasis on parental resources, while in older adults, measurements should target cumulative wealth or financial assets.[18]

Principles from social epidemiology can provide insights into identifying and addressing disparities in hearing health. Whether an upstream or downstream factor,

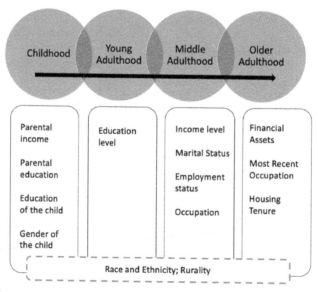

FIGURE 12.2

Examples of indicators used to identify and measure disparities in hearing healthcare across the life course.

health is determined by not only biologic factors but social factors as well, including within hearing health.

Review of disparities in hearing health

In order to understand how disparities affect different populations, one must understand the complex relationship between social factors and health outcomes. Within hearing health, we will explore the influence of education, employment and income, race and ethnicity, and rurality in order to understand existing disparities and their potential underlying mechanisms.

Education

Education influences health across numerous conditions, with lower educational attainment often and consistently associated with poorer health outcomes.[24] Individuals with lower educational levels are more likely to have lower health literacy levels and lower rates of healthcare utilization.[15,25] As with other conditions, educational level can influence hearing care at an individual, family, and societal level. Within hearing-related research, education is commonly used as a measurement for SEP and often as a covariate in statistical models. Across the life course, less education has been associated with worse hearing health outcomes.[18]

In younger populations, individuals with hearing loss have up to three times higher odds of lower educational attainment than normal hearing peers.[4] Those with hearing loss were less likely to graduate high school, and individuals with a mild hearing loss were found to be half as likely to obtain a college degree as individuals with normal hearing.[4,26] With lower education, people with hearing loss may have less potential earned income and lower-level employment opportunities, which will be discussed in the following section.

Level of education has also been associated with hearing aid use and hearing care service utilization more broadly. Mahmoudi et al. (2018) retrospectively analyzed a nationally representative cohort in the US and found older adults with hearing loss and lower educational attainment were less likely to wear a hearing aid than those with higher educational attainment.[27] Higher levels of education are also associated with individuals reporting recent hearing testing and wearing a hearing aid regularly.[28] Maternal education is important in hearing care as well, as delayed identification and diagnosis of hearing loss in a child is four times higher with mothers who have less than a high school education compared to mothers with at least a bachelor's degree.[29] These studies show both the potential upstream and downstream effects of education on individuals with hearing loss.

Employment and income

Hearing loss has been consistently associated with both unemployment and low income. Disparities in employment and income are often related to the downstream effects of education, especially for people with hearing loss, which may be secondary to communication barriers and reduced employment opportunities.[30,31] Studies assessing large populations ($n > 900,000$) have shown that individuals with hearing loss are more likely to be unemployed or underemployed.[4,32,33] Emmett et al. (2015) found people with hearing loss to have almost two times higher odds of being unemployed.[4] Hearing loss has also been associated with lower income, where individuals with hearing loss are have 1.5 times higher odds of having low-income than those with normal hearing.[4,32,34] Evidence suggests that individuals with low income and low SEP are less likely to use hearing aids and are less likely to have seen an audiologist.[35–40] Individuals with hearing loss may have fewer options for employment and may only qualify for lower paying jobs due to low educational attainment and communication skills necessary to perform job duties.

Individuals with hearing loss that are employed often have differences in job satisfaction, employment-related injuries, and income. Research based in Canada has shown that individuals who identify as deaf and/or hard of hearing were more likely to report being less satisfied with their job than those without hearing loss.[41] Higher levels of work-related stress, including an increase in sick days related to stress, are more common for people with hearing loss, who often report frustration and fatigue related the listening demands.[31,32,41] Hearing loss also increases the likelihood of occupational injuries, with one study finding individuals with combined high frequency hearing loss and tinnitus to be at higher risk for acute work-related injuries.[41,42] People with untreated hearing loss have also been shown to have an increase in annual healthcare expenditures, spending an average of over $20,000 more per year than normal hearing individuals.[8] Individuals with hearing loss also tend to make less money, with Jung and Bhattacharyya (2012) reporting the mean wage income being $8000 less for those with hearing loss than for those without.[32] Early retirement is also more common in individuals with hearing loss, which can create financial strain caused by a fixed income.[43]

The cost of hearing care services creates a barrier for individuals with hearing loss and low SEP. The cost of hearing aids is high, with an average price for a pair ranging from $2000 to $7000.[44] They are often not covered by insurance nor are the related audiology services for fitting and maintaining the devices.[40] The high cost makes hearing care unaffordable for an estimated 77% of Americans, particularly creating a large barrier for people of low SEP.[45] Coverage of hearing care through Medicaid varies by state[46]; however, audiologists were found to be less likely to practice in states with Medicaid coverage of hearing aids, which may exacerbate the ability of individuals of low SEP to find a hearing care provider.[47]

Race and ethnicity

Race is a social construct that, from an interpersonal to a systemic level, has been associated with differences in health outcomes, including hearing health.[20] Racial and ethnic disparities exist due to the lasting effects of segregation and racism systemically grounded in policies and healthcare delivery, including implicit bias.[20]

Multiple studies from various nationally representative datasets have demonstrated differences in hearing aid use by race and ethnicity. Individuals who identify as Black and Hispanic are less likely to report wearing hearing aids and to wear them less regularly than individuals who identify as White.[27,28,35,37,39,48] Studies have also shown Mexican American individuals are less likely to have had a recent hearing test compared to White American individuals, though Black American individuals were more likely to report recent testing.[28]

Other ethnic minorities and immigrant populations have expressed barriers to care including language barriers during healthcare visits, lack of education materials appropriate for their culture and language, and scarcity of culturally appropriate hearing interventions.[49,50] For Spanish-speaking individuals, there is a shortage of Spanish-speaking audiologists in the US, with only 2.6% of audiologists providing hearing health care in Spanish.[51] In focus groups consisting of Spanish-speaking Hispanic adults with hearing loss, some reported initial testing with an audiologist was not completed in Spanish and caused confusion and frustration.[50] For older Korean Americans, language difficulties and limited healthcare access can lead to differences in hearing outcomes, but insurance due to immigration status may also limit the ability to apply for Medicare, leading to further barriers to receiving covered audiological evaluations.[50,52]

Not only do hearing care outcomes and challenges vary by race and ethnicity but also differences in inclusion in current research are found. In a systematic review examining representation by race and ethnicity in clinical trials in the US related to management of hearing loss, only 16 out of 125 trials (12.8%) reported race and ethnicity; in addition, inclusion of participants from racial and ethnic minorities in those trials was small, with a median of nine participants in trials and a mean of total participants reaching to 80.[53] Trials reporting on race and ethnicity were more likely to be published in hearing or geriatric journals and were more likely to be funded through government funds, foundations, or nonprofits.[53] Lack of research with appropriate representation of the diverse races and ethnicities that make up the US population can limit advances in hearing care and exacerbate disparities in already underserved populations.

Rurality

The current model of hearing care is centralized around a hearing care professional, either an audiologist or hearing instrument specialist, along with an otolaryngologist to diagnose and manage hearing loss. Audiologists and hearing aid dispensers have traditionally been the primary gatekeepers for hearing aids, making the majority of devices only to be bought, fit, and serviced through clinic-based settings. This centralized approach can contribute to differential access for many individuals, as there are not enough hearing care professionals to provide services for the US population. Furthermore, a large proportion of hearing care professionals practice in urban areas. Although over-the-counter hearing aids promise to disrupt this model of care, clinic-based hearing care remains the dominant model of care for the foreseeable future.[54]

In the US, the number and geographic distribution of audiologists and hearing aid dispensers vary by state. The US Bureau of Labor Statistics reported there were 13,240 audiologists[55] and 10,790 hearing aid dispensers[56] estimated to be providing hearing care in 2021. For a US population of over 331 million people[57] and a range of population densities across states, access to hearing care providers can be a challenge. This is especially true for individuals living in less populated areas and in rural communities away from a large metropolis.

A spatial and economic analysis of the supply and availability of audiologists in the US was completed in 2019 by Planey.[47] In this analysis, audiologists practiced primarily in wealthy, urban communities with an overall younger population demographic.[47] The lowest number of audiologists per 100,000 people was found to be in Southern and Western states, including Alabama, Georgia, Nevada, and Idaho.[47] At the county level, audiologists were found to only practice in 43.4% of all US counties, leaving over half of all counties in the country without at least one practicing audiologist.[47] In rural parts of the US, the closest audiologist could be several hours away creating a barrier to get to and from the multiple appointments often needed for hearing testing and fitting of hearing aids. Public transportation is often lacking or nonexistent in rural areas. Those older adults with low income and without their own means of transportation, including for those who have ceased to drive as they age, may be less likely to receive or have delays in receiving needed hearing care.

Disparities in hearing care continue to affect millions of Americans, including differences based on education, employment, income, race, ethnicity, and rurality. While the disparities presented in this chapter have been well documented, their underlying mechanisms, and therefore potential targets for intervention, have often been less well characterized. As a result, the list of disparities affecting hearing health outcomes and access to care is likely more extensive. Hearing care professionals must work to identify disparities in their clinic populations and strive to address these in clinical practice.

Approaches to addressing hearing health

The current hearing care model leaves many individuals in the US without access to ear and hearing care, especially care that is of high-quality and culturally responsive. Several approaches to hearing health have been used increasingly over the last decade, including models of care that partner with CHWs, hearing care programs that employ telehealth, policy advances, and individual clinicians taking intentional steps to deliver more inclusive patient care.

Community health worker models

CHWs have played a large role in providing healthcare services across diverse settings nationally and globally and are considered vital members of healthcare teams. CHWs are nonspecialized members of a healthcare team that often work on the frontlines of care and have gone by various titles, such as community health aides, peer counselors, and public health aids.[58] In the face of inadequate health resources, including a lack of healthcare professionals, especially in low-resource settings, CHWs partner with healthcare professionals via task sharing. Task sharing entails the appropriate redistribution of tasks to trained CHWs under supervision by professionals.[59] Task sharing in partnership with CHWs has been employed in diverse areas of health care, including maternal and reproductive health, family planning and contraception, as well as mental health, cardiovascular health, cancer screenings, and primary care.[60–65] As of May 2021, there were an estimated 61,000 paid CHWs working in the US across various health-related fields, though this estimate does not include CHWs in the US that are volunteers, and likely add an additional 20,000 CHWs to the workforce.[66] CHW duties are often culturally tailored to their community, making their responsibilities variable depending on the region and communities in which they work.

Hearing healthcare professionals have partnered with CHWs to provide care to individuals who may have limited access to the traditional hearing care system. In a scoping review on the roles of CHWs in addressing ear and hearing care globally, CHWs were found to participate in various components of hearing health care, including screening, diagnosis, and management of hearing loss and ear diseases.[67] Services provided by CHWs included newborn hearing screenings, school screenings, otoscopy, diagnostic audiometry, fitting and maintaining hearing aids, and other community-driven acts, such as raising awareness regarding hearing loss and encouraging preventative measures, such as vaccinations to prevent hearing loss.[67] CHWs were trained at several levels from basic to advanced, with heterogeneity in training duration, modalities, and curriculum.[67] Training evaluations were commonly completed using pretraining and posttraining knowledge assessments or by assessing the change in practice following training.[67] Ongoing supervision by healthcare professionals trained in the supervision of CHWs and continued education for the CHWs are also critical in any task sharing program involving CHWs.[68]

Within the US, two studies highlight partnerships with CHWs to increase access to hearing care in a culturally responsive way to reach traditionally underserved racial and ethnic minority populations: HEARS (Hearing health Equity through Accessible Research and Solutions) and Oyendo Bien (Hearing Well). HEARS is a theory-driven intervention that was delivered in the community to urban-dwelling, low-income older adults in Baltimore, Maryland.[69] In this intervention, CHWs, specifically older adult peer mentors, met one-on-one with an older adult with hearing loss and completed a structured program that included selection of a personal sound amplification device (PSAP), education on age-related hearing loss, and aural rehabilitation using communication strategies and expectations around device use and management of hearing loss.[69] Findings from the initial pilot study demonstrated the HEARS intervention to be safe, feasible, and acceptable in improving communication, decreasing communication difficulties, and reducing depressive symptoms.[69] Recent data from a randomized controlled trial (RCT) to assess the efficacy of the HEARS intervention demonstrated participants reported a significant improvement in communication function three months postintervention as compared to a waitlist control.[70] To the authors' knowledge, this is the first RCT of a hearing care intervention delivered by CHWs for older adults that included provision of amplification. Furthermore, the trial represents the largest hearing-related trial to date of African American older adults and low-income older adults in the US.[70]

The second intervention, Oyendo Bien, is an audiological intervention that aims to address disparities in hearing care among older individuals in rural Arizona along the border of the US and Mexico.[71] This intervention included a culturally adapted aural rehabilitation program in Spanish delivered by CHWs in a federally qualified health center using group sessions to provide education on hearing loss and foster group discussions to increase support from peers.[71] Evaluation of the pilot intervention study indicated interventional audiology programs that are tailored to be culturally relevant and in the common language spoken of that population can improve quality of life and empower individuals to manage their hearing loss through family and peer support.[71]

CHW-delivered models of care can benefit individuals with hearing loss and can help in addressing a number of disparities in hearing care. Although interventions partnering with CHWs are promising, many areas lack interventions designed for the range of communities seen throughout the US. More research on CHW-delivered models of hearing care is needed to understand important questions around the sustainability and scalability of these approaches and their ultimate role in potentially decreasing hearing care disparities among older adults.

Teleaudiology

Telehealth is the use of telecommunications technology to provide health care remotely and provide a line of communication from patients to various healthcare providers in real time without direct contact.[59,72] Telehealth has recently come to the forefront of healthcare during the COVID-19 pandemic and has been an effective method of healthcare delivery, creating accessible and cost-effective options for patients.[59,73] Benefits of this type of care delivery for patients have been shown as it can save personal time and money from driving long distances to clinician visits, provide less time lost at work from taking off for appointments, and can save on costs of childcare needed during visits.[74] However, disparities in access and use of telehealth have been seen for individuals with low health literacy, low income, and low digital literacy, as well as for those without access to technology.[75] These disparities often disproportionately affect racial and ethnic minority populations and older adults.[75]

As many specialty healthcare services have begun to provide telehealth services, including radiology, psychiatry, and dermatology, the same can be seen in otolaryngology and audiology. Teleotology to provide remote diagnosis, treatment, and management of ear disease has long been used in the US.[76,77] In a systematic review assessing telehealth in otolaryngology, findings suggest that the delivery of services through telemedicine provided adequate imaging, high patient and provider satisfaction, and accurate diagnosis through telemedicine in comparison to in-person otology visits.[76] Teleaudiology has also been used frequently to diagnose and treat hearing loss in various populations for several services, including infant hearing screenings, diagnostic hearing evaluations, adult hearing aid fittings, cochlear implant mapping, tinnitus management, and aural rehabilitation.[78–80] To provide these services, a patient may use a mobile device or computer, or they may meet with a trained facilitator at an offsite location (e.g., mobile clinic, community clinic).[81] Facilitators are trained to assist the audiologist during the appointment by performing video otoscopy to obtain images, placing headphones on patients, and performing other audiology specific duties.[81]

Several approaches to provide hearing health care in remote areas using tele-health have been developed. The Alaska Community Health Aide Program provides telehealth services to children in remote villages of Alaska using community health aides trained in ear and hearing, as well as emergency and primary care, as facilitators.[82,83] History of ear disease and hearing loss are taken by the community health aide and ear examinations and hearing screenings are performed.[83] These re-sults are then forwarded on to an audiologist at a distant clinic or hospital through a store-and-forward technology, where recommendations regarding care plans and re-ferrals to necessary providers can be made.[83] This telehealth model paired with com-munity health aides has helped bring specialized otology and audiology care to areas that have long been without ear and hearing care.

Alaska is not the only state to deliver ear and hearing care using telehealth and trained paraprofessional site facilitators. A feasibility study of partnering with CHWs as site facilitators for teleaudiology in a remote area has also been conducted in Southern Arizona with a large Hispanic population with high rates of unemploy-ment and individuals with low income.[84] Coco, Piper, and Marrone (2021) demon-strated CHWs were efficacious in delivering teleaudiology duties including performing otoscopy and assisting with hearing aid fitting procedures for a remote audiologist, with an intensive multilevel training program.[84] Not only does this in-crease access to hearing care services in remote areas but it also has the potential to deliver care in a culturally responsive manner.

As telehealth technologies continue to develop, there will be an increase in remote access to services in otology and audiology more broadly as well as for un-derserved populations. Addressing barriers and disparities in hearing health care through telehealth may allow individuals across the US to receive services that were once out of reach.

Policy

One of the most important ways to make lasting change in addressing hearing care disparities is through changes in policy at both the federal and state levels. As the US population continues to age, health of older adults is becoming increasingly relevant to policy makers and driving legislation to address issues related to disparities in healthcare services. Hearing health professionals have recently collaborated with policy makers to address disparities in care for age-related hearing loss in older adults. Legislation was passed in 2017 to increase access to hearing aids through the passage of the Over-the-Counter (OTC) Hearing Aid Act, which allows conventional markets, such as big box stores, to sell hearing aids directly to consumers who have perceived mild-to-moderate hearing loss.[85] This new regulated category of devices promises to disrupt the current hearing care model and hearing aid market as older adults will no longer be required to go through a hearing care clinician to obtain a hearing aid. The US Food and Drug Administration released the regulatory guidelines for OTC hearing aids in August 2022, and increasing numbers of OTC devices are anticipated to enter the market.

Although hearing aids will be more accessible, disparities in hearing care will likely persist due to the lack of insurance coverage for hearing aid services provided by audiologists or hearing aid dispensers. Hearing aids require routine maintenance, as well as adjustments over time as age-related hearing loss progresses. Especially for older adults with fixed incomes or of low SEP, these necessary services may remain inaccessible without insurance coverage. To address this issue, the Biden administration pushed to include hearing aid services and aural rehabilitation as part of Medicare expansion in the Build Back Better Act in 2021.[86] This bill was passed in the House of Representatives in November 2021 but failed to progress. Medicare reform efforts are expected to continue. Without increased insurance coverage for hearing aid services, many older adults will likely remain without access to affordable hearing care.

Personal role in addressing disparities in clinical practice

Social epidemiological concepts can be applied directly to clinical practice and can aid practitioners in identifying opportunities to intervene. When reading new or past literature in hearing health and interpreting findings, readers should pay special attention to the population included in the study, including reported variables, their measurement, and associated limitations. Social and demographic variables and their measurements, as well as assessing whether authors were inclusive in sampling their population, must be considered by readers to understand the generalizability of results and the study's limitations. For clinicians providing hearing care, consideration for diagnosis and treatment must not only focus on the individual and their symptoms but also on the various social factors that may influence their hearing health. Clinicians should look to electronic health records and other sources for information regarding measures related to a patient's SDOH and work with the patient to determine what treatment options may be the most effective for that individual. Following patient outcomes with considerations for SDOH may also help identify areas where differences exist, and a targeted intervention may be necessary. Finally, education and literature on racism in health care, including hearing health care, and the various forms of racism should be sought, including an understanding of the historical contexts of the community and organization in which one works. As both consumers of current literature and as clinicians directly providing patient care, more can be done to consider SDOH, provide high-quality care for each patient, and work toward greater hearing health equity.

Conclusion

Hearing care professionals must strive to provide inclusive and equitable care that addresses the needs of individuals from diverse backgrounds, including communities that have traditionally gone unserved by hearing health care. Without addressing disparities, large differences in hearing health care based on educational level, employment and income, race, ethnicity, and rurality will persist. Consideration of new and complementary approaches of hearing care is needed to address these disparities, extend access to quality care, and improve health outcomes for individuals with hearing loss.

References

1. Haile LM, Kamenov K, Briant PS, et al. Hearing loss prevalence and years lived with disability, 1990–2019: findings from the global burden of disease study 2019. *Lancet.* 2021;397(10278):996–1009. https://doi.org/10.1016/S0140-6736(21)00516-X.
2. Goman AM, Lin FR. Prevalence of hearing loss by severity in the United States. *Am J Public Health.* 2016;106(10):1820–1822. https://doi.org/10.2105/AJPH.2016.303299.
3. Bowl MR, Dawson SJ. Age-related hearing loss. *Cold Spring Harb Perspect Med.* 2019. https://doi.org/10.1101/cshperspect.a033217.
4. Emmett SD, Francis HW. *The Socioeconomic Impact of Hearing Loss in U.S. Adults.* 2015.
5. Tomblin JB, Harrison M, Ambrose SE, Walker EA, Oleson JJ, Moeller MP. language outcomes in young children with mild to severe hearing loss HHS public access. *Ear Hear.* 2015;36(1):76–91. https://doi.org/10.1097/AUD.0000000000000219.
6. Deal JA, Betz J, Yaffe K, et al. Hearing impairment and incident dementia and cognitive decline in older adults: the health ABC study. *J Gerontol Ser A.* 2017;72(5):703–709. https://doi.org/10.1093/GERONA/GLW069.
7. Reed NS, Boss EF, Lin FR, Oh ES, Willink A. Satisfaction with quality of health care among Medicare beneficiaries with functional hearing loss. *Med Care.* 2021;59(1):22–28. https://doi.org/10.1097/MLR.0000000000001419.
8. Reed NS, Altan A, Deal JA, et al. Trends in health care costs and utilization associated with untreated hearing loss over 10 years. *JAMA Otolaryngol Head Neck Surg.* 2019;145(1):27–34. https://doi.org/10.1001/JAMAOTO.2018.2875.
9. Shukla A, Harper M, Pedersen E, et al. Hearing loss, loneliness, and social isolation: a systematic review. *Otolaryngol Head Neck Surg.* 2020;(5):622–633. https://doi.org/10.1177/0194599820910377.
10. Ferguson MA, Kitterick PT, Chong LY, Edmondson-Jones M, Barker F, Hoare DJ. Hearing aids for mild to moderate hearing loss in adults. *Cochrane Database Syst Rev.* 2017;2017(9). https://doi.org/10.1002/14651858.CD012023.PUB2/PDF/CDSR/CD012023/CD012023.PDF.
11. Frérot M, Lefebvre A, Aho S, et al. What is epidemiology? Changing definitions of epidemiology 1978–2017. *PloS One.* 2018. https://doi.org/10.1371/journal.pone.0208442.
12. Krieger N. A glossary for social epidemiology. *J Epidemiol Community Health.* 2001;55(10):693–700. https://doi.org/10.1136/jech.55.10.693.

13. Krieger N. Theories for social epidemiology in the 21st century: an ecosocial perspective. *Int J Epidemiol.* 2001;30(4):668–677.

14. Closing the Gap in a Generation: Health Equity Through Action on the Social ... - WHO Commission on Social Determinants of Health, World Health Organization - Google Books. https://books.google.com/books?hl=en&lr=&id=zc_VfH7wfV8C&oi=fnd&pg=PA1&dq=Commission+on+the+Social+Determinants+of+Health.+Closing+the+Gap+in+a+Generation,+2008.&ots=4x6jFjVffL&sig=MfVWhmcD8NsoL7HEvVefqmOH7so#v=onepage&q&f=false. Accessed 2 October 2022.

15. Bergmark RW, Sedaghat AR. Disparities in health in the United States: an overview of the social determinants of health for otolaryngologists. *Laryngoscope Investig Otolaryngol.* 2017. https://doi.org/10.1002/lio2.81.

16. Braveman P. Health disparities and health equity: concepts and measurement introduction and background: WHY discuss these concepts? *Annu Rev Public Health.* 2006;27:167–194. https://doi.org/10.1146/annurev.publhealth.27.021405.102103.

17. Penman-Aguilar A, Talih M, Huang D, Moonesinghe R, Bouye K, Beckles G. Measurement of health disparities, health inequities, and social determinants of health to support the advancement of health equity HHS public access. *J Public Health Manag Pract.* 2016;22(1):33–42. https://doi.org/10.1097/PHH.0000000000000373.

18. Nieman CL, Suen JJ, Dean LT, Chandran A. Foundational approaches to advancing hearing health equity: a primer in social epidemiology. *Ear Hear.* 2022;43(Supplement 1):5S–14S. https://doi.org/10.1097/AUD.0000000000001149.

19. Flanagin A, Frey T, Christiansen SL. Updated guidance on the reporting of race and ethnicity in medical and science journals. *JAMA.* 2021;326(7):621–627. https://doi.org/10.1001/JAMA.2021.13304.

20. Bailey ZD, Krieger N, Agénor M, Graves J, Linos N, Bassett MT. Structural racism and health inequities in the USA: evidence and interventions. *Lancet.* 2017;389(10077):1453–1463. https://doi.org/10.1016/S0140-6736(17)30569-X.

21. Lin FR, Maas P, Chien W, Carey JP, Ferrucci L, Thorpe R. Association of skin color, race/ethnicity, and hearing loss among adults in the USA. *JARO J Assoc Res Otolaryngol.* 2012;13(1):109–117. https://doi.org/10.1007/S10162-011-0298-8/TABLES/3.

22. Sun DQ, Zhou X, Lin FR, Francis HW, Carey JP, Chien WW. Racial difference in cochlear pigmentation is associated with hearing loss risk. *Otol Neurotol.* 2014;35(9):1509–1514. https://doi.org/10.1097/MAO.0000000000000564.

23. Hammer MS, Swinburn TK, Neitzel RL. Commentary environmental noise pollution in the United States: developing an effective public health response. *Environ Health Perspect.* 2014;122(2). https://doi.org/10.1289/ehp.1307272.

24. Schuh MR, Bush ML. Evaluating equity through the social determinants of hearing health. *Ear Hear.* 2022;43(Supplement 1):15S–22S. https://doi.org/10.1097/AUD.0000000000001188.

25. Berkman ND, Sheridan SL, Donahue KE, Halpern DJ, Crotty K. Low health literacy and health outcomes: an updated systematic review. *Ann Intern Med.* 2011;155(2):97–107. https://doi.org/10.7326/0003-4819-155-2-201107190-00005/SUPPL_FILE/155_2_97_SUPPLEMENT.PDF.

26. Idstad M, Engdahl B. Childhood sensorineural hearing loss and educational attainment in adulthood: results from the HUNT study. *Ear Hear.* 2019;40(6):1359–1367. https://doi.org/10.1097/AUD.0000000000000716.

27. Mahmoudi E, Zazove P, Meade M, McKee MM. Association between hearing aid use and health care use and cost among older adults with hearing loss. *JAMA Otolaryngol Head Neck Surg.* 2018;144(6):498–505. https://doi.org/10.1001/JAMAOTO.2018.0273.

28. Nieman CL, Marrone N, Szanton SL, Thorpe Jr RJ, Lin FR, Hopkins J. Racial/ethnic and socioeconomic disparities in hearing health care among older Americans. *J Aging Health*. 2016;28(1):68−94. https://doi.org/10.1177/0898264315585505.

29. Noblitt B, Alfonso KP, Adkins M, Bush ML. Barriers to rehabilitation care in pediatric cochlear implant recipients HHS public access. *Otol Neurotol*. 2018;39(5):307−313. https://doi.org/10.1097/MAO.0000000000001777.

30. Järvelin MR, Mäki-Torkko E, Sorri MJ, et al. Effect of hearing impairment on educational outcomes and employment up to the age of 25 years in Northern Finland. *Br J Audiol*. 1997;31(3):165−175. https://doi.org/10.3109/03005364000000019.

31. Kramer SE, Kapteyn TS, Houtgast T. Occupational performance: comparing normally-hearing and hearing-impaired employees using the Amsterdam Checklist for Hearing and Work/Desempeño laboral: Comparación de empleados con audición normal o alterada usando el Listado Amsterdam para Audición y Trabajo. *Int J Audiol*. 2009. https://doi.org/10.1080/14992020600754583.

32. Jung D, Bhattacharyya N. Association of hearing loss with decreased employment and income among adults in the United States. *Rhinol Laryngol*. 2012;121(12):771−775.

33. Shan A, Ting JS, Price C, et al. Hearing loss and employment: a systematic review of the association between hearing loss and employment among adults. *J Laryngol Otol*. 2022. https://doi.org/10.1017/S0022215120001012.

34. Mamo SK, Nieman CL, Lin FR. Prevalence of untreated hearing loss by income among older adults in the United States. *J Health Care Poor Underserved*. 2016;27(4):1812−1818. https://doi.org/10.1353/hpu.2016.0164.

35. Assi L, Reed NS, Nieman CL, Willink A. Factors associated with hearing aid use among medicare beneficiaries. *Innov Aging*. 2021;5(3). https://doi.org/10.1093/geroni/igab021.

36. Helvik AS, Krokstad S, Tambs K. How sociodemographic and hearing related factors were associated with use of hearing aid in a population-based study: the HUNT Study. *BMC Ear Nose Throat Disord*. 2016;16(1):1−9. https://doi.org/10.1186/S12901-016-0028-2/TABLES/2.

37. Reed NS, Garcia-Morales EG, Willink A. Trends in hearing aid ownership among older adults in the United States from 2011 to 2018. *JAMA Intern Med*. 2021;181(3):383−385. https://doi.org/10.1001/JAMAINTERNMED.2020.5682.

38. Wells TS, Nickels LD, Rush SR, et al. Characteristics and health outcomes associated with hearing loss and hearing aid use among older adults. *Article J Aging Health*. 2019;32:7−8. https://doi.org/10.1177/0898264319848866.

39. Yi JS, Garcia Morales EE, Betz JF, et al. Individual life-course socioeconomic position and hearing aid use in the atherosclerosis risk in communities study. *J Gerontol Ser A*. 2022;77(3):647−655. https://doi.org/10.1093/GERONA/GLAB273.

40. Willink A, Reed NS, Swenor B, Leinbach L, Dugoff EH, Davis K. Dental, vision, and hearing services: access, spending, and coverage for medicare beneficiaries. *Health Aff*. 2020;39(2):297−304. https://doi.org/10.1377/hlthaff.2019.00451.

41. Woodcock K, Pole JD. Educational attainment, labour force status and injury: a comparison of Canadians with and without deafness and hearing loss. *Int J Rehabil Res*. 2008;31(4):297−304. https://doi.org/10.1097/MRR.0B013E3282FB7D4D.

42. Cantley LF, Galusha D, Cullen MR, et al. Does tinnitus, hearing asymmetry, or hearing loss predispose to occupational injury risk? 2015;54:S30−S36. https://doi.org/10.3109/14992027.2014.981305.

43. Helvik AS, Krokstad S, Tambs K. Hearing loss and risk of early retirement. The HUNT study. *Eur J Public Health*. 2013;23(4):617−622. https://doi.org/10.1093/EURPUB/CKS118.

44. Whitson HE, Lin FR. Hearing and vision care for older adults: sensing a need to update medicare policy. *JAMA*. 2014;312(17):1739−1740. https://doi.org/10.1001/JAMA.2014.13535.

45. Jilla AM, Johnson CE, Huntington-Klein N. Hearing aid affordability in the United States. *Disabil Rehabil Assist Technol*. 2023. https://doi.org/10.1080/17483107.2020.1822449.

46. Arnold ML, Hyer K, Chisolm T. Medicaid hearing aid coverage for older adult beneficiaries: a state-by-state comparison. *Health Aff*. 2017;36:8. https://doi.org/10.1377/hlthaff.2016.1610.

47. Planey AM. Audiologist availability and supply in the United States: a multi-scale spatial and political economic analysis. *Social Sci Med*. 2019. https://doi.org/10.1016/j.socscimed.2019.01.015.

48. Arnold ML, Hyer K, Small BJ, et al. Hearing aid prevalence and factors related to use among older adults from the Hispanic community health study/study of Latinos. *JAMA Otolaryngol Head Neck Surg*. 2019;145(6):501−508. https://doi.org/10.1001/JAMAOTO.2019.0433.

49. Choi JS, Shim KS, Kim K, et al. Understanding hearing loss and barriers to hearing health care among Korean American older adults: a focus group study. *J Appl Gerontol*. 2018;37(11):1344−1367. https://doi.org/10.1177/0733464816663554.

50. Arnold ML, Reyes CA, Lugo-Reyes N, Sanchez VA. Hispanic/Latino perspectives on hearing loss and hearing healthcare: focus group results. *Ear Hear*. 2022. https://doi.org/10.1097/AUD.0000000000001268.

51. American Speech-Language-Hearing Association. *Demographic profile of ASHA members providing bilingual services year-end 2020*; 2021. https://www.asha.org/siteassets/surveys/demographic-profile-bilingual-spanish-service-members.pdf. Accessed September 15, 2022.

52. Gubernskaya Z, Bean FD, van Hook J. (Un)Healthy immigrant citizens: naturalization and activity limitations in older age. *J Health Soc Behav*. 2013;54(4):427−443. https://doi.org/10.1177/0022146513504760/ASSET/IMAGES/LARGE/10.1177_00221 46513504760-FIG2.JPEG.

53. Pittman CA, Roura R, Price C, Lin FR, Marrone N, Nieman CL. Racial/ethnic and sex representation in US-based clinical trials of hearing loss management in adults: a systematic review. *JAMA Otolaryngol Head Neck Surg*. 2021;147(7):656−662. https://doi.org/10.1001/jamaoto.2021.0550.

54. Food and Drug Administration. Medical devices; ear, nose, and throat devices; establishing over-the-counter hearing aids. *Fed Regist*. 2022;87(158):50698−50762. www.regulations.gov. Accessed October 16, 2022.

55. Audiologists. https://www.bls.gov/oes/current/oes291181.htm#st. Accessed 28 April 2022.

56. Hearing Aid Specialists. https://www.bls.gov/oes/current/oes292092.htm. Accessed 28 April 2022.

57. U.S. Census Bureau QuickFacts: United States. https://www.census.gov/quickfacts/fact/table/US/PST045221. Accessed 1 May 2022.

58. Katigbak C, van Devanter N, Islam N, Trinh-Shevrin C. Partners in health: a conceptual framework for the role of community health workers in facilitating patients' adoption of healthy behaviors. *Am J Public Health*. 2015;105(5):872−880. https://doi.org/10.2105/AJPH.2014.302411.

59. World Report on Hearing; 2021.

60. Anand TN, Joseph LM, Geetha Av, Prabhakaran D, Jeemon P. Task sharing with non-physician health-care workers for management of blood pressure in low-income and middle-income countries: a systematic review and meta-analysis. *Lancet Glob Health*. 2019;7(6):e761−e771. https://doi.org/10.1016/S2214-109X(19)30077-4.

61. Dawson AJ, Buchan J, Duffield C, Homer CSE, Wijewardena K. Task shifting and sharing in maternal and reproductive health in low-income countries: a narrative synthesis of current evidence. *Health Policy Plan*. 2014;29(3):396−408. https://doi.org/10.1093/HEAPOL/CZT026.

62. Hartzler AL, Tuzzio L, Hsu C, Wagner EH. Roles and functions of community health workers in primary care. *Ann Fam Med*. 2018;16(3):240−245. https://doi.org/10.1370/AFM.2208.

63. Naslund JA, Shidhaye R, Patel V. Digital technology for building capacity of non-specialist health workers for task-sharing and scaling up mental health care globally HHS public access. *Harv Rev Psychiatry*. 2019;27(3):181−192. https://doi.org/10.1097/HRP.0000000000000217.

64. Wadler BM, Judge CM, Prout M, Allen JD, Geller AC. Improving breast cancer control via the use of community health workers in South Africa: a critical review. *J Oncol*. 2011. https://doi.org/10.1155/2011/150423.

65. World Health Organization. Task sharing to improve access to family planning/contraception summary information problem. 2017. https://apps.who.int/iris/bitstream/handle/10665/259633/WHO-RHR-17.20-eng.pdf. Accessed September 26, 2022.

66. Community Health Workers. *U.S. Bureau of Labor Statistics*; 2021. https://www.bls.gov/oes/current/oes211094.htm. Accessed September 22, 2022.

67. O'Donovan J, Verkerk M, Winters N, Chadha S, Bhutta MF. The role of community health workers in addressing the global burden of ear disease and hearing loss: a systematic scoping review of the literature. *BMJ Glob Health*. 2019;4(2), e001141. https://doi.org/10.1136/BMJGH-2018-001141.

68. Suen JJ, Bhatnagar K, Emmett SD, et al. Hearing care across the life course provided in the community. *Bull World Health Organ*. 2019;97(10):681. https://doi.org/10.2471/BLT.18.227371.

69. Nieman CL, Marrone N, Mamo SK, et al. The Baltimore HEARS pilot study: an affordable, accessible, community-delivered hearing care intervention. *Gerontol*. 2017;57(6):1173−1186. https://doi.org/10.1093/geront/gnw153.

70. Nieman CL, Betz J, Garcia Morales EE, et al. Effect of a community health worker−delivered personal sound amplification device on self-perceived communication function in older adults with hearing loss: a randomized clinical trial. *JAMA*. 2022;328(23):2324−2333. https://doi.org/10.1001/JAMA.2022.21820.

71. Marrone N, Ingram M, Somoza M, et al. Interventional audiology to address hearing health care disparities: Oyendo bien pilot study. *Semin Hear*. 2017. https://doi.org/10.1055/s-0037-1601575.

72. Telemedicine | Medicaid. https://www.medicaid.gov/medicaid/benefits/telemedicine/index.html. Accessed 25 September 2022.

73. Sun R, Blayney DW, Hernandez-Boussard T. Health management via telemedicine: learning from the COVID-19 experience. *J Am Med Inf Assoc*. 2021;28(11):2536−2540. https://doi.org/10.1093/JAMIA/OCAB145.

74. Shah ED, Siegel CA. Systems-based strategies to consider treatment costs in clinical practice. *Clin Gastroenterol Hepatol*. 2020;18:1010−1014. https://doi.org/10.1016/j.cgh.2020.02.030.

75. Nouri S, Khoong EC, Lyles CR, Karliner L. Addressing equity in telemedicine for chronic disease management during the Covid-19 pandemic. *NEJM Catal Innov Care Deliv.* 2020;1(3). https://doi.org/10.1056/CAT.20.0123.

76. Ning AY, Cabrera CI, D'Anza B. Telemedicine in otolaryngology: a systematic review of image quality, diagnostic concordance, and patient and provider satisfaction. *Ann Otol Rhinol Laryngol.* 2021;130(2):195—204. https://doi.org/10.1177/0003489420939590/ASSET/IMAGES/LARGE/10.1177_0003489420939590-FIG1.JPEG.

77. Fang CH, Smith RV. COVID-19 and the resurgence of telehealth in otolaryngology tele-health in the COVID-19 pandemic. *Oper Tech Otolaryngol.* 2022;33:158—164. https://doi.org/10.1016/j.otot.2022.04.012.

78. Muñoz K, Nagaraj NK, Nichols N. Applied tele-audiology research in clinical practice during the past decade: a scoping review. *Int J Audiol.* 2020. https://doi.org/10.1080/14992027.2020.1817994.

79. Bush ML, Thompson R, Irungu C, Ent M, Ayugi J. The role of telemedicine in auditory rehabilitation: a systematic review. *Otol Neurotol.* 2016;37(10):1466—1474. https://doi.org/10.1097/MAO.0000000000001236.

80. Tao KFM, Brennan-Jones CG, Capobianco-Fava DM, et al. Teleaudiology services for rehabilitation with hearing aids in adults: a systematic review. *J Speech Lang Hear Res.* 2018. https://doi.org/10.23641/asha.

81. Coco L, Davidson A, Marrone N. The role of patient-site facilitators in teleaudiology: a scoping review. *Am J Audiol.* 2020;29:661—675. https://doi.org/10.23641/asha.

82. Emmett SD, Robler SK, Gallo JJ, Wang NY, Labrique A, Hofstetter P. Hearing Norton Sound: mixed methods protocol of a community randomised trial to address childhood hearing loss in rural Alaska. *BMJ Open.* 2019;9(1), e023081. https://doi.org/10.1136/BMJOPEN-2018-023081.

83. Kokesh J, Ferguson AS, Patricoski C. The Alaska experience using store-and-forward telemedicine for ENT care in Alaska. *Otolaryngol Clin North Am.* 2011;44(6): 1359—1374. https://doi.org/10.1016/J.OTC.2011.08.010.

84. Coco L, Piper R, Marrone N. Feasibility of community health workers as teleaudiology patient-site facilitators: a multilevel training study. *Int J Audiol.* 2021. https://doi.org/10.1080/14992027.2020.1864487.

85. H.R.2430 - 115th Congress (2017—2018): FDA Reauthorization Act of 2017 | Congress.gov | Library of Congress. https://www.congress.gov/bill/115th-congress/house-bill/2430. Accessed 1 May 2022.

86. Text - H.R.5376 - 117th Congress (2021—2022): Build Back Better Act | Congress.gov | Library of Congress. https://www.congress.gov/bill/117th-congress/house-bill/5376/text. Accessed 28 April 2022.

Disparities in cochlear implantation: summary and recommendations

13

Amanda G. Davis[1], Marissa Schuh[1], Karen Hawley[2], Matthew L. Bush[1,3]

[1]*Department of Otolaryngology—Head and Neck Surgery, University of Kentucky, Lexington, KY, United States;* [2]*Pediatric Otolaryngology, Division of Otolaryngology—Head and Neck Surgery, Department of Surgery, University of New Mexico, Albuquerque, NM, United States;* [3]*UK College of Medicine Endowed Chair in Rural Health Policy, Department of Otolaryngology—Head and Neck Surgery, University of Kentucky, Lexington, KY, United States*

Introduction

Cochlear implantation is a surgical procedure that aims to restore hearing for individuals with qualifying hearing loss through the implantation of an electrode array into the cochlea, intended to provide direct stimulation of the cochlear nerve. As a neuro-prosthetic device, a cochlear implant (CI) communicates auditory information to the cochlear nerve through electrical stimulation rather than traditional acoustic stimulation. The system is composed of two components: an internal device that includes the electrode array and an external sound processor. Together, these devices work to convert acoustic sounds into electrical information that is presented to the brain through the cochlear nerve. In general, recipients of a CI can expect that the device increases the perception to and recognition of acoustic sound in their surroundings. Restoring functional hearing through a CI requires consistent use of the device by the patient along with collaborative programming and adjustment of the device between the patient and providers. This process requires extensive time, resources, and rehabilitation efforts, but can be a rewarding experience that greatly improves an individual's functional hearing along with their quality of life.[1,2]

Originally, CIs were approved by the Food and Drug Administration (FDA) in 1984, but the treatment was reserved only for adults with bilateral profound sensorineural hearing loss.[3] However, through time and research, candidacy criteria for those who are eligible to receive a CI have expanded significantly. Today, candidates for CIs take many forms, including adults with bilateral moderate to profound sensorineural hearing loss who do not demonstrate benefit from traditional amplification, children over the age of two with bilateral severe to profound sensorineural hearing loss, children as young as nine months with bilateral profound sensorineural hearing loss, and individuals over the age of five who have single-sided deafness (SSD) or asymmetric hearing loss (AHL).[3,4]

Despite the expansions in candidacy criteria and research supporting the benefits of the use of CIs, the penetration of cochlear implantation into the population of patients who are likely candidates remains disparagingly low in the United States. Recent studies have estimated the range of CI utilization in the United States at around 2.1%—12.7% of those who could benefit from the device.[5–7] A wide variety of social factors have the potential to impact access to and utilization of cochlear implantation, thus it is useful to consider the social determinants of health (SDoH) model to characterize the factors that influence health outcomes. SDoH are henceforth defined as "the conditions in the environments where people are born, live, learn, work, play, worship, and age that affect a wide range of health, functioning, and quality of life outcomes and risks."[8] Broadly, they are classified into the following domains: economic stability, education access and quality, healthcare access and quality, neighborhood and built environment, and social and community context.[8] The SDoH represents an expansive model on the different categories of factors that may influence health outcomes, and within each SDoH domain, there are barriers and facilitators that impact these outcomes. Structural racism and other forms of systematic oppression may impact each of these domains separately and result in health disparities that disproportionately affect marginalized and vulnerable populations. Extrinsic factors, such as laws and policies, can further perpetuate healthcare inequities in cochlear implantation. These factors should be viewed from an intersectional lens; therefore, this chapter aims to address inequity related to cochlear implantation within the framework of adult and pediatric patients' SDoH and other contributive factors.

Disparities in adult cochlear implantation
Disparities in adult diagnosis of hearing loss

The cochlear implantation journey is complex and typically begins with the diagnosis of hearing loss (Fig. 13.1). Goman and Lin[9] estimate that 23% of Americans aged 12 and older have some degree of hearing loss in at least one ear. Historically, literature has suggested that there are sex and racial/ethnic differences in the prevalence of hearing loss, with males generally having a higher prevalence of hearing loss than females, and White and Hispanic patients having a higher prevalence of hearing loss than Black patients across the lifespan.[9–11] Some of these racial differences in hearing loss prevalence have been analyzed from a biological perspective assessing protective factors related to skin pigmentation.[12] However, there is also a critical need to obtain a deeper understanding of hearing loss prevalence in relation to sociodemographic factors, as many of these aspects, such as employment status and type, low socioeconomic status, and low education levels, may disproportionally impact vulnerable populations. An understanding of inequitable access to cochlear implantation cannot be fully grasped until hearing loss is better understood from a social epidemiologic lens.[12]

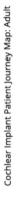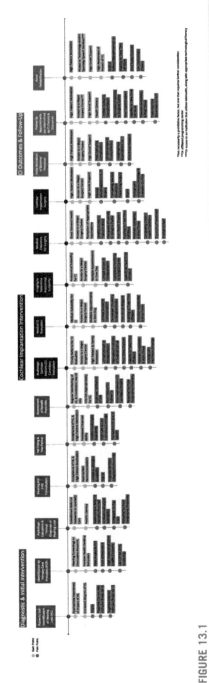

Cochlear Implant Patient Journey Map: Adult

FIGURE 13.1

Journey map illustrating the process of adult cochlear implantation and follow-up care. Elements illustrated in green represent "gain points," or attributes that may facilitate the process, whereas elements illustrated in red represent "pain points," or points that may act as barriers that deter patient success.

Of the estimated 23% of Americans with hearing loss, approximately 2.5% of those individuals have a hearing loss classified as severe to profound in at least one ear—potentially qualifying for a CI.[9] However, the factors influencing patients' behaviors to seek cochlear implantation candidacy remain poorly understood. Most patients who pursue CI candidacy evaluations have much more severe hearing loss than is needed to be considered a candidate, thus, this suggests that patients with hearing loss who are being evaluated for CIs could likely be evaluated and receive this care much sooner.[13] The delays in the utilization of CI are related to limitations in access to diagnostic services. Barriers in access to diagnostic services for potential CI candidates can be classified broadly into two categories: provider-related and patient-related factors. The culmination of these factors creates disproportionate barriers to timely identification and intervention for severe to profound hearing loss across patients from various backgrounds.

Provider factors

Access to hearing healthcare depends, in part, on variables related to the availability and accessibility of hearing healthcare providers. Many patients rely on referral networks from primary care providers to appropriate professionals for intervention services. Further, some insurance payers require a referral for a patient to be seen by a specialist—such as an otolaryngologist or audiologist. However, there are few established standards in monitoring hearing loss in primary care settings that would consistently lead to such referrals, especially for adults. Lack of consistent routine hearing screenings for adult patients in primary care offices, and other more widely accessible settings, is commonly cited as a reason for poor utilization of hearing healthcare.[5,7,14,15] When conversations regarding hearing loss are not initiated by the provider, patients may be less likely to discuss their hearing difficulties with providers due to underestimation of the impact of hearing loss, stigma, or other factors.[14,15] As patients progress to a hearing loss that may qualify for cochlear implantation, there is an increased likelihood that they will discuss the impact of their hearing loss with providers sooner.[16] However, when the progression of hearing loss is gradual over time, patients may experience a longer duration of untreated hearing loss, increasing the potential time for auditory deprivation, social withdrawal, socioeconomic decline, and other negative health impacts.[17–19] When patients do present with concerns for hearing, it is critical that primary care providers are knowledgeable about appropriate referral networks to hearing healthcare specialists. At present, it is estimated that less than 5% of patients referred for cochlear implantation evaluation by their primary care physician actually follow-through with the referral visit.[5] This lack of guidance leaves many patients left unsure about avenues for the next steps in hearing intervention and may leave them vulnerable to misconceptions about CI candidacy.

When referrals are made to hearing healthcare specialists, the supply, location, and availability of those providers may present as a barrier to timely care. Unfortunately, there are presently not enough audiologists to provide treatment for those with hearing loss,[16,20] and even fewer who specialize in CI programming—

estimated at approximately 11% in 2018.[21] In a study of the widespread availability of audiologists across the United States, Planey[20] found that audiologists are only found in approximately 44% of counties, more often in urban/metro counties with higher general socioeconomic status. These provider factors create and perpetuate barriers in access to care, as patients from rural areas may have to travel greater distances to receive audiologic treatment, placing strain on time and financial resources. Similar to that of primary care providers, research has found that there is a low referral rate for cochlear implantation candidacy evaluations even among hearing healthcare providers, such as audiologists and otolaryngologists.[13,15,22]

Patient factors

There are several domains of the SDoH that are associated with inequitable access to diagnostic hearing healthcare, and each of these domains may be influenced by sociodemographic factors such as race, geographic location, socioeconomic status, and education. At present, there is a limited body of research on racial disparities in access to diagnostic hearing healthcare. Some research indicates that Mexican American populations are less likely to interact with diagnostic hearing healthcare services,[23] but Black Americans are more likely to have had a recent hearing evaluation as compared to White Americans.[24] Lower education levels are also commonly cited as an intersectional factor when assessing patients' interaction with diagnostic hearing health services. Patients with lower education levels are less likely to have received a recent hearing evaluation despite having a higher incidence of hearing loss due to noise exposure.[24,25] Several studies cite lower socioeconomic status as an inhibitor to patients receiving timely hearing healthcare services.[26–28] Patient insurance status is closely related to socioeconomic status and access to hearing healthcare, as there is inequitable coverage of audiologic services across state Medicaid programs.[20,29] Geographic location, as previously mentioned, may also influence timing of audiologic intervention. There is a greater time to diagnosis of hearing loss among those who live in rural areas as compared to patients in more urban areas.[27,30] Other barriers to hearing healthcare include negative societal attitudes toward aging, disability, and hearing loss that perpetuate stigma among communities.[26,31] The impact of these negative attitudes is seen across a diverse range of ethnic and racial backgrounds, but is especially prominent in minority communities.[32,33]

Access to hearing aids

The impact of inequitable access to diagnostic hearing healthcare further influences access to timely audiologic intervention with amplification. Before cochlear implantation is considered, many centers require that patients have utilized appropriately fit amplification devices, such as hearing aids, to evaluate for possible benefit. Similar to CIs, the market penetration of hearing aids is generally low across the adult population.[34] While amplification utilization rates for individuals with severe to profound hearing loss are higher,[35] those patients may still have delays in obtaining amplification. Nieman et al.[24] found that there are racial and socioeconomic factors that influence access to amplification; while Black Americans were more likely to have had recent diagnostic hearing testing, White patients were more likely to obtain hearing aids. This factor is critical, as the duration of auditory deprivation may serve as a predictor for postlingually deafened adults who undergo cochlear implantation; outcomes decline with increased delays.[36,37] These SDoH-related factors contributing to delay in traditional amplification may have subsequent effects that disproportionately influence outcomes with CIs.

Cochlear implant evaluations

After the diagnosis of hearing loss has been established, the process of obtaining a CI begins with a candidacy evaluation involving several medical professionals. Candidacy is determined by an extensive audiologic evaluation and a medical evaluation from an otolaryngologist who performs cochlear implantation. Preoperative medical evaluations may involve primary care and/or specialist assessments with diagnostic testing to provide clearance for surgery. CI candidates typically undergo a radiographic imaging procedure, as well as appropriate vaccinations prior to surgery. Appointments with other specialists to determine suitability for anesthesia may also be warranted. This complex series of appointments can be taxing on a patient's time and finances and can place a high demand on limited resources even prior to implantation. Many of these specialist appointments are localized to major cities,[20,21] with limited availability and longer wait times.

There are a variety of factors influencing patterns of referrals for cochlear implantation evaluation, many of which are related to patients' SDoH. When considering the preoperative presentation of patients who are pursuing cochlear implantation, several studies observe significant differences in evaluation based on race, with minority populations referred at disproportionately lower rates.[13,38] When referred, Black patients had worse preoperative scores for both pure tones and speech discrimination indicating more advanced degrees of hearing loss and that they were likely candidates for CI much earlier.[38] Tolisano et al.[39] found that of the patients who present for cochlear implantation candidacy determination, the majority of patients assessed that personally owned hearing aids were White individuals, potentially indicating a shorter duration of auditory deprivation. Disparities are also seen in patients based on geographic location; in addition to the delay in amplification, Hixon et al.[27] found that there are significantly greater time intervals between diagnosis of hearing loss and cochlear implantation among patients in rural areas compared with those from urban areas.

Further, standards for audiometric qualification for cochlear implantation vary based on the insurance coverage. At present, Medicare has a stricter set of requirements for CI candidacy, poorly aligned compared to those of private insurance companies who may more frequently update their coverage regulations.[3,40] Interestingly, Tolisano et al.[41] found that the majority of patients present for CI evaluation with public insurance, particularly Medicare. Given stricter requirements for candidacy in the context of expanded indications for cochlear implantation, there may be many patients for whom insurance restrictions prohibit timely intervention.[13]

Disparities in adult CI surgery

Once candidacy has been determined, the patient may then elect to undergo cochlear implantation surgery. Cochlear implantation is a process and not a transaction, thus the decision to proceed with surgery and CI rehabilitation involves complex considerations on the part of the patient. Historically, there has been a long duration of untreated severe to profound hearing loss before adult patients elect to pursue surgery, greater than 10 years on average.[15] This delay, in part, may be due to several of the factors already discussed within the context of this chapter, compounding over time.

Several major cochlear implantation centers have found similar patterns in patients who present for surgery. Of those who present for evaluation, surgical centers have found that approximately 62%–82% of adult patients who qualified for cochlear implantation elected to undergo surgery.[13,38,41] Generally, the average profile for these patients is White, non-Hispanic individuals in their fifth and 6th decade of life, with English as their primary language.[41–43] With surgical centers existing primarily in urban environments, some studies have found the majority of patients live at a median of 30.8 miles away from their surgery center.[41] Other studies have found that rural patients reside typically within 100 miles (71%) of the implanting institution.[43] These discrepancies are likely dependent on the regional composition of the state.

Factors associated with patients' SDoH have been found to influence access to cochlear implantation. Interestingly, Mahendran et al.[38] found that of patients who are referred, Black and White patients undergo cochlear implantation at the same rate. However, preoperative presentation of those patients differed significantly in degree of hearing loss and preoperative speech discrimination scores, with Black patients having significantly worse scores.[38] However, Dornhoffer et al.[43] found that non-White patients were half as likely as White patients to pursue cochlear implantation after candidacy was determined, and found that non-White patients and those with increased age had an increased time from diagnosis of hearing loss to cochlear implantation.[43] Additionally, these patients had worse degrees of hearing loss as measured by their pure-tone average, were less likely to use hearing aids prior to surgery, and generally had lower scores on speech discrimination metrics used to determine candidacy for implantation.[43] Geographic location also presents barriers to cochlear implantation, as greater travel distances correlate with older age at cochlear implantation.[42] Further, social and community variables, such as health literacy and misconception regarding cochlear implantation, the impact of societal attitudes toward disability, and the stigma surrounding cochlear implantation, may also deter patients from pursuing surgical intervention.[44–46]

Discrepancies in insurance coverage also present as a potential barrier to cochlear implantation. Under current regulations, Medicare covers 80% of surgical costs, leaving patients with an additional 20% responsibility.[3,40] Given the high costs of cochlear implantation, this financial responsibility may be too substantial for patients from lower socioeconomic backgrounds, especially if there is no secondary insurance to aid. Additionally, patients with Medicaid undergo cochlear implantation at a lower rate, partially due to issues with obtaining authorization for surgery and a more stringent reimbursement rate for the procedure and other related services.[47] While cochlear implantation centers are already sparse across the United States, there are even fewer facilities that accept Medicaid insurance coverage for cochlear implantation due to low reimbursement rates.[20,47]

Disparities in adult CI outcomes

Generally, there is a limited body of research investigating follow-up patterns for adult CI recipients, making factors that either facilitate or deter attendance poorly understood. There is little evidence that describes the variation in performance outcomes for adults, especially in relation to SDoH-related factors. Some literature suggests that there may be a significant effect of insurance status on speech discrimination outcomes on both CNC words and AzBio sentences, indicating that patients with public insurance (e.g., Medicare and Medicaid) have poorer scores on both metrics, even when age at implantation is a controlled variable.[40] Mahendran et al.[38] found that Black patients who pursued a CI had significantly worse scores on speech discrimination outcomes, as measured by performance on AzBio sentences, than White patients. The impact of other elements of patients' SDoH on outcomes with CI, such as geographic location, education status, and other factors, has not been extensively studied.

Several studies have suggested that time to implantation and duration of auditory deprivation have a significant impact on postoperative outcomes.[36,37,43] As discussed in the diagnostic section of this chapter, there are several factors related to patients' SDoH that delay time to cochlear implantation. More research is needed to determine the degree to which these factors are influencing patients' timeline to cochlear implantation and their subsequent outcomes if they elect to pursue surgery.

Aural rehabilitation

Generally, recommendations for adult aural rehabilitation after cochlear implantation are inconsistent, as there is no defined protocol for best practice, despite the observation of benefits from extensive aural rehabilitation after cochlear implantation documented in the literature.[48] Hjaldahl et al.[49] identified several demographic factors related to patients who are more likely to elect to participate in extensive aural rehabilitation, including younger age, female sex, earlier onset of hearing loss, worse degree of preoperative hearing loss, self-perception of the impact of hearing loss, and ability to utilize sick leave from work. Patients' success with aural rehabilitation increased with familiarity with electronic tablets, a common source of informal auditory rehabilitation exercises, in-home familial support, and consultation with a trained auditory rehabilitation therapist.[50] Participation in aural rehabilitation as related to SDoH factors is not well known, but serves as an area for more research in order to equitably optimize the outcomes of CI recipients.

Summary and recommendations

Overall, barriers that impede adult patients' ability to pursue cochlear implantation begin at the diagnostic evaluation of hearing loss and persist throughout the surgical and rehabilitative process. These barriers are deeply intersectional and multifactorial, existing at the individual patient level by way of SDoH, the institutional level, and broad-scale systemic levels. The first step in ameliorating these barriers begins at a more universal awareness of their existence and potential impact. Creative and intentional solutions to these barriers may include (1) more expansive education regarding hearing loss, cochlear implantation, and CI candidacy criteria for primary care providers and specialty providers involved in hearing healthcare, (2) implementation of routine hearing screenings for the adult population, (3) utilization of telemedicine for cochlear implantation preoperative counseling and follow-up mapping to decrease travel burdens, and (4) targeted identification and intervention for vulnerable populations.

Disparities in pediatric cochlear implantation

Evidence also demonstrates that there are growing disparities among cochlear implantation rates as well as speech and language outcomes after implantation in the pediatric population.[51] The process of pediatric cochlear implantation can also be complex, and multiple barriers at various timepoints may prevent timely care delivery (Fig. 13.2). These disparities are, in part, a result of the SDoH and the interplay between them. These factors determine if and when a child receives a CI, what outcomes they will experience, and how those outcomes will impact the child's quality of life. Cochlear implantation in the pediatric population may provide unique challenges for each child and family; however, health disparities can magnify these challenges with respect to diagnosis, surgical access, and outcomes.

Disparities in pediatric diagnosis of hearing loss

Hearing loss in the pediatric population may either be congenital, acquired, or progressive over time. Further, the origins of hearing loss may be genetic in nature, or secondary to nongenetic factors, such as congenital infection, exposure to intrauterine toxins, or other elements. Congenital hearing loss is present in one to two per 1000 infants and increases significantly among babies who are admitted into the neonatal intensive care unit (NICU). The incidence of congenital hearing loss increases in children who are socioeconomically disadvantaged and in those who are non-White race.[52–54] Congenital CMV (cCMV) is the most common nonhereditary cause of congenital hearing loss, and it is the most common intrauterine viral infection. Independent of race, cCMV has a higher prevalence in women living in neighborhoods with lower socioeconomic status.[52,55] In addition to higher cCMV prevalence, children born with other risk factors for congenital hearing loss,

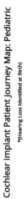

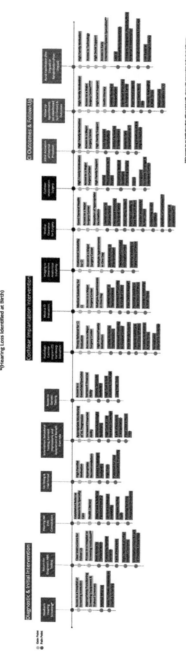

FIGURE 13.2

Journey map illustrating the process of pediatric cochlear implantation and follow-up care. Elements illustrated in green represent "gain points," or attributes that may facilitate the process, whereas elements illustrated in red represent "pain points," or points that may act as barriers that deter patient success.

including lower birth weight and family history of deafness are also found in populations who are socioeconomically disadvantaged.[53,56]

When considering hearing losses related to genetic factors, GJB2 is the most common genetic cause of nonsyndromic hearing loss, is the most frequently studied gene associated with hearing loss, and is less commonly identified in Black patients. Furthermore, Chan et al.[57] found that Asian children were more likely to have genetic mutations in GJB2 associated with hearing loss compared to White and Hispanic children. The discrepancies in identification of genes related to hearing loss across racial and ethnic groups in may be secondary to fewer instances of genetic testing completed in minority populations, as will be discussed subsequently in this chapter. Further studies are needed to identify genetic causes of hearing loss in Black and Hispanic children.[58]

There is well-established literature suggesting that earlier diagnosis and management of children with any level of hearing loss can greatly benefit speech and language outcomes, educational performance, and quality-of-life measures.[54,59,60] In order to accomplish these goals, the Joint Commission on Infant Hearing (JCIH) recommends infants are screened for hearing loss no later than one month of age, undergo diagnostic audiometric testing by three months of age, and have access to early intervention (EI) by six months of age.[61] The first step in the diagnosis of pediatric hearing loss is the universal newborn hearing screening (NBHS) that is conducted shortly after birth. For those newborns who fail the NBHS, more comprehensive follow-up diagnostic testing is recommended; however, the testing is underutilized. In 2019, although greater than 98% of infants born in the United States received a newborn hearing screen, 27.5% of infants who referred on their NBHS were lost to follow-up (LTF) and did not undergo the appropriate audiological work-up.[62] Of the infants who were diagnosed with a hearing loss, more than 20% of them were diagnosed after the age of three months, in poor accordance with JCIH guidelines. Infants who were publicly insured were more likely to experience delays nearly twice as long in obtaining comprehensive diagnostic testing compared to those insured privately.[63,64] Risk factors for a delay in diagnosis have been identified by studying national EHDI (Early Hearing Detection and Intervention) data. Infants who have had a delayed diagnosis of hearing loss are more likely to be of non-White race, have a lower birthweight, public insurance, live outside a metropolitan area, and have a mother with lower level of education or a mother <25 years of age.[64–67]

Addressing the issue of infants with hearing loss who are LTF has been a recent priority. Historically, approximately two-thirds of infants who referred on their NBHS did not have audiological diagnostic testing documented in the EHDI system in 2005; therefore, yielding an LTF rate of approximately 67%.[62] The Hearing Screening Follow up Survey (HSFS) was developed to improve documentation and further clarify the causes of LTF. Four categories pertaining to systemic barriers in adhering to the JCIH 1-3-6 goals were identified. These included (a) lack of service system capacity, (b) lack of provider knowledge, (c) challenges to families obtaining services, and (d) information gaps. Efforts have been made to improve the timing, completeness, and accuracy of data recording within the EHDI system. Therefore, enhancements in EHDI-IS (EHDI-Information Systems) have yielded an improved rate for LTF in the EHDI Database from 68.1% in 2005 to 27.5% in 2019.[62] This development suggests that with more complete and accurate data, we are now able to better understand the underlying patient and systemic issues related to LTF, but more work is needed to continue to improve the LTF ratio and better address the underlying causes for LTF.

Data is not consistently recorded with respect to maternal demographics, which could help elucidate underlying patient factors related to LTF. In states that do have a higher rate of maternal demographic data, it has been shown that an increased risk of LTF is associated with younger maternal age, mothers with less than a high school degree, race identified as non-White, carrying public health insurance, and living in a rural community.[54,68] Additionally, LTF rates are higher among infants with conductive hearing loss compared to those with sensorineural hearing loss.[68] Infants with unilateral hearing loss also had higher LTF rates compared to infants with bilateral hearing loss.[68]

Further increasing the critical nature of addressing LTF, the JCIH guidelines recommend follow-up audiometric testing in children with specific risk factors for progressive hearing loss or delayed onset hearing loss; however, these data are not well tracked. Approximately 25% of children with significant permanent childhood hearing loss in an Australian study developed their hearing loss in the postnatal period and therefore were not detected with NBHS.[69] Children with progressive hearing loss must be monitored, as they may eventually qualify for cochlear implantation. Young et al.[69] studied 391 pediatric CI recipients and found that nearly 30% passed their NBHS, suggesting that their hearing loss progressed over time. Children who passed their NBHS but eventually pursued cochlear implantation were significantly older at the time of initial diagnosis of hearing loss, diagnosis of severe to profound hearing loss, and age at implantation.

Following the diagnosis, it is recommended that a child with qualifying hearing loss is medically evaluated prior to cochlear implantation. This evaluation typically includes, but is not limited to, physical evaluation, subsequent audiological evaluation to determine CI candidacy when age appropriate, medical history (i.e., cCMV or NICU), laboratory testing, electrocardiogram, imaging (i.e., CT or MRI), and genetic testing.[70] The consensus statement from the International Pediatric Otolaryngology Group recommends genetic testing for patients with bilateral sensorineural hearing loss as it is felt to add diagnostic and prognostic value.[71] A study assessing a private insurance database identified over 65,000 unique children with sensorineural hearing loss and found that Black children or children that come from a family with an annual income under $100,000 may be less likely to undergo genetic testing or MRI.[72] Interestingly, those who do undergo genetic testing are more likely to have a definitive diagnosis if they are Asian or White (26% and 46%) children and less likely if they are Black or Hispanic (10% and 13%) children.[71]

Access to hearing aids and early intervention

Following the diagnosis of hearing loss, a child must then have immediate access to EI, amplification, and medical evaluation for optimal development of spoken language.[66,73] The SDoH can influence if and when a child receives amplification and EI. Children who are diagnosed with a hearing loss and receive amplification by six months of age have been shown to have better language outcomes at two, three, four, five, and six years of age when compared to peers who were amplified later.[73] Bush et al.[74] found that children who reside in rural areas are delayed in receiving amplification compared to their urban peers. This delay could be due to limited access to hearing healthcare services and poorer health outcomes in rural regions. Additionally, insurance coverage may influence when and if a child receives a hearing aid. Children who are privately insured face greater financial distress and poor reimbursement of hearing aids compared to those covered by Medicaid.[75] However, one study found that children who have public insurance reported increased difficulty in acquiring hearing aids.[63] Research found that lower levels of maternal education are associated with delays in hearing aid fitting and EI.[67] In 2019, only 61.7% of children with a diagnosed hearing loss were enrolled in EI, and 44.7% of children with a hearing loss were enrolled before six months of age.[62] SDoH can greatly impact the utilization of EI services, and unfortunately, parents with a lower level of education and income, as well as ethnic minority status have greater challenges in accessing EI.[76]

Cochlear implant evaluations

Overall, the implementation of the universal NBHS program has allowed for an earlier age of diagnosis and audiologic management of congenital hearing loss.[60,69] As a child progresses in age, hearing sensitivity should continue to be monitored to ensure timely intervention with cochlear implantation, if applicable. Research indicates that early implantation allows for optimal speech outcomes and auditory performance,[77–79] though this timing relies on prompt diagnosis and management as outlined by the JCIH. These findings supported the FDA's approval of cochlear implantation in children with bilateral profound sensorineural hearing loss aged nine months and older in 2020. To support equitable optimal outcomes for all children, it is essential that systemic barriers to cochlear implantation are identified and addressed.

The primary goals for cochlear implantation include the acquisition of sound and the ability to use spoken language for communication. Several factors can determine the language outcomes for children with congenital hearing loss or prelingual deafness. The Children's Implant Profile (CHIP) outlines 11 variables commonly assessed when deciding on whether or not a child is a good candidate for a CI (See Table 13.1).[80] Although a few of these variables directly reflect upon family and educational support structures, most of the variables are affected indirectly by health inequities.[81] Children with sociodemographic disadvantages have confounding variables which may contribute to poorer outcomes in cochlear implantation (See Disparities in Pediatric CI Outcomes).

Table 13.1 Journey map of adult cochlear implant process.

Children's implant profile (ChIP) variables	
Chronological age	Duration of deafness
Medical/radiological abnormalities	Multiple handicaps
Functional hearing	Speech and language abilities
Family structure/support	Expectations: parents and child
Educational environment	Availability: support service
Cognitive/learning style	

Disparities in pediatric CI surgery

The SDoH also influence which children are receiving cochlear implantation surgery and when that surgery takes place during their lifetime. Some of those determinants are influenced by racial and ethnic status, parental education, household income, insurance status, and geographic location. These factors can also interact with one another to cause further disparities related to cochlear implantation.

A child's race and ethnicity may play a role in their likelihood to not only receive a CI but also when the implantation occurs. Pediatric patients from minority races or ethnicities are underrepresented compared to White children when it comes to implantation surgery.[82] For example, rates of cochlear implantation among White children are three times higher compared to Hispanic children and 10 times higher compared to African American children.[83] White and Asian children are twice as likely to be implanted compared to Black or Hispanic children.[84,85] In addition to reduced implantation rates, non-White pediatric patients also face delays from time of diagnosis to surgical intervention, which has downstream effects on developmental outcomes. Black and Hispanic children are less likely to get implanted before age 2, and the gap is further exacerbated when looking at cochlear implantation before 1 year of age.[86] Additionally, Liu et al.[86] found that 0% of Black children were implanted before 12 months of age and that White children who were Medicaid-insured were more likely to get implanted before 2 years of age compared to Black children with private insurance. Some of these race and ethnicity-based disparities could be a result of the intersection of multiple SDoH.

Household income and parental education may also influence the timeline for if and when a child receives CI surgery. Research shows that children who receive CIs are more likely to come from families whose household income is $100,000 or greater.[82] Furthermore, children from lower income households tend to be premature and have poorer health or complex comorbidities that can delay implantation.[85,87] Families with lower incomes experience a lack of access to educational resources or social support services, and greater difficulty in attending appointments, which can be barriers resulting in missed or delayed appointments that affect the timing of implantation as well.[77,85] Moreover, lower income families are associated with lower educational attainment, which affects when a child undergoes implantation.[85] For instance, research shows that delays in pediatric cochlear implantation were correlated with parents of lower educational level.[87] Fujiwara et al.[88] also found that higher maternal education resulted in increased rates of cochlear implantation before 2 years of age. Similar to race and ethnicity, household income and parental education can affect and interact with other SDOH, such as insurance, to exacerbate disparities.

The impact of insurance status on pediatric cochlear implantation disparities has been well described in the literature. Most children who undergo implantation come from families with private insurance versus Medicaid.[63,83,89] This disparity could be due to the different Medicaid coverage and reimbursement rates for cochlear implantation. Despite coverage for CIs under Medicaid in all 50 states for pediatric patients, states vary in their coverage and services, including reimbursement for surgery and services, equipment replacement, limitations on amount of therapy, and authorization for CI procedures and services.[47] These restrictions greatly affect low-income families, who already encounter other barriers as previously mentioned. The lack of Medicaid coverage also affects how healthcare providers care for their pediatric patients. In one study, clinics reported that poor reimbursement of CIs from Medicaid is a major challenge to providing care.[47] Insurance status also affects whether or not a child receives unilateral or bilateral implants. Chang et al.[90] found that implanted children insured by Medicaid were half as likely to receive sequential bilateral CIs compareed to children with private insurance. In some states, Medicaid will only reimburse for one implant of a bilateral surgery, which forces the family to undergo and pay for a second surgery to receive the additional implant.[47] Delayed or nonexistent bilateral implantation can negatively impact language, social, and educational development, as well as vestibular and balance functioning in children.[91–95] Insurance also the timing of CI placement in children. For example, research found that those with private insurance are more likely to get implanted at a younger age and within a year of diagnosis.[85] The same study found that uninsured or delays in obtaining insurance resulted in delays of cochlear implantation.[85] Additionally, Medicaid-insured children have a longer time period between diagnosis and implantation.[96] These children also are less likely to receive CIs before the age of two years, which can have a negative downstream effect on language development.[88] In addition to the coverage limitations, publicly insured families reported a lack of communication as the most common barrier to CI care compared to privately insured families who reported taking time off of work as the biggest barrier to care.[96] There is substantial evidence demonstrating the need for states to change reimbursement rates for CIs in order to close the gap in pediatric disparities.

Alongside the other aforementioned SDoH, where a child lives predisposes their access to cochlear implantation surgery. Stern et al.[83] found that most children who received implants lived in areas where the population was composed of White individuals with higher education and greater wealth. The study also noted that most children were implanted at urban hospitals, given the lack of otolaryngologists in rural communities.[83] Reduced availability of providers in rural areas may play a role in when pediatric patients receive their CIs. Research shows that children from rural areas are delayed in cochlear implantation compared to children from urban areas despite more rural children having bilateral CIs compared to their urban counterparts.[74,79] This finding is not surprising, given that those rural families have to travel a greater distance to attend appointments, both before and after implantation, compared to those from urban ones.[74,79] Increasing availability of providers in rural communities may reduce geographic disparities among children receiving a CI.

Disparities in pediatric CI outcomes

The SDoH not only affects if and when a child receives a CI but also the outcomes postsurgery. These outcomes include surgical, auditory, and speech and language development, which can play a role in a child's overall development and quality of life. For example, insurance status is associated with postsurgery complications in pediatric patients. One study found that implanted children who were Medicaid-insured were five times more likely to have postoperative complications, both minor and major, than those who were privately insured.[90] Additionally, pediatric patients from rural areas are more likely to undergo revision implant surgery due to increased rates of trauma and infection.[97] In some cases, children may experience issues with their CI devices after surgery and those who are publicly insured face barriers to getting the device issues resolved. A survey of audiologists reported that children from Medicaid-insured families experience more broken equipment than those who are privately insured.[51] Medicaid rules make it challenging for patients to receive equipment upgrades or replacements, such as new processors or batteries for devices.[47] This lack of coverage could result in those pediatric patients becoming nonusers due to nonworking devices, which could affect other developmental outcomes.

Auditory outcomes, as well as speech and language outcomes, differ among pediatric CI patients due to a variety of SDoH. A systematic review observed that poor auditory performance in children postimplantation was associated with lower income.[98] Children from low income families also experience worse speech and language outcomes postimplantation.[51,82,99] These negative outcomes could be due to lower self-efficacy among parents of low-income families on how to navigate the healthcare systems.[51] Additionally, insurance type affects speech and hearing outcomes among pediatric patients. Research shows that Medicaid-insured children were not only less likely to receive therapy but also had significant delays in postimplantation sound recognition via the Ling-6 sound test.[63,100] This may result in further speech and language delays, which can affect academic performance and employment opportunities down the line.[101] These same children also experience worse language outcomes, regardless of unilateral or bilateral implantation.[94] This pediatric population faces greater disparity when it comes to speech and language outcomes due to delays in implantation. Research found that children who are implanted at a later age have poorer speech and language outcomes and a lesser quality of life postimplantation compared to those implanted at an earlier age.[77,102–104] In addition to household income and insurance status influences, children from non-English-speaking families encounter similar delays in language development compared to those from English speaking families.[105,106] These non-English-speaking children face greater difficulty in accessing interventions and educational accommodations compared to English-speaking families, and most of the time the accommodations are not in the child's native language.[63] Furthermore, studies have found that higher maternal education resulted in better or improved language development and auditory progress among pediatric CI recipients.[98,107,108] CI providers need to consider how the SDoH will affect a child's outcomes postimplantation and incorporate this into preoperative counseling as well as postoperative expectations.

Aural rehabilitation

Postsurgery rehabilitation and follow-up compliance are shaped by the SDoH as well. Access to rehabilitation services postimplantation varies for different pediatric populations. For instance, research indicates that limited education and economic resources have the greatest influence on access to rehabilitation services in pediatric patients.[51] This finding is reflected in the evidence that children from low-income families are less likely to receive appropriate rehabilitation information when not provided by early intervention services.[82] Noblitt et al.[109] found that low-income families experience a lack of local speech services for their child. The same study noted that lower parental education was also associated with a lack of local speech services and a reduced utilization of those services.[109] This absence and poor utilization of services can further worsen the speech and language outcomes among low-income children as stated previously. Insurance type also influences if and where pediatric patients can receive rehabilitation services postimplantation. Medicaid places limitations on the amount of coverage for CI rehabilitation services, preventing children from receiving sufficient therapy.[47,102] For example, one clinic reported that the Medicaid managed care organization restricted therapy sessions to 5–10 per year despite medical recommendations for weekly sessions for the first one–two years postsurgery.[47]

The location of where children attend or access rehabilitation services is governed by the SDoH. Children from rural areas who receive a CI are more likely to use the school services for speech therapy compared to children residing in urban areas due to a lack of providers in their communities.[109] Additionally, implanted children who are privately insured are more likely to attend schools with specialized hearing loss services compared to Medicaid-insured children. This lack of access to specialized services (i.e., therapist with CI expertise) can play a role in the language, auditory, and educational delays and subsequent poor outcomes in Medicaid-insured children.[102] Pediatric patients who are both Medicaid-insured and reside in rural areas have historically faced limited or no coverage for teletherapy for cochlear implant care.[47]

Follow-up appointments

The issue of accessibility of services results in the likelihood that these pediatric patients may not have adequate follow-up. Medicaid-insured patients are more likely to miss or cancel appointments postsurgery compared to privately insured patients.[90] Another study noted that missing mapping appointments was associated with later age of implantation, which typically happens among children insured by Medicaid.[110] The same patients are also more likely to no-show for consecutive follow-up appointments, which indicates that those Medicaid-insured patients have longer intervals between follow-up appointments.[90] Alongside insurance, rurality affects attendance to follow-up appointments. Dham et al.[97] found that CI patients from rural areas were more likely to drop out of rehabilitation services compared to their urban counterparts, which may result in pediatric patients becoming nonusers. Among Medicaid-insured patients, those with postsurgery complications were less compliant with follow-up compared to privately insured patients.[90] Furthermore, one study of audiologists found that a greater proportion of children from low-income families tend to be non-compliant users.[51] These two findings are significant as noncompliant users from these populations have a greater risk for suboptimal speech and language outcomes as well as severe medical outcomes.[110]

Summary and recommendations

There is clear evidence that the SDoH and the interactions among them create disparities among pediatric CI recipients. However, future work remains to address and alleviate the current disparities. Information on cochlear implantation for children needs to be widely disseminated among all families regardless of race, ethnicity, geographic location, or socioeconomic status.[82,90] Increasing access and utilization of services among underserved populations will help make CIs equitable to all and allow for better outcomes. Specifically, research supports increasing access to spoken language therapy among low-income families as well as non-English-speaking families.[63,82] Moreover, there is a great need to increase the amount of CI providers and therapists, as well as expand on the diversity of those providers to create an inclusive environment for minority and non-English-speaking populations.[90] Insurance coverage of pediatric CI through Medicaid should be expanded across states with current lower-coverage rates to reduce disparity among access and implantation between privately and Medicaid-insured patients. This recommendation may warrant researchers to further analyze pediatric implantation data by each state given the varying reimbursement rates. Lastly, providers should alter pediatric CI care plans to promote self-efficacy and compliance among disadvantaged families. Some changes could include further education and training for families, additional social support, automated appointment reminders, and hands-on longitudinal care.[77] Overall, future research needs to continue to analyze how SDoH exacerbate disparities that affect diagnosis, implantation, and outcomes among pediatric CI patients and then develop programs or interventions to address those disparities.

Telehealth in the setting of cochlear implantation

As reviewed in this chapter, one major barrier related to adult and pediatric CI work-up, management, and follow-up is distance to specialized services. Telehealth has been an expanding entity within the healthcare delivery system over the last two-and-a-half decades, with exponential growth during the COVID-19 pandemic.[111] This service offers opportunities to provide tertiary care services to patients who have travel limitations related to physical disabilities, distance, or time. It has also been found to be desirable to patients living in rural communities and to providers who are able to offer such services.[112–114]

Telehealth has been adapted into the field of audiology, to be known as "tele-audiology." Tele-audiology services can be implemented in a number of ways, including home-based otoscopy using a smart phone-based device, or local office-based hearing screenings or diagnostic evaluations conducted with distortion product otoacoustic emissions (dpOAEs) or tympanometry completed with an on-site facilitator and interactive video and screen sharing software.[113] Expanding technology allows for differentiation between types of hearing loss, but these systems are limited by levels of background noise and accuracy with a mixed hearing loss.[113,115] Similarly, diagnostic auditory brainstem response (ABR) tests can be accomplished with an audiologist interpreting and guiding the testing from a remote location, where the set up and test delivery are collaboratively carried out by an on-site facilitator. This has been studied in both the pediatric and adult population, demonstrating tele-ABR to have results comparable to in-person ABR.[113,114,116] Encouragingly, Dharmar et al.[114] was able to demonstrate tele-ABR can decrease the LTF rates for infants who refer on their NBHS. Outside of the scope of diagnostics, tele-audiology can also be used for the remote programming of hearing aids and remote mapping of cochlear implants. This generally requires specialized equipment, and thus an on-site trained facilitator is required in addition to an experienced audiologist who can work with the patient via teleconferencing.[113,117–119] Future work is needed to determine the equity in access to these tele-audiology services in regard to insurance coverage and state guidelines.

As discussed earlier in this chapter, speech therapy and aural rehabilitation are key factors when discussing the outcomes for CI patients. Similar to audiology services, long distance travel can limit a patient's access to specialized speech services. Such services have been demonstrated as feasible when provided in a remote manner. The evidence to support the use of telehealth for speech and language therapy is encouraging, but quality studies are still limited.[120]

With the rapid expansion of telephone and internet access, telehealth provides a promising delivery system for those who are limited by distance or travel to specialty services. However, limitations still exist for this patient population, and some propose that telehealth may in fact widen disparities due to "the digital divide."[113,121] The same SDoH leading to healthcare disparities may also provide challenges for patients attempting to access and navigate the telehealth delivery model. These factors may include language barriers, poverty, lower digital literacy, limited access to sufficient broadband, and difficulty in accessing a secure and private space for teleconferencing. Although around 7% of Americans overall do not have access to an internet speed of 25mbps/3mbps (the speed deemed necessary for telehealth communication), up to 50% of patients in rural or tribal households do not have broadband access.[113,121,122] The quality of broadband necessary for complex diagnostic tele-audiology is likely greater than this minimal speed.[113] Additionally, people with an income of less than $30,000 are more likely to be reliant on smart phones for internet usage, and these devices are significantly more limited in the context of tele-audiology services.[121] Several studies have looked at populations who have shown a reduced utilization of telehealth services when compared to the general population; at risk groups included non-White patients, patients with public insurance, patients with less than a college degree, and patients with lower income.[121,123] These are populations which have been demonstrated to be marginalized within other sections of this chapter.

Telehealth offers a promising modality to improve access to tertiary care. Through tele-audiology and remote speech rehabilitation, many of the steps to becoming a successful cochlear implant user may be achieved. However, we must use caution in assuming the access and utilization of digital technology is not affected by the SDoH. Further research into these health disparities, along with programmatic development to improve access is warranted.

Summary and future directions

This chapter reveals how the SDoH influence and interact to create disparities among adult and pediatric patients undergoing cochlear implantation. These SDoH factors affect if, when, and how a patient receives a CI. Some of these determinants include insurance coverage, educational attainment, household income, access to healthcare services and providers, and discrimination. Those from underserved populations, including minority races or non-English-speaking individuals, face greater disparities in access and utilization of CIs. While systemic changes need to be made to address some of the SDoH (i.e., equitable insurance coverage for CIs), hearing healthcare providers and the research community should continue to study the impact of SDoH on CI disparities across all populations. There are current validated measures and tools that investigators or practitioners can use to collect SDoH information from their patients. Collecting and analyzing SDoH data among the CI patient population could lead to the development of interventions, programs, or policies that could alleviate current disparities and promote equity in cochlear implantation.

References

1. Waltzman SB, Cohen NL, Shapiro WH. The benefits of cochlear implantation in the geriatric population. *Otolaryngol Head Neck Surg*. April 1993;108(4):329—333. https://doi.org/10.1177/019459989310800404.

2. Loy B, Warner-Czyz AD, Tong L, Tobey EA, Roland PS. The children speak: an examination of the quality of life of pediatric cochlear implant users. *Otolaryngol Head Neck Surg*. February 2010;142(2):247—253. https://doi.org/10.1016/j.otohns.2009.10.045.

3. Zwolan TA, Basura G. Determining cochlear implant candidacy in adults: limitations, expansions, and opportunities for improvement. *Semin Hear*. November 2021;42(4): 331—341. https://doi.org/10.1055/s-0041-1739283.

4. Gifford R. *Cochlear Implant Patient Assessment: Evaluation of Candidacy, Performance, and Outcomes*. 2nd ed. Plural Publishing Inc; 2020.

5. Sorkin DL. Cochlear implantation in the world's largest medical device market: utilization and awareness of cochlear implants in the United States. *Cochlear Implants Int*. March 2013;14 Suppl 1(Suppl 1):S4—S12. https://doi.org/10.1179/1467010013z.00000000076.

6. Nassiri AM, Sorkin DL, Carlson ML. Current estimates of cochlear implant utilization in the United States. *Otol Neurotol*. June 1, 2022;43(5):e558—e562. https://doi.org/10.1097/mao.0000000000003513.

7. Sorkin DL, Buchman CA. Cochlear implant access in six developed countries. *Otol Neurotol*. February 2016;37(2):e161—e164. https://doi.org/10.1097/mao.0000000000000946.

8. U.S. Department of Health and Human Services OoDPaHP. Social Determinants of Health; https://health.gov/healthypeople/priority-areas/social-determinants-health.

9. Goman AM, Lin FR. Prevalence of hearing loss by severity in the United States. *Am J Publ Health*. October 2016;106(10):1820—1822. https://doi.org/10.2105/ajph.2016.303299.

10. Agrawal Y, Platz EA, Niparko JK. Prevalence of hearing loss and differences by demographic characteristics among US adults: data from the National Health and Nutrition Examination Survey, 1999—2004. *Arch Intern Med*. July 28, 2008;168(14): 1522—1530. https://doi.org/10.1001/archinte.168.14.1522.

11. Lin FR, Thorpe R, Gordon-Salant S, Ferrucci L. Hearing loss prevalence and risk factors among older adults in the United States. *J Gerontol A Biol Sci Med Sci*. May 2011; 66(5):582—590. https://doi.org/10.1093/gerona/glr002.

12. Nieman CL, Suen JJ, Dean LT, Chandran A. Foundational approaches to advancing hearing health equity: a primer in social epidemiology. *Ear Hear*. Jul-Aug 01 2022; 43(Suppl 1):5s—14s. https://doi.org/10.1097/aud.0000000000001149.

13. Holder JT, Reynolds SM, Sunderhaus LW, Gifford RH. Current profile of adults presenting for preoperative cochlear implant evaluation. *Trends Hear*. Jan-Dec 2018;22:1—16. https://doi.org/10.1177/2331216518755288.

14. Schneider JM, Gopinath B, McMahon CM, et al. Role of general practitioners in managing age-related hearing loss. *Med J Aust*. January 4, 2010;192(1):20—23. https://doi.org/10.5694/j.1326-5377.2010.tb03395.x.

15. Nassiri AM, Marinelli JP, Sorkin DL, Carlson ML. Barriers to adult cochlear implant care in the United States: an analysis of health care delivery. *Semin Hear*. November 2021;42(4):311—320. https://doi.org/10.1055/s-0041-1739281.

16. Pratt SR. Profound hearing loss: addressing barriers to hearing healthcare. *Semin Hear.* November 2018;39(4):428−436. https://doi.org/10.1055/s-0038-1670708.

17. Jung D, Bhattacharyya N. Association of hearing loss with decreased employment and income among adults in the United States. *Ann Otol Rhinol Laryngol.* December 2012; 121(12):771−775. https://doi.org/10.1177/000348941212101201.

18. Li CM, Zhang X, Hoffman HJ, Cotch MF, Themann CL, Wilson MR. Hearing impairment associated with depression in US adults, national health and nutrition examination survey 2005-2010. *JAMA Otolaryngol Head Neck Surg.* April 2014;140(4):293−302. https://doi.org/10.1001/jamaoto.2014.42.

19. Dalton DS, Cruickshanks KJ, Klein BE, Klein R, Wiley TL, Nondahl DM. The impact of hearing loss on quality of life in older adults. *Gerontol.* October 2003;43(5): 661−668. https://doi.org/10.1093/geront/43.5.661.

20. Planey AM. Audiologist availability and supply in the United States: a multi-scale spatial and political economic analysis. *Soc Sci Med.* February 2019;222:216−224. https://doi.org/10.1016/j.socscimed.2019.01.015.

21. American Speech-Language-Hearing Association. *Audiology Survey Report: Clinical Focus Patterns 2014−2018;* 2019. https://www.asha.org/siteassets/surveys/2018-audiology-survey-clinical-focus-patterns-trends.pdf.

22. Looi V, Bluett C, Boisvert I. Referral rates of postlingually deafened adult hearing aid users for a cochlear implant candidacy assessment. *Int J Audiol.* December 2017;56(12): 919−925. https://doi.org/10.1080/14992027.2017.1344361.

23. Crowson MG, Schulz K, Tucci DL. Access to health care and hearing evaluation in US adults. *Ann Otol Rhinol Laryngol.* September 2016;125(9):716−721. https://doi.org/10.1177/0003489416649972.

24. Nieman CL, Marrone N, Szanton SL, Thorpe Jr RJ, Lin FR. Racial/ethnic and socioeconomic disparities in hearing health care among older Americans. *J Aging Health.* February 2016;28(1):68−94. https://doi.org/10.1177/0898264315585505.

25. Cruickshanks KJ, Nondahl DM, Tweed TS, et al. Education, occupation, noise exposure history and the 10-yr cumulative incidence of hearing impairment in older adults. *Hear Res.* June 1, 2010;264(1−2):3−9. https://doi.org/10.1016/j.heares.2009.10.008.

26. Barnett M, Hixon B, Okwiri N, et al. Factors involved in access and utilization of adult hearing healthcare: a systematic review. *Laryngoscope.* May 2017;127(5):1187−1194. https://doi.org/10.1002/lary.26234.

27. Hixon B, Chan S, Adkins M, Shinn JB, Bush ML. Timing and impact of hearing healthcare in adult cochlear implant recipients: a rural-urban comparison. *Otol Neurotol.* October 2016;37(9):1320−1324. https://doi.org/10.1097/mao.0000000000001197.

28. Mamo SK, Nieman CL, Lin FR. Prevalence of untreated hearing loss by income among older adults in the United States. *J Health Care Poor Underserved.* 2016;27(4): 1812−1818. https://doi.org/10.1353/hpu.2016.0164.

29. Arnold ML, Hyer K, Chisolm T. Medicaid hearing aid coverage for older adult beneficiaries: a state-by-state comparison. *Health Aff.* August 1, 2017;36(8):1476−1484. https://doi.org/10.1377/hlthaff.2016.1610.

30. Hay-McCutcheon MJ, Yuk MC, Yang X. Accessibility to hearing healthcare in rural and urban populations of Alabama: perspectives and a preliminary roadmap for addressing inequalities. *J Community Health.* August 2021;46(4):719−727. https://doi.org/10.1007/s10900-020-00943-4.

31. Nieman CL, Lin FR. Increasing access to hearing rehabilitation for older adults. *Curr Opin Otolaryngol Head Neck Surg*. October 2017;25(5):342−346. https://doi.org/10.1097/moo.0000000000000386.

32. McKee MM, Choi H, Wilson S, DeJonckheere MJ, Zazove P, Levy H. Determinants of hearing aid use among older Americans with hearing loss. *Gerontol*. November 16, 2019;59(6):1171−1181. https://doi.org/10.1093/geront/gny051.

33. Laplante-Lévesque A, Hickson L, Worrall L. Predictors of rehabilitation intervention decisions in adults with acquired hearing impairment. *J Speech Lang Hear Res*. October 2011;54(5):1385−1399. https://doi.org/10.1044/1092-4388(2011/10-0116.

34. Nassiri AM, Ricketts TA, Carlson ML. Current estimate of hearing aid utilization in the United States. *Otol Neurotol Open*. 2021;1(1). https://doi.org/10.1097/ONO.0000000000000001.

35. Bainbridge KE, Ramachandran V. Hearing aid use among older U.S. adults; the national health and nutrition examination survey. *2005−2006 and 2009−2010. Ear Hear*. May-Jun 2014;35(3):289−294. https://doi.org/10.1097/01.aud.0000441036.40169.29.

36. Green KM, Bhatt Y, Mawman DJ, et al. Predictors of audiological outcome following cochlear implantation in adults. *Cochlear Implants Int*. March 2007;8(1):1−11. https://doi.org/10.1179/cim.2007.8.1.1.

37. Blamey P, Arndt P, Bergeron F, et al. Factors affecting auditory performance of postlinguistically deaf adults using cochlear implants. *Audiol Neurootol*. Sep-Oct 1996;1(5):293−306. https://doi.org/10.1159/000259212.

38. Mahendran GN, Rosenbluth T, Featherstone M, Vivas EX, Mattox DE, Hobson CE. Racial disparities in adult cochlear implantation. *Otolaryngol Head Neck Surg*. June 2022;166(6):1099−1105. https://doi.org/10.1177/01945998211027340.

39. Tolisano AM, Fang LB, Kutz Jr JW, Isaacson B, Hunter JB. Better defining best-aided condition: the role of hearing aids on cochlear implantation qualification rates. *Am J Otolaryngol*. May-Jun 2020;41(3):102431. https://doi.org/10.1016/j.amjoto.2020.102431.

40. Miller SE, Anderson C, Manning J, Schafer E. Insurance payer status predicts postoperative speech outcomes in adult cochlear implant recipients. *J Am Acad Audiol*. October 2020;31(9):666−673. https://doi.org/10.1055/s-0040-1717137.

41. Tolisano AM, Schauwecker N, Baumgart B, et al. Identifying disadvantaged groups for cochlear implantation: demographics from a large cochlear implant program. *Ann Otol Rhinol Laryngol*. April 2020;129(4):347−354. https://doi.org/10.1177/0003489419888232.

42. Nassiri AM, Holcomb MA, Perkins EL, et al. Catchment profile of large cochlear implant centers in the United States. *Otolaryngol Head Neck Surg*. September 2022;167(3):545−551. https://doi.org/10.1177/01945998211070993.

43. Dornhoffer JR, Holcomb MA, Meyer TA, Dubno JR, McRackan TR. Factors influencing time to cochlear implantation. *Otol Neurotol*. February 2020;41(2):173−177. https://doi.org/10.1097/mao.0000000000002449.

44. Entwisle LK, Warren SE, Messersmith JJ. Cochlear implantation for children and adults with severe-to-profound hearing loss. *Semin Hear*. November 2018;39(4):390−404. https://doi.org/10.1055/s-0038-1670705.

45. Balachandra S, Tolisano AM, Qazi S, Hunter JB. Self-identified patient barriers to pursuit of cochlear implantation. *Otol Neurotol*. December 1, 2021;42(10s):S26−s32. https://doi.org/10.1097/mao.0000000000003376.

46. Zhang L, Ding AS, Xie DX, Creighton FX. Understanding public perceptions regarding cochlear implant surgery in adults. *Otol Neurotol*. March 1, 2022;43(3):e331−e336. https://doi.org/10.1097/mao.0000000000003439.

47. Sorkin DL. Impact of Medicaid on cochlear implant access. *Otol Neurotol*. March 2019; 40(3):e336−e341. https://doi.org/10.1097/mao.0000000000002142.

48. Fu QJ, Galvin 3rd JJ. Maximizing cochlear implant patients' performance with advanced speech training procedures. *Hear Res*. August 2008;242(1−2):198−208. https://doi.org/10.1016/j.heares.2007.11.010.

49. Hjaldahl J, Widén S, Carlsson P-I. Severe to profound hearing impairment: factors associated with the use of hearing aids and cochlear implants and participation in extended audiological rehabilitation. *Hearing, Balance Communication*. 2017;15(1):6−15. https://doi.org/10.1080/21695717.2016.1242250.

50. Tang L, Thompson CB, Clark JH, Ceh KM, Yeagle JD, Francis HW. Rehabilitation and psychosocial determinants of cochlear implant outcomes in older adults. *Ear Hear*. Nov/Dec 2017;38(6):663−671. https://doi.org/10.1097/aud.0000000000000445.

51. Kirkham E, Sacks C, Baroody F, et al. Health disparities in pediatric cochlear implantation: an audiologic perspective. *Ear Hear*. October 2009;30(5):515−525. https://doi.org/10.1097/AUD.0b013e3181aec5e0.

52. Lantos PM, Maradiaga-Panayotti G, Barber X, et al. Geographic and racial disparities in infant hearing loss. *Otolaryngol Head Neck Surg*. October 9, 2018;159(6):1051−1057. https://doi.org/10.1177/0194599818803305.

53. Kubba H, MacAndie C, Ritchie K, MacFarlane M. Is deafness a disease of poverty? The association between socio-economic deprivation and congenital hearing impairment. *Int J Audiol*. March 2004;43(3):123−125. https://doi.org/10.1080/14992020400 050017.

54. Nicholson N, Rhoades EA, Glade RE. Analysis of health disparities in the screening and diagnosis of hearing loss: early hearing detection and intervention hearing screening follow-up survey. *Am J Audiol*. May 25, 2022:1−25. https://doi.org/10.1044/ 2022_aja-21-00014.

55. Lantos PM, Hoffman K, Permar SR, et al. Neighborhood disadvantage is associated with high cytomegalovirus seroprevalence in pregnancy. *J Racial Ethn Health Disparities*. August 2018;5(4):782−786. https://doi.org/10.1007/s40615-017-0423-4.

56. Emmett SD, Francis HW. The socioeconomic impact of hearing loss in U.S. adults. *Otol Neurotol*. March 2015;36(3):545−550. https://doi.org/10.1097/mao.000000000 0000562.

57. Chan DK, Schrijver I, Chang KW. Diagnostic yield in the workup of congenital sensorineural hearing loss is dependent on patient ethnicity. *Otol Neurotol*. January 2011; 32(1):81−87. https://doi.org/10.1097/MAO.0b013e3181fc786f.

58. Florentine MM, Rouse SL, Stephans J, et al. Racial and ethnic disparities in diagnostic efficacy of comprehensive genetic testing for sensorineural hearing loss. *Hum Genet*. April 2022;141(3−4):495−504. https://doi.org/10.1007/s00439-021-02338-4.

59. Infant Hearing T. Year 2019 Position Statement: principles and guidelines for early hearing detection and intervention programs. *J Early Hearing Detect Interv*. 2019; 4(2):1−44. https://doi.org/10.15142/fptk-b748.

60. Philips B, Corthals P, De Raeve L, et al. Impact of newborn hearing screening: comparing outcomes in pediatric cochlear implant users. *Laryngoscope*. May 2009; 119(5):974−979. https://doi.org/10.1002/lary.20188.

61. (JCIH) JCoIH. Year 2019 position statement: principles and guidelines for early hearing detection and intervention programs. In: *The Journal of Early Hearing Detection and Intervention*. 2 ed 2019:1–44.

62. Centers for Disease Control and Prevention. *Annual Data: Early Hearing Detection and Intervention (EHDI) Program*; July 20, 2022. https://www.cdc.gov/ncbddd/hearingloss/ehdi-data.html.

63. Su BM, Park JS, Chan DK. Impact of primary language and insurance on pediatric hearing health care in a multidisciplinary clinic. *Otolaryngol Head Neck Surg*. October 2017;157(4):722–730. https://doi.org/10.1177/0194599817725695.

64. Zhang L, Links AR, Boss EF, White A, Walsh J. Identification of potential barriers to timely access to pediatric hearing aids. *JAMA Otolaryngol Head Neck Surg*. January 1, 2020;146(1):13–19. https://doi.org/10.1001/jamaoto.2019.2877.

65. Meyer AC, Marsolek M, Brown N, Coverstone K. Delayed identification of infants who are deaf or hard of hearing - Minnesota, 2012–2016. *MMWR Morb Mortal Wkly Rep*. March 20, 2020;69(11):303–306. https://doi.org/10.15585/mmwr.mm6911a6.

66. Bush ML, Bianchi K, Lester C, et al. Delays in diagnosis of congenital hearing loss in rural children. *J Pediatr*. February 2014;164(2):393–397. https://doi.org/10.1016/j.jpeds.2013.09.047.

67. Holte L, Walker E, Oleson J, et al. Factors influencing follow-up to newborn hearing screening for infants who are hard of hearing. *Am J Audiol*. December 2012;21(2):163–174. https://doi.org/10.1044/1059-0889(2012/12-0016.

68. Spivak L, Sokol H, Auerbach C, Gershkovich S. Newborn hearing screening follow-up: factors affecting hearing aid fitting by 6 months of age. *Am J Audiol*. June 2009;18(1):24–33. https://doi.org/10.1044/1059-0889(2008/08-0015.

69. Young NM, Reilly BK, Burke L. Limitations of universal newborn hearing screening in early identification of pediatric cochlear implant candidates. *Arch Otolaryngol Head Neck Surg*. March 2011;137(3):230–234. https://doi.org/10.1001/archoto.2011.4.

70. Chen MM, Oghalai JS. Diagnosis and management of congenital sensorineural hearing loss. *Curr Treat Options Pediatr*. September 2016;2(3):256–265. https://doi.org/10.1007/s40746-016-0056-6.

71. Liming BJ, Carter J, Cheng A, et al. International Pediatric Otolaryngology Group (IPOG) consensus recommendations: hearing loss in the pediatric patient. *Int J Pediatr Otorhinolaryngol*. November 2016;90:251–258. https://doi.org/10.1016/j.ijporl.2016.09.016.

72. Qian ZJ, Chang KW, Ahmad IN, Tribble MS, Cheng AG. Use of diagnostic testing and intervention for sensorineural hearing loss in US children from 2008 to 2018. *JAMA Otolaryngol Head Neck Surg*. March 1, 2021;147(3):253–260. https://doi.org/10.1001/jamaoto.2020.5030.

73. Grey B, Deutchki EK, Lund EA, Werfel KL. Impact of meeting early hearing detection and intervention benchmarks on spoken language. *J Early Interv*. September 2022;44(3):235–251. https://doi.org/10.1177/10538151211025210.

74. Bush ML, Osetinsky M, Shinn JB, et al. Assessment of Appalachian region pediatric hearing healthcare disparities and delays. *Laryngoscope*. July 2014;124(7):1713–1717. https://doi.org/10.1002/lary.24588.

75. Ostrowski T, Mouzakes J. Financial distress experienced by privately insured pediatric hearing aid patients: a pilot study. *Clin Pediatr (Phila)*. October 2022;61(9):596–604. https://doi.org/10.1177/00099228221090362.

76. Sapiets SJ, Totsika V, Hastings RP. Factors influencing access to early intervention for families of children with developmental disabilities: a narrative review. *J Appl Res Intellect Disabil*. May 2021;34(3):695–711. https://doi.org/10.1111/jar.12852.

77. Sharma S, Bhatia K, Singh S, Lahiri AK, Aggarwal A. Impact of socioeconomic factors on paediatric cochlear implant outcomes. *Int J Pediatr Otorhinolaryngol*. November 2017;102:90–97. https://doi.org/10.1016/j.ijporl.2017.09.010.

78. Fitzpatrick EM, Ham J, Whittingham J. Pediatric cochlear implantation: why do children receive implants late? *Ear Hear*. Nov-Dec 2015;36(6):688–694. https://doi.org/10.1097/aud.0000000000000184.

79. Bush ML, Burton M, Loan A, Shinn JB. Timing discrepancies of early intervention hearing services in urban and rural cochlear implant recipients. *Otol Neurotol*. December 2013;34(9):1630–1635. https://doi.org/10.1097/MAO.0b013e31829e83ad.

80. Hellman SA, Chute PM, Kretschmer RE, Nevins ME, Parisier SC, Thurston LC. The development of a children's implant profile. *Am Ann Deaf*. April 1991;136(2):77–81. https://doi.org/10.1353/aad.2012.1077.

81. Sharma SD, Cushing SL, Papsin BC, Gordon KA. Hearing and speech benefits of cochlear implantation in children: a review of the literature. *Int J Pediatr Otorhinolaryngol*. June 2020;133:109984. https://doi.org/10.1016/j.ijporl.2020.109984.

82. Sorkin DL, Zwolan TA. Parental perspectives regarding early intervention and its role in cochlear implantation in children. *Otol Neurotol*. February 2008;29(2):137–141. https://doi.org/10.1097/mao.0b013e3181616c88.

83. Stern RE, Yueh B, Lewis C, Norton S, Sie KC. Recent epidemiology of pediatric cochlear implantation in the United States: disparity among children of different ethnicity and socioeconomic status. *Laryngoscope*. January 2005;115(1):125–131. https://doi.org/10.1097/01.mlg.0000150698.61624.3c.

84. Tampio AJF, Schroeder Ii RJ, Wang D, Boyle J, Nicholas BD. Trends in sociodemographic disparities of pediatric cochlear implantation over a 15-year period. *Int J Pediatr Otorhinolaryngol*. December 2018;115:165–170. https://doi.org/10.1016/j.ijporl.2018.10.003.

85. Armstrong M, Maresh A, Buxton C, et al. Barriers to early pediatric cochlear implantation. *Int J Pediatr Otorhinolaryngol*. November 2013;77(11):1869–1872. https://doi.org/10.1016/j.ijporl.2013.08.031.

86. Liu X, Rosa-Lugo LI, Cosby JL, Pritchett CV. Racial and insurance inequalities in access to early pediatric cochlear implantation. *Otolaryngol Head Neck Surg*. March 2021;164(3):667–674. https://doi.org/10.1177/0194599820953381.

87. Ozcebe E, Sevinc S, Belgin E. The ages of suspicion, identification, amplification and intervention in children with hearing loss. *Int J Pediatr Otorhinolaryngol*. August 2005;69(8):1081–1087. https://doi.org/10.1016/j.ijporl.2005.03.002.

88. Fujiwara RJT, Ishiyama G, Ishiyama A. Association of socioeconomic characteristics with receipt of pediatric cochlear implantations in California. *JAMA Netw Open*. January 4, 2022;5(1):e2143132. https://doi.org/10.1001/jamanetworkopen.2021.43132.

89. Wiley S, Meinzen-Derr J. Access to cochlear implant candidacy evaluations: who is not making it to the team evaluations? *Int J Audiol*. February 2009;48(2):74–79. https://doi.org/10.1080/14992020802475227.

90. Chang DT, Ko AB, Murray GS, Arnold JE, Megerian CA. Lack of financial barriers to pediatric cochlear implantation: impact of socioeconomic status on access and outcomes. *Arch Otolaryngol Head Neck Surg*. July 2010;136(7):648–657. https://doi.org/10.1001/archoto.2010.90.

91. Griffin AM, Poissant SF, Freyman RL. Speech-in-Noise and quality-of-life measures in school-aged children with normal hearing and with unilateral hearing loss. *Ear Hear.* Jul/Aug 2019;40(4):887−904. https://doi.org/10.1097/aud.0000000000000667.

92. Appachi S, Specht JL, Raol N, et al. Auditory outcomes with hearing rehabilitation in children with unilateral hearing loss: a systematic review. *Otolaryngol Head Neck Surg.* October 2017;157(4):565−571. https://doi.org/10.1177/0194599817726757.

93. Sokolov M, Gordon KA, Polonenko M, Blaser SI, Papsin BC, Cushing SL. Vestibular and balance function is often impaired in children with profound unilateral sensori-neural hearing loss. *Hear Res.* February 2019;372:52−61. https://doi.org/10.1016/j.heares.2018.03.032.

94. Eskridge HR, Park LR, Brown KD. The impact of unilateral, simultaneous, or sequential cochlear implantation on pediatric language outcomes. *Cochlear Implants Int.* July 2021;22(4):187−194. https://doi.org/10.1080/14670100.2020.1871267.

95. Yoshinaga-Itano C, Sedey AL, Wiggin M, Mason CA. language outcomes improved through early hearing detection and earlier cochlear implantation. *Otol Neurotol.* December 2018;39(10):1256−1263. https://doi.org/10.1097/mao.0000000000001976.

96. Yang CQ, Reilly BK, Preciado DA. Barriers to pediatric cochlear implantation: a parental survey. *Int J Pediatr Otorhinolaryngol.* January 2018;104:224−227. https://doi.org/10.1016/j.ijporl.2017.11.026.

97. Dham R, Dharmarajan S, Kurkure R, Sampath Kumar RN, Kameswaran M. Socio-demographic profile and its influences on rehabilitation in children undergoing revision cochlear implantation - MERF experience. *Int J Pediatr Otorhinolaryngol.* December 2021;151:110919. https://doi.org/10.1016/j.ijporl.2021.110919.

98. Omar M, Qatanani AM, Douglas NO, et al. Sociodemographic disparities in pediatric cochlear implantation outcomes: a systematic review. *Am J Otolaryngol.* August 16, 2022;43(5):103608. https://doi.org/10.1016/j.amjoto.2022.103608.

99. Geers A, Brenner C. Background and educational characteristics of prelingually deaf children implanted by five years of age. *Ear Hear.* February 2003;24(1 Suppl): 2s−14s. https://doi.org/10.1097/01.Aud.0000051685.19171.Bd.

100. Tolan M, Serpas A, McElroy K, et al. Delays in sound recognition and imitation in un-derinsured children receiving cochlear implantation. *JAMA Otolaryngol Head Neck Surg.* January 1, 2017;143(1):60−64. https://doi.org/10.1001/jamaoto.2016.2730.

101. Catts HW, Fey ME, Tomblin JB, Zhang X. A longitudinal investigation of reading out-comes in children with language impairments. *J Speech Lang Hear Res.* December 2002;45(6):1142−1157. https://doi.org/10.1044/1092-4388(2002/093.

102. Dev AN, Nahas G, Pappas A, et al. Underinsurance in children is associated with wors-ened quality of life after cochlear implantation. *Int J Pediatr Otorhinolaryngol.* June 2022;157:111119. https://doi.org/10.1016/j.ijporl.2022.111119.

103. Niparko JK, Tobey EA, Thal DJ, et al. Spoken language development in children following cochlear implantation. *JAMA.* April 21, 2010;303(15):1498−1506. https://doi.org/10.1001/jama.2010.451.

104. Panda S, Sikka K, Singh V, et al. Comprehensive analysis of factors leading to poor per-formance in prelingual cochlear implant recipients. *Otol Neurotol.* July 2019;40(6): 754−760. https://doi.org/10.1097/mao.0000000000002237.

105. Vukkadala N, Perez D, Cabala S, Kapur C, Chan DK. Linguistic and behavioral perfor-mance of bilingual children with hearing loss. *Int J Pediatr Otorhinolaryngol.* September 2018;112:34−38. https://doi.org/10.1016/j.ijporl.2018.06.020.

106. Wu D, Woodson EW, Masur J, Bent J. Pediatric cochlear implantation: role of language, income, and ethnicity. *Int J Pediatr Otorhinolaryngol*. May 2015;79(5):721−724. https://doi.org/10.1016/j.ijporl.2015.02.030.

107. Marnane V, Ching TY. Hearing aid and cochlear implant use in children with hearing loss at three years of age: predictors of use and predictors of changes in use. *Int J Audiol*. August 2015;54(8):544−551. https://doi.org/10.3109/14992027.2015.1017660.

108. Szagun G, Stumper B. Age or experience? The influence of age at implantation and social and linguistic environment on language development in children with cochlear implants. *J Speech Lang Hear Res*. December 2012;55(6):1640−1654. https://doi.org/10.1044/1092-4388(2012/11-0119.

109. Noblitt B, Alfonso KP, Adkins M, Bush ML. Barriers to rehabilitation care in pediatric cochlear implant recipients. *Otol Neurotol*. June 2018;39(5):e307−e313. https://doi.org/10.1097/mao.0000000000001777.

110. Choo D, Dettman SJ. What can long-term attendance at programming appointments tell us about pediatric cochlear implant recipients? *Otol Neurotol*. March 2017;38(3):325−333. https://doi.org/10.1097/mao.0000000000001299.

111. Bashshur RL, Goldberg MA. The origins of telemedicine and e-Health. *Telemed J e Health*. March 2014;20(3):190−191. https://doi.org/10.1089/tmj.2014.9996.

112. Bush ML, Hardin B, Rayle C, Lester C, Studts CR, Shinn JB. Rural barriers to early diagnosis and treatment of infant hearing loss in Appalachia. *Otol Neurotol*. January 2015;36(1):93−98. https://doi.org/10.1097/mao.0000000000000636.

113. D'Onofrio KL, Zeng FG. Tele-audiology: current state and future directions. *Front Digit Health*. 2021;3:788103. https://doi.org/10.3389/fdgth.2021.788103.

114. Dharmar M, Simon A, Sadorra C, et al. Reducing loss to follow-up with tele-audiology diagnostic evaluations. *Telemed J e Health*. February 2016;22(2):159−164. https://doi.org/10.1089/tmj.2015.0001.

115. Swanepoel de W, Clark JL, Koekemoer D, et al. Telehealth in audiology: the need and potential to reach underserved communities. *Int J Audiol*. March 2010;49(3):195−202. https://doi.org/10.3109/14992020903470783.

116. Ramkumar V, Nagarajan R, Shankarnarayan VC, Kumaravelu S, Hall JW. Implementation and evaluation of a rural community-based pediatric hearing screening program integrating in-person and tele-diagnostic auditory brainstem response (ABR). *BMC Health Serv Res*. January 3, 2019;19(1):1. https://doi.org/10.1186/s12913-018-3827-x.

117. Evans T, Nejman T, Stewart E, Windmill I. Increasing pediatric audiology services via telehealth. *Semin Hear*. May 2021;42(2):136−151. https://doi.org/10.1055/s-0041-1731694.

118. Hughes ML, Sevier JD, Choi S. Techniques for remotely programming children with cochlear implants using pediatric audiological methods via telepractice. *Am J Audiol*. November 19, 2018;27(3s):385−390. https://doi.org/10.1044/2018_aja-imia3-18-0002.

119. Bush ML, Thompson R, Irungu C, Ayugi J. The role of telemedicine in auditory rehabilitation: a systematic review. *Otol Neurotol*. December 2016;37(10):1466−1474. https://doi.org/10.1097/mao.0000000000001236.

120. Wales D, Skinner L, Hayman M. The efficacy of telehealth-delivered speech and language intervention for primary school-age children: a systematic review. Int J Telerehabil. *Spring*. 2017;9(1):55−70. https://doi.org/10.5195/ijt.2017.6219.

121. Saeed SA, Masters RM. Disparities in health care and the digital divide. *Curr Psychiatr Rep.* July 23, 2021;23(9):61. https://doi.org/10.1007/s11920-021-01274-4.
122. Hirko KA, Kerver JM, Ford S, et al. Telehealth in response to the COVID-19 pandemic: implications for rural health disparities. *J Am Med Inf Assoc.* November 1, 2020;27(11): 1816–1818. https://doi.org/10.1093/jamia/ocaa156.
123. Luo J, Tong L, Crotty BH, et al. Telemedicine adoption during the COVID-19 pandemic: gaps and inequalities. *Appl Clin Inf.* August 2021;12(4):836–844. https://doi.org/10.1055/s-0041-1733848.

Health disparities in head and neck cancer

14

Sunshine Dwojak-Archambeau

Northwest Permanente Medicine, Portland, OR, United States

Introduction

In the United States (US), racial inequality is our national inheritance. This is our history and our truth, and historically marginalized populations suffer disproportionately as a result. My great-grandparents were taken from reservations as children—my great-grandmother from the Rosebud Sioux reservation in South Dakota and my great-grandfather from Anadarko, Oklahoma—and grew up in residential boarding schools. My grandparents attended segregated Indian high schools. As a result of violence, discrimination, and government policies that deprived them of their land, my grandparents and my parents endured poverty, addiction, and mental illness. They lived in poor health for much of their adult lives and suffered early deaths. These experiences drove me to pursue a medical degree with the intention of helping people like my mother and her family.

While working on my master's degree in public health as an otolaryngology resident, I studied disparities in head and neck cancer among the American Indian community and quickly found that this was almost impossible to do from the outset. For example, the requirement for large sample sizes in order to demonstrate statistical significance among disparate outcome measures means that many minorities are excluded from major influential studies—the numbers just simply are not there. American Indian, Alaska Native and Asian American individuals are combined into a category of "Other," or they are simply excluded from the dataset entirely due to their small numbers. What is this, other than another form of cultural assimilation? We cease to be identified because there are too few of us, and because we aren't identified, we are erased from the literature altogether.

Let us look at the current data on head and neck cancer through this lens. Head and neck cancer includes cancer of the oral cavity, pharynx, larynx, nasopharynx, salivary glands, and thyroid. This group of diseases has different etiologies, treatments, and outcomes; therefore, we will look at the data for each of them separately and see what larger trends emerge when looking at all these cancers together. We will review the current literature which focuses on differences in presentation, treatment, and outcomes in head and neck cancer, and as we do so, I ask that you think about who and what are left out of the data, and what implications that has on the conclusions drawn from that data.

Healthcare Disparities in Otolaryngology. https://doi.org/10.1016/B978-0-443-10714-6.00004-3

253

Thyroid cancer

Thyroid cancer is the seventh most common cancer in women, with 73% of thyroid cancers diagnosed in women. There will be approximately 43,000 new cases in 2022 with 2230 associated deaths.[1] The majority of thyroid cancers are well-differentiated papillary and follicular cancers. After a dramatic 211% increase in incidence from 1975 to 2013, attributed to over detection from increased scans and ultrasounds, incidence rates are starting to decline.[2,3] Several studies have shown that incidence rates for thyroid cancer go up with increasing levels of health insurance. As a result, incidence rates of thyroid cancer in the US are highest in White American individuals and lowest in Black American individuals.[4,5]

Presentation

Minority patients with differentiated thyroid cancer present with larger and more aggressive tumors. Surveillance, Epidemiology, and End Result (SEER) data show that White American individuals were more likely to have classic papillary thyroid carcinoma (62%) compared to Black American individuals who were more likely to present with the more aggressive follicular variant papillary thyroid carcinoma (41%). Black patients present with larger tumors and were more likely to present with lymph node metastases.[6] In a retrospective review of the California Cancer Registry, Black, Hispanic, and Asian patients were more likely to present with metastatic disease.[7]

Treatment

The primary treatment for thyroid cancer is surgery. Postoperative radioactive iodine (RAI) is prescribed when high-risk features are present.[8] There is a significant body of research showing that thyroid surgery outcomes improve with surgeon volume.[9,10] However, minority patients are more likely to have surgery by low-volume surgeons. Compared to White patients, Black patients have less access to intermediate and high-volume surgeons (49% vs. 45% and 19% vs. 16%, $P < .001$). Hispanic patients have the least access to high-volume surgeons (13%).[11] Sosa et al. confirmed this in a review of Nationwide Inpatient Sample (NIS) data, showing that the majority of Hispanic (55%) and Black (52%) patients had surgery by the lowest-volume surgeons (1–9 cases per year), compared with only 44% of White patients. They found that 90% of the patients for the highest volume surgeons (>100 cases per year) were White.[12]

This discrepancy results in Black and Hispanic patients having poorer surgical outcomes from thyroidectomy. Black patients undergoing thyroidectomy had longer length of stay, higher surgical complication rates, and higher total cost.[12] Hispanic and Black patients had the highest 30-day hospital readmission rate.[13] While mortality from thyroidectomy remains low, 30- and 90-day mortality rates were highest for Black patients (0.2% and 0.4% $P < .001$).[12,14]

Minority patients with thyroid cancer are also more likely to be undertreated. Black patients have lower odds of receiving appropriate extent of thyroid surgery (OR 0.78 CI 0.71−0.87).[13] Black patients were significantly less likely to undergo central neck dissection (OR 0.468 CI 0.45−0.48).[15] Uninsured, lower socioeconomic status (SES), and Black post-op thyroidectomy patients were less likely to receive RAI. The likelihood of RAI undertreatment was higher for all races compared to White patients, who were more likely to be overtreated with RAI.[3,13,15,16]

Outcomes

These differences in presentation and treatment affect overall survival. Data from both SEER and the National Cancer Database (NCDB) show a survival disparity for Black patients with thyroid cancer. Black patients have reduced 5- and 10-year overall survival (94% vs. 93% and 87% vs. 84%, $P < .001$).[13,17] After adjusting for sex, marital status, age, year of diagnosis, multifocal disease, and type of surgery, Black patients still had an increased risk of death from thyroid carcinoma with a hazard ratio (HR) of 2.59.[18]

Medullary and anaplastic thyroid carcinomas

These disparities in presentation, treatment, and outcomes persist in rarer, more aggressive forms of thyroid cancer. In a SEER review of patients with medullary thyroid carcinoma, Hispanic and Black patients were more likely to present with higher-stage disease. Black patients were less likely to undergo lymph node examination in surgery (OR 0.61 CI 0.39−0.93), as were patients living in counties below poverty level (OR 0.76 CI 0.59−0.9). Black patients had lower five-year overall survival (74.8% vs. 83.4%) and lower five-year disease-specific survival (79.6% vs. 86.1%). Additionally, increasing tumor size at the time of presentation was directly associated with increased risk of death.[19]

In an analysis of patients with anaplastic thyroid carcinoma in the SEER database, there were no differences in stage at disease presentation, but non-White patients were more likely to not receive any treatment (OR 0.29 CI 0.16−0.54). Both non-White patients and patients living in high poverty areas were also less likely to receive radiation therapy (RT) (OR 0.55 CI 0.35−0.88; OR, 0.47 CI 0.23−0.99). Non-White patients with anaplastic thyroid cancer had worse overall survival at 20 months (15.5% vs. 20.8%). Differences in treatment led to a dramatic effect on overall survival, as patients who received radiation in this cohort were half as likely to die as those who did not (five-year overall survival [OS] 12.0% vs. 5.2%, $P < .0001$.)[20]

Oral cavity cancer

Oral cavity cancer encompasses tumors of the tongue, lips, gingiva, and buccal mucosa. There will be an estimated 35,100 cases of oral cavity cancer in 2022 with an

associated 13,060 deaths.[1] The primary risk factors for oral cavity cancer are tobacco use and alcohol consumption. There has been a decline in the incidence of
some oral cavity cancer due to public health efforts to decrease smoking.[21] However,
data show that Black and American Indian individuals have increased exposure to
tobacco and alcohol. Data from the Behavioral Risk Factor Surveillance System
(BRFSS) show that American Indian individuals reported higher rates of binge
drinking, and that American Indian and Black individuals reported the highest rates
of current smoking (28.1% and 21.1%, $P < .001$), making them particularly vulnerable to these cancers.[22]

Presentation

Prognosis for oral cavity cancer is worse for increasing stage at presentation. Several
reviews of national cancer databases show that minority patients with oral cavity
cancer are more likely to present with late-stage disease.[23,24] The NCDB for oral
cavity cancers shows that Black patients were younger, of lower SES, more likely
to have Medicaid, and to present with more advanced tumors. Compared to 32%
of White patients, 58% of Black patients presented with stage IV disease. SEER
data show that Black individuals have a significantly higher proportion of tongue
cancers that were >4 cm in diameter at time of diagnosis (59% vs. 44%;
$P < .001$). In addition, most Black patients presented with regional metastasis or
to a distant site at diagnosis (70% vs. 53%, $P < .001$).[23,25]

Treatment

Primary surgery is recommended for oral cavity cancers, as it leads to superior clinical outcomes for all stages of disease.[26] Adjuvant radiation or adjuvant chemoradiation is recommended for adverse features. Studies show that minority patients are
less likely to receive appropriate surgical treatment. American Indian individuals
with oral cavity cancer were 9% less likely to receive surgery than White patients
with similar disease and stage.[24] Black patients are significantly less likely to
have surgery recommended (HR 1.42 CI 1.31–1.54), despite not being more likely
to have contraindications to surgery and are much less likely to receive surgery
(64.2% vs. 82.3%, $P < .001$). White patients are more likely to receive surgery
regardless of SES or insurance status. Overall, it was found that Black patients
were 11% less likely to receive surgery when controlling for potential confounders
and tumor size.[25,27]

Outcomes

Patients with upfront surgery experience better overall survival at one and five years
(87% and 60% compared to 64% and 27%, $P < 0.001$). Black patients treated surgically had poorer one-year and five-year survival compared to White patients (84%
vs. 87% and 50% vs. 60%). American Indian individuals with oral cavity cancer had

an increased HR for death compared to White patients (HR 1.3, $P = 0.05$). This HR became insignificant after adding in stage and treatment effects, suggesting that late stage and less surgery significantly affects survival.[24,27]

Oropharynx cancer

There will be an estimated 54,000 cancers of the oral cavity and pharynx in 2022 with an approximately 11,230 deaths.[1] With the decline in the incidence of oral cavity cancers beginning in the 1980s, there has been a significant increase in the incidence rates of oropharyngeal cancers (OPCs). Changing behaviors in the population, the decrease in tobacco and alcohol use, and the risk of human papillomavirus (HPV) are driving this increase. HPV is now responsible for about 80% of oropharynx cancers. HPV-related tumors have a higher sensitivity to chemoradiation. Patients with HPV-related OPC have improved survival regardless of stage at presentation.[28,29] This differential response to treatment complicates disparity research in the oropharynx subsite, as the rate of HPV-related OPC has been found to be different among the Black American population.

This differential rate of HPV-related OPC was first reported by Settle, who found lower rates of HPV-positivity in Black patients with OPC in a review of the TAX 324 trial.[30] Subsequent studies have confirmed this. A large review of OPC patients treated at Mt. Sinai from 1995 to 2013 found that their population, demographics, smoking, and alcohol history were all similar. However, they found a significantly higher incidence of HPV-positive OPC in White patients (84.2% vs. 62% for minorities $P = .017$.)[31] A recent review of OPC in the NCDB found that 67.6% of White patients were HPV-positive compared to 42.3% of Black patients and 57.1% of Hispanic patients ($P < .001$).[32,33]

Presentation

In addition to differential tumor biology, several studies show that minority patients present with higher stages of oropharyngeal disease. A 2018 study by Albert et al., found that Black patients in Mississippi were more likely to present with advanced disease (33% AJCC 7th ed stage IV vs. 8%) and more likely to present with HPV-negative disease (67.6% vs. 26.9%, $P = .002$).[34] In Megwalu's review of the SEER database, Black patients had a higher risk of presenting with AJCC 7 locally advanced stage III or IV tumors (OR 2.55, 95% CI 2.29–2.84), distant metastasis (OR 2.25, 95% CI 1.8–2.70), and unresectable tumors (OR 2.0, 95% CI 1.76–2.29).[35]

Treatment

Treatment for early stage OPCs is unimodality therapy, either surgery or primary radiation. Advanced stage disease is treated with multimodality treatment, namely concurrent chemoradiation.[26] In a review of the NCDB, Black patients were significantly less likely to receive surgery (28.1% vs. 39.1%). This was most signif-icant for early stage HPV-negative disease (47.2% vs. 63%, $P = 0.0001$), but held across all stages. Surgical treatment was more often found in patients with high SES. Additional studies show that Black patients have longer times before the start of chemotherapy, longer times between diagnosis and the start and end of radiation, and higher likelihood of incomplete radiation treatment.[34,36]

Outcomes

These disparities in presentation and treatment affect survival for minority patients with OPCs. Rotsides's review of the NCDB found that Black patients had worse sur-vival after controlling for age, stage, and treatment (HR 1.22, 95% CI 1.11−1.34). After controlling for HPV status, survival was worse for Black patients and those of lower SES. Survival disparities were most pronounced for Black patients in the lowest SES and with HPV-negative disease (three-year survival was 44% vs. 74%). Black patients with HPV-positive disease also experienced a worse survival outcome (58.5% vs. 86.6%).[33] SEER data also show that Black patients have worse disease-specific survival than other racial groups (HR 1.67, $P < .0001$). But impor-tantly, SEER at that time did not include HPV status.[37] In addition, Black patients had worse survival for HPV-related OPC when radiation was prolonged >50 days (HR 1.77, 95% CI 1.03−3.05).[36]

Two separate systematic reviews attempted to sort out the survival disparity with relation to race and HPV status. A meta-analysis of five studies performed by Lenze and colleagues revealed a pooled HR of death for Black patients with OPC of 1.45 (95% CI 0.87−2.40) after adjusting for HPV status.[38] Stein et al. also performed a meta-analysis of four studies looking at overall survival. Their pooled data showed an HR of 1.10 (CI 0.96−1.23) for HPV-positive disease. HPV-negative pooled data showed an HR of 1.50 (CI 1.12−1.88), suggesting that survival disparities exist by race and are more significant among patients with HPV-negative disease.[39]

Laryngeal cancer

Laryngeal cancer includes cancers of the larynx and includes the subsites of the supraglottis, glottis, and subglottis. Hypopharyngeal cancers are also frequently included in these analyses. In 2022, data projected approximately 12,470 laryngeal cancers and 3820 deaths.[1] Risk factors for laryngeal cancer include cigarette smoke and alcohol use.

Presentation

A 2015 SEER database review found that Black patients were more likely to be diag-nosed at a younger age, with nodal metastasis, and with advanced stage disease.[40] An updated SEER study in 2020 confirmed that Black patients were more likely to present with AJCC 7th ed stage III or IV disease for laryngeal cancer.[41]

Treatment

Current guidelines for laryngeal cancer treatment include single-modality treatment for early stage tumors, either surgery or radiation. Multimodality treatment with surgery, chemotherapy, and radiation is reserved for late-stage disease.[26] Within this paradigm, there is room for variation in treatment based on patient preferences for voice outcomes and the feasibility of larynx preservation. However, even within this variation, patterns of racial disparity emerge from the data.

Misono et al. found that for early glottic tumors, surgery conferred a survival benefit and that Black patients were more likely to receive radiation. Black race was associated with a greater likelihood of receiving radiation only and a lower likelihood of undergoing surgical resection.[42] Black patients are also significantly less likely to undergo larynx preservation. SEER data show that Black patients with early stage disease were more likely to undergo total laryngectomy, a surgery reserved for advanced tumors, compared with White patients (stage T1-2, 8.2% vs. 4.3%; $P < .001$).[40] This racial disparity persisted on multivariate analysis, even when controlling for age, sex, year of diagnosis, stage, and subsite (OR 0.78 CI 0.63−0.96).[43] For patients with stage T4 disease, where the indications for laryngectomy are clearer, rates of primary radiotherapy among Black patients were higher (40.5% vs. 35.7%; $P = .015$). Black patients were also more likely not to receive any treatment (8.4% vs. 6.5% $P < 0.001$.) Additionally, they had higher rates of nonstandard treatment with chemotherapy only (3.1% vs. 1.7% $P < 0.001$), chemoradiotherapy (30.3% vs. 25.1% $P < 0.001$), and triple modality therapy (9.7% vs. 7.5% $P < 0.001$).[41]

Outcomes

SEER data show disparities in survival for laryngeal cancer. Rates of five-year survival are significantly different between White (60.6%), Black (52.7%), Hispanic (59.5%), and Asian (65.7%) patients ($P < .001$). This significant five-year OS difference by race persisted regardless of age, gender, year of diagnosis, primary treatment, nodal status, or tumor grade. On multivariate analysis, race remained an independent prognostic factor for overall survival.[40] In Chen's later review, overall mortality was significantly higher for Black patients (51.7% vs. 42.0%). In the study, there was a multivariable overall mortality HR 1.10 (CI 1.02−1.18). This disparity persisted in cancer specific mortality (HR 1.22, 95% CI 1.09−1.35) but disappeared on multivariable analysis when stage was added to the model, suggesting that late-stage presentation is a driving factor in worse disease-specific survival for Black patients.[41]

Salivary gland cancer

Salivary gland malignancies make up a small portion of head and neck cancers, 5%−10%. Most of the tumors arise in the parotid glands, and other sites include the submandibular glands and other minor salivary glands. The literature on disparities in these subsites is sparse. Iwata et al. performed a retrospective review within the Henry Ford Health system from 1990 to 2015. In their analysis of 217 salivary gland tumors, they found that overall survival was 66.5% at 5 years and 50% at 10 years. Age, gender, comorbidities, and stage at presentation all influenced this outcome. Race alone was not associated with survival outcomes on univariate analysis. However, they found that lack of education and living in a neighborhood with a high percentage of poverty was associated with Black race. Every 10% increase in proportion of the population with less than a high school education was associated with a 28% increase in the hazard of death at 5 years.[44]

Larger studies of salivary gland malignancies from the SEER database show that Black and Hispanic patients are younger at the time of diagnosis. Black patients receive significantly less surgery for squamous cell carcinoma of the salivary glands (58.26 vs. 76.94%, $P < 0.001$).[45]

Multivariate modeling of all tumor subtypes revealed a worse disease-specific survival for Black patients after controlling for tumor characteristics and treatment (HR 1.34 $P < 0.001$). When looking at specific subtypes of salivary gland malignancies, multivariate modeling showed worse disease-specific survival for Black patients with mucoepidermoid carcinoma (HR 1.56 $P = 0.03$) and for squamous cell carcinoma (HR 1.58, $P = 0.05$). There were no detected survival differences for adenoid cystic carcinoma or adenocarcinoma, and there were too few cases for acinic cell carcinoma for analysis.[45]

Nasopharyngeal cancer

Nasopharyngeal cancer (NPC) is relatively rare in the US, making up only 2% of all head and neck cancers.[46] Risk factors include Epstein–Barr virus (EBV) infection, smoking, inhalant exposure, consumption of nitrosamine-containing foods, and decreased fresh fruit and vegetable intake. NPC is divided into three different subtypes: keratinizing squamous cell carcinoma (WHO type 1) that is not associated with EBV infection; nonkeratinizing squamous cell carcinoma (WHO type 2) and undifferentiated or poorly differentiated carcinoma (WHO type 3) that are both associated with EBV. Nonkeratinizing histologies respond better to treatment and portend improved survival.[47]

Presentation

Even here, with an incidence of <1/100,000 in the US, disparities in presentation, care, and outcomes have been identified. Asian American individuals have the highest incidence rates of NPC. When looking further into Asian American subpopulations, Chinese American individuals have the highest rates of NPC in the US.[48] Black, Hispanic, and Asian patients with NPC are diagnosed at younger ages than White American individuals. Black patients present with larger tumors and have the highest percentage of regional metastasis on presentation. White and Black patients most often present with keratinizing squamous histology, while Asian American patients most often present with undifferentiated, nonkeratinizing histology.[46,49]

Treatment

Treatment for NPC is with radiotherapy. Chemotherapy is given for stage II disease, and induction chemotherapy or adjuvant chemotherapy is recommended for advanced stage III or IV NPC.[50] For localized tumors, Asians American patients have a much higher rate of radiation (85.9%) compared to White (61.2%), Hispanic (57.7%), and Black patients (70.2%).[48]

Outcomes

Black, Hispanic, and American Indian patients with NPC have worse survival. Multivariate modeling shows increased hazard for death for Black (HR 1.26, 95% CI 1.07−1.49) and Hispanic (HR 1.27, 95% CI 1.01−1.61) individuals.[49] In a review of SEER data looking at outcomes for American Indian individuals, it was found that American Indian and Alaska Native patients with NPC had the worst cause-specific survival of all racial groups (HR 2.63, 95% CI 1.67−4.13).[51]

Wang stratified outcomes by histologic type and found that Asian American individuals with keratinizing squamous cell carcinoma had the best survival rate (57.1%) compared to other racial groups (32.7%). For differentiated nonkeratinizing squamous cell carcinoma, Black patients had the second-best (58.9%) survival rate, with other races still having the worst (45.2%). For undifferentiated nonkeratinizing squamous cell carcinoma, White individuals had the second-best survival rate (65.9%). When looking at all subtypes together, five-year survival was 67%, 73%, and 70% for White, Black, and Hispanic, respectively. Survival appeared statistically superior for Black and Asian patients compared to White patients on univariate analysis; however, this was lost when controlling for sex and age. Therefore, it represents the effect of older age of White patients at presentation for NPC in the US.[48]

Given the higher prevalence of NPC in Asian American individuals, Wang reviewed the outcomes for subgroups of patients in the US. They found that NPC incidence rates were higher among Laotian and Chinese subgroups. Laotian individuals had an 18-fold higher incidence rate and presented with the highest proportion of distant disease (53%), thought to be due to the high prevalence of smoking among the Laotian community. Chinese American patients had a 27% higher risk of NPC-specific mortality than White patients. Higher mortality was also found in Vietnamese, Laotian, and Cambodian patients.[52]

Mediators of disparity in head and neck cancer

The previous studies reveal the presence of disparities in historically marginalized patients with head and neck cancer. The following data attempt to answer why these disparities exist. I think of them as factors either exerting influence prior to or at the time of entry into the medical system, or factors within the medical system itself, influencing diagnostic and treatment decisions.

Poverty and lack of education

Poverty, or low SES, has been linked to poor survival for head and neck cancer. In a prospective, observational study of head and neck cancer at all Michigan hospitals, low-income patients and patients without a high school education had the worst overall survival. Analysis showed that lowest quartile income (HR 1.5, 95% CI 1.1–2.0) and high school education or less (HR 1.4, 95% CI 1.1–1.9) predicted both overall survival and disease-specific survival. The lowest income quartile had a 48% increased hazard of dying and 40% increased hazard of disease recurrence. They noted that this held true in a system with fairly equal access to care.[53]

In a meta-analysis from 2020, Black patients with head and neck cancer had higher levels of poverty. They were found to have lower overall survival for all subsites (HR 1.27, 95% CI 1.18–1.36) while controlling for SES, tumor stage, and treatment modality. This disparity was also shown in oral cavity (HR 1.29, 95% CI 1.11–1.33) and oropharynx (HR 1.29, 95% CI 1.20–1.57) regions. Once SES was controlled for, there was a reduction in the survival disparity, suggesting that poverty directly impacts overall survival for head and neck cancer patients.[54]

Location and ability to travel

In a review of the NCDB, long travel distance was associated with treatment at academic and high-volume centers. Black and Hispanic patients and those with Medicaid who were treated nonsurgically were less likely to travel long distances. Traveling long distances (defined as 50 to 249 miles) was associated with improved overall survival (HR 0.93, 95% CI 0.89–0.96). This survival benefit persisted despite controlling for facility type, volume, age, race, insurance, and treatment modality. Multivariate models show Black, rural patients have the highest risk of mortality (HR 1.30, 95% CI 1.27–1.33). Black patients treated at community hospitals had the lowest survival.[55]

These data were replicated by another retrospective cohort from NCDB that looked at the interaction between geography and race in outcomes for hypopharynx, larynx, and oral cavity cancer. They found that the highest five-year survival was among White, urban patients (67.0 months, 95% CI 66–67.9), followed by White, rural patients (59.1 months, 95% CI 57.2–60), Black urban patients (43.1 months, 95% CI 41.1–44.5), and Black rural patients (35.1 months 95% CI 31.9–39).[56] In our study of American Indians in South Dakota, distance from a cancer center of more than 60 miles was also shown to affect survival.[57]

In addition, minority patients are less likely to be treated at high-quality hospitals. Megwalu & Ma reviewed the California Care registry for all oral cavity cancers and found that treatment in a high-quality hospital was associated with improved survival for oral cavity cancer (HR 0.86, 95% CI 0.76–0.98). High-quality definition was based on volume of oral cavity cases treated per year, percentage of stage III/IV patients who were treated with postoperative radiotherapy, percentage who received a quality lymph node dissection, and accreditation by National Comprehensive Cancer Network, National Cancer Institute, and American College of Surgeons. However, Black patients are significantly less likely to be treated in those hospitals (OR 0.87, 95% CI 0.77−0.98).[58]

Health insurance

In 2020, 31.6 million (9.7%) Americans lacked health insurance. Minority patients are more likely to be uninsured or have public health insurance; 45% of Black patients are uninsured or have Medicaid.[59] SEER data from 2010 to 2015 show that Black patients with head and neck cancer are more likely to be uninsured (OR 2.11, 95% CI 1.64−2.69) or more likely to have Medicaid (OR 3.31, 95% CI 2.84−3.85). These patients are more likely to present with unresectable disease and distant metastasis. Disease-specific survival is worse for Black patients, and insurance was found to account for a significant part of the disparity (HR 1.16, 95% CI 1.03−1.31).[60] SEER data from 2007 to 2013 show that uninsured patients with head and neck cancer have reduced five-year overall survival (48.5% vs. 62.5%; difference of 14.0%; 95% CI, 12.8%−15.2%) and five-year disease-specific survival compared with insured patients (56.6% vs. 72.2%; difference of 15.6%; 95% CI, 14.0%−17.2%).[61] Agarwal et al. in a recent SEER review showed that Medicaid patients with oral cavity cancer were more likely to present with later-stage disease, larger tumor size, more distant metastases, and more lymph node involvement. They were less likely to receive surgery and more likely to receive chemoradiation. This resulted in Medicaid patients having worse cancer-specific survival for oral cavity cancer (HR 1.87, 95% CI 1.72−2.04).[62]

The Affordable Care Act (ACA) went into effect in 2013, expanding access to health insurance for low-income individuals. Several studies show that it has been effective at decreasing those uninsured with head and neck cancer. There was an increase after implementation of the ACA in the percentage of patients enrolled in Medicaid and private insurance. In addition, there was a large decrease in the rate of uninsured patients after implementation of the ACA (3.0% after vs. 6.2% before, 95% CI 2.9%−3.5%). These changes more significantly affected patients in low-income zip codes.[61,63]

Not all states chose to participate in Medicaid expansion under the ACA. In a SEER comparison of states that did or did not enact the ACA, the uninsured rate decreased significantly in those states that chose to expand. Between 2011 and 2014, the uninsured rate decreased by 2.6% in nonexpanded states and by 63.8% in expanded states. Rates of Medicaid patients increased by 4.71% in nonexpanded states and increased by 23.76% in expanded states. When stratified by race, there was a significant decrease in the uninsured Hispanic population (10.4% vs. 4.4%, $P < .001$) versus no change in nonexpanded states. There was a decrease in the uninsured rate by 73% in the Black population (9.0%−2.4%, $P < .001$) compared to a nonsignificant increase in the uninsured population in nonexpanded states.[64]

Health system factors

Treatment delays

Delay in the start of cancer treatment is known to affect survival.[65] Liao et al. performed an in-depth review of all patients presenting to New York City hospitals and the time-to-treatment initiation (TTI). TTI was defined as days between histopathological diagnosis and first treatment; median TTI was 40 days. They found that the threshold for effect on survival was 60 days; 31.2% of Black patients and 22% of Hispanic patients had TTI >60 days. Those patients were more likely to have Medicaid insurance (38.2% vs. 24.6%) and SES in the bottom quartile (30% vs. 21.9%). The two most common reasons for delay were missed appointments and extensive pretreatment workup, including dental visits, tooth extractions, medical clearance for surgery, and unknown primary workup. Overall five-year survival was 60.9% for all patients and 47% for patients with TTI exceeding the threshold. These patients also had a higher likelihood of recurrence (OR 1.77). The HR was greater for local stage cancers (1.94 vs.1.47), likely because of stage migration due to treatment delay.[66]

These data were replicated in Florida, with a retrospective review of head and neck cancer at Moffitt cancer center from 1998 to 2013. Black patients were more likely to present with stage T4 disease and more often had >45 days disease until treatment initiation (61% vs. 49%, $P = .028$). Black race was associated with lower locoregional control at three years (65% vs. 81% and OS 43% vs. 69%) after adjusting for tobacco status, stage, and socioeconomic factors, even while being treated at an academic center. This indicates that minority patients and patients with less access to resources are more likely to have difficulty completing all the necessary tasks prior to initiation of treatment.[67]

Total treatment package time, or the time from surgery to the completion of radiation, is known to affect survival outcomes from head and neck cancer.[68] A review of the NCDB found that uninsured patients and those with Medicaid had longer treatment times. Mean treatment package time was 100 days with a standard deviation (SD) of 23 days. Mean time of surgery to start radiation was 47 days (SD 21 days). After controlling for variables, Medicaid patients were 7.52 days longer ($P < .001$, SD 6.23–8.81), low-income areas 3.77 days (SD 2.36–5.18), and African American patients 4.77 days (SD 2.84–6.71). Package time was an independent variable. Each week increase in package time resulted in an average 4% risk of death 1.04 (1.03–1.05). Longer total treatment time is directly related to coordination of care.[69]

Uninsured patients and those with Medicaid are more likely to have treatment interruptions during RT. The overall percentage of treatment interruptions was 18.5% for uninsured patients, 12.9% for Medicaid, and 8.1% for private insurance ($P = 0.001$). No show appointments were more than doubled for Medicaid and uninsured patients. This counted for approximately a week of missed radiation appointments.[70]

Treatment variation

A recent review of NCDB from 2004 to 2014 found that Black patients were significantly less likely to receive surgery and more likely to not be offered surgery for head and neck cancer. Oral cavity patients were 13% less likely to receive surgery, and 38% more likely to not have surgery offered. Black patients were also more likely to refuse surgery at all sites. Patients receiving surgery had significantly greater survival than those not offered surgery (HR 0.61). For all sites, those declining surgery had significantly poorer survival. They did note that this trend improved from 2001 to 2014.[71]

This was confirmed in two studies of SEER data in reviews of all sites of head and neck cancer where primary surgery is recommended. They found a higher proportion of Black patients (14% vs. 7%) and Asian patients (7% vs. 4.8%) refused surgery. Black race was significantly predictive (OR: 1.71, 95% CI: 1.37–2.13) of surgery refusal. This translated to a higher risk of death. The risk of dying was 2.16 higher (95% CI 2.02–2.30) for those who chose nonsurgical treatment. Minority patients and uninsured patients with head and neck cancer were also found to have higher in-hospital mortality when they did undergo surgery. In general, 3.8% of patients with head and neck cancer died within 90 days. Those who were uninsured, Medicaid, or Black race were more likely to die within 90 days of their hospitalization.[72–74]

Conclusion

The victims of systemic oppression in the US need more: more access, more support, and more treatment. We need research and interventions targeted to our needs. The above research represents just the beginning of what tackling these systems looks like. We see from the cited studies that minority patients present with later-stage disease for all subsites of head and neck cancer. They experience delays in treatment initiation, have fewer effective treatments offered, and choose different treatments. They are more likely to be treated at low-volume centers with inexperienced providers. These differences result in poorer outcomes from surgery and radiation, as well as worse disease-specific survival. Lack of insurance, poverty, and low levels of education are some mediators that have been examined in prior studies.

One of the most actionable items that these data show is that minority patients are most frequently uninsured or have public health care and that directly results in worse outcomes for head and neck cancer. With the expansion of insurance through the ACA, we saw that patients in expansion states with head and neck cancer gained insurance and had improved access to care as a result. Universal health care is a necessary step to lower barriers to care and improve outcomes for minority patients.

Missing from the current research, though, are studies that answer the deeper question of why these disparities persist in head and neck cancer. The current data examine trends in large databases, but we are limited by how much we can extrapolate from that information. Qualitative methods of research, such as structured interviews and focus groups, are designed to get at the patient's point of view. These methods examine the patient's experience of their health and treatment and can answer some of the "Why" that contributes to disparities. These methods can be tailored to include small populations and build community by engaging the very people who need it most.

My own personal experience sitting with community members and talking about their conceptions of health and cancer care was both wonderful and heartbreaking. It was the first time some people had ever been able to give voice to their thoughts and opinions about a system from which they frequently felt excluded. They left feeling empowered. But the stories they told were of missed diagnosis, late-stage cancers, and lack of money and gas for travel to appointments.

Also missing from the research are intervention studies. Intervention studies have the potential to bridge the gap between the medical system and minority patients. I worked within a nurse navigation program in Indian Country. The published data from that program showed that American Indian patients receiving nurse navigation had fewer radiation treatment interruptions.[75] But more than that, everyone in the community knew the navigators and the doctors. Everyone knew that they could count on help with a ride to the clinic for a treatment or an appointment. Interventions build trust that communities can see. When the program was disbanded due to lack of funding, the community felt the loss. These systems-level interventions have been shown to eliminate disparities in cancer treatment and outcomes.[76]

Also missing from the research are minority populations too small to show statistical significance using multivariate modeling. For most studies, this includes Indigenous American, Native Hawaiian, and Pacific Islander populations. Middle Eastern American individuals are never mentioned. Where and how we as physicians direct our attention matters. As individuals, it is unlikely that we can shift such large and historical forces like poverty and poor health outcomes in our lifetimes. We can, however, pay attention to our vulnerable populations. We can ask them directly what they need. And with them in mind, we can design studies and direct the flow of material resources within our purview.

References

1. Siegel RL, Miller KD, Fuchs HE, Jemal A. Cancer statistics, 2022. *CA Cancer J Clin.* 2022;72(1):7–33. https://doi.org/10.3322/caac.21708.
2. Vaccarella S, Franceschi S, Bray F, Wild CP, Plummer M, Dal Maso L. Worldwide thyroid-cancer epidemic? The increasing impact of overdiagnosis. *N Engl J Med.* 2016;375(7):614–617. https://doi.org/10.1056/NEJMp1604412.
3. Lim H, Devesa SS, Sosa JA, Check D, Kitahara CM. Trends in thyroid cancer incidence and mortality in the United States, 1974–2013. *JAMA.* 2017;317(13):1338. https://doi.org/10.1001/jama.2017.2719.
4. Weeks KS, Kahl AR, Lynch CF, Charlton ME. Racial/ethnic differences in thyroid cancer incidence in the United States, 2007–2014. *Cancer.* 2018;124(7):1483–1491. https://doi.org/10.1002/cncr.31229.

5. Morris LGT, Sikora AG, Myssiorek D, DeLacure MD. The basis of racial differences in the incidence of thyroid cancer. *Ann Surg Oncol.* 2008;15(4):1169–1176. https://doi.org/10.1245/s10434-008-9812-6.

6. Tang J, Kong D, Cui Q, et al. Racial disparities of differentiated thyroid carcinoma: clinical behavior, treatments, and long-term outcomes. *World J Surg Oncol.* 2018;16:45. https://doi.org/10.1186/s12957-018-1340-7.

7. Harari A, Li N, Yeh MW. Racial and socioeconomic disparities in presentation and outcomes of well-differentiated thyroid cancer. *J Clin Endocrinol Metab.* 2014;99(1):133–141. https://doi.org/10.1210/jc.2013-2781.

8. Orosco RK, Hussain T, Noel JE, et al. Radioactive iodine in differentiated thyroid cancer: a national database perspective. *Endocr Relat Cancer.* 2019;26(10):795–802. https://doi.org/10.1530/ERC-19-0292.

9. Meltzer C, Klau M, Gurushanthaiah D, et al. Surgeon volume in thyroid surgery: surgical efficiency, outcomes, and utilization. *Laryngoscope.* 2016;126(11):2630–2639. https://doi.org/10.1002/lary.26119.

10. Al-Qurayshi Z, Robins R, Hauch A, Randolph GW, Kandil E. Association of surgeon volume with outcomes and cost savings following thyroidectomy: a national forecast. *JAMA Otolaryngol Head Neck Surg.* 2016;142(1):32. https://doi.org/10.1001/jamaoto.2015.2503.

11. Noureldine SI, Abbas A, Tufano RP, et al. The impact of surgical volume on racial disparity in thyroid and parathyroid surgery. *Ann Surg Oncol.* 2014;21(8):2733–2739. https://doi.org/10.1245/s10434-014-3610-0.

12. Sosa JA, Mehta PJ, Wang TS, Yeo HL, Roman SA. Racial disparities in clinical and economic outcomes from thyroidectomy. *Ann Surg.* 2007;246(6):1083–1091. https://doi.org/10.1097/SLA.0b013e31812eecc4.

13. Shah SA, Adam MA, Thomas SM, et al. Racial disparities in differentiated thyroid cancer: have we bridged the gap? *Thyroid.* 2017;27(6):762–772. https://doi.org/10.1089/thy.2016.0626.

14. Al-Qurayshi Z, Randolph GW, Srivastav S, Kandil E. Outcomes in endocrine cancer surgery are affected by racial, economic, and healthcare system demographics. *Laryngoscope.* 2016;126(3):775–781. https://doi.org/10.1002/lary.25606.

15. Jaap K, Campbell R, Dove J, et al. Disparities in the care of differentiated thyroid cancer in the United States: exploring the national cancer database. *Am Surg.* 2017;83(7):739–746.

16. Haymart MR, Banerjee M, Stewart AK, Koenig RJ, Birkmeyer JD, Griggs JJ. Use of radioactive iodine for thyroid cancer. *JAMA.* 2011;306(7):721–728. https://doi.org/10.1001/jama.2011.1139.

17. Nnorom SO, Baig H, Akinyemi OA, et al. Persistence of disparity in thyroid cancer survival after adjustments for socioeconomic status and access. *Am Surg.* 2022;88(7):1484–1489. https://doi.org/10.1177/00031348221082282.

18. Megwalu UC, Saini AT. Racial disparities in papillary thyroid microcarcinoma survival. *J Laryngol Otol.* 2017;131(1):83–87. https://doi.org/10.1017/S0022215116009737.

19. Roche AM, Fedewa SA, Chen AY. Association of socioeconomic status and race/ethnicity with treatment and survival in patients with medullary thyroid cancer. *JAMA Otolaryngol Head Neck Surg.* 2016;142(8):763–771. https://doi.org/10.1001/jamaoto.2016.1051.

20. Roche AM, Fedewa SA, Shi LL, Chen AY. Treatment and survival vary by race/ethnicity in patients with anaplastic thyroid cancer. *Cancer.* 2018;124(8):1780—1790. https://doi.org/10.1002/cncr.31252.

21. LeHew CW, Weatherspoon DJ, Peterson CE, et al. The health system and policy implications of changing epidemiology for oral cavity and oropharyngeal cancers in the United States from 1995 to 2016. *Epidemiol Rev.* 2017;39(1):132—147. https://doi.org/10.1093/epirev/mxw001.

22. Dwojak S, Bhattacharyya N. Racial disparities in preventable risk factors for head and neck cancer. *Laryngoscope.* 2017;127(5):1068—1072. https://doi.org/10.1002/lary.26203.

23. Shiboski CH, Schmidt BL, Jordan RCK. Racial disparity in stage at diagnosis and survival among adults with oral cancer in the US. *Community Dent Oral Epidemiol.* 2007;35(3):233—240. https://doi.org/10.1111/j.0301-5661.2007.00334.x.

24. Dwojak SM, Sequist TD, Emerick K, Deschler DG. Survival differences among American Indians/Alaska natives with head and neck squamous cell carcinoma. *Head Neck.* 2013;35(8):1114—1118. https://doi.org/10.1002/hed.23089.

25. Lewis CM, Ajmani GS, Kyrillos A, et al. Racial disparities in the choice of definitive treatment for squamous cell carcinoma of the oral cavity. *Head Neck.* 2018;40(11): 2372—2382. https://doi.org/10.1002/hed.25341.

26. National Comprehensive Cancer Network. Head and Neck Cancers. V 2.2022-April 26 2022. https://www.nccn.org/professionals/physician_gls/pdf/head-and-neck.pdf. Accessed 15 October 2022.

27. Weng Y, Korte JE. Racial disparities in being recommended to surgery for oral and oropharyngeal cancer in the United States. *Community Dent Oral Epidemiol.* 2012; 40(1):80—88. https://doi.org/10.1111/j.1600-0528.2011.00638.x.

28. Ang KK, Harris J, Wheeler R, et al. Human papillomavirus and survival of patients with oropharyngeal cancer. *N Engl J Med.* 2010;363(1):24—35. https://doi.org/10.1056/NEJMoa0912217.

29. Fakhry C, Zhang Q, Nguyen-Tan PF, et al. Human papillomavirus and overall survival after progression of oropharyngeal squamous cell carcinoma. *J Clin Oncol.* 2014; 32(30):3365—3373. https://doi.org/10.1200/JCO.2014.55.1937.

30. Settle K, Posner MR, Schumaker LM, et al. Racial survival disparity in head and neck cancer results from low prevalence of human papillomavirus infection in black oropharyngeal cancer patients. *Cancer Prev Res.* 2009;2(9):776—781. https://doi.org/10.1158/1940-6207.CAPR-09-0149.

31. Ramer I, Varier I, Zhang D, et al. Racial disparities in incidence of human papillomavirus-associated oropharyngeal cancer in an urban population. *Cancer Epidemiol.* 2016;44:91—95. https://doi.org/10.1016/j.canep.2016.07.004.

32. Liederbach E, Kyrillos A, Wang CH, Liu JC, Sturgis EM, Bhayani MK. The national landscape of human papillomavirus-associated oropharynx squamous cell carcinoma. *Int J Cancer.* 2017;140(3):504—512. https://doi.org/10.1002/ijc.30442.

33. Rotsides JM, Oliver JR, Moses LE, et al. Socioeconomic and racial disparities and survival of human papillomavirus-associated oropharyngeal squamous cell carcinoma. *Otolaryngol Head Neck Surg.* 2021;164(1):131—138. https://doi.org/10.1177/0194599820935853.

34. Albert A, Giri S, Kanakamedala M, et al. Racial disparities in tumor features and outcomes of patients with squamous cell carcinoma of the tonsil. *Laryngoscope.* 2019; 129(3):643—654. https://doi.org/10.1002/lary.27395.

35. Megwalu UC, Ma Y. Racial disparities in oropharyngeal cancer stage at diagnosis. *Anticancer Res.* 2017;37(2):835−839. https://doi.org/10.21873/anticanres.11386.
36. Zhu D, Wong A, Oh EJ, et al. Impact of treatment parameters on racial survival differences in oropharyngeal cancer: national cancer database study. *Otolaryngol Head Neck Surg.* 2022;166(6):1134−1143. https://doi.org/10.1177/01945998211035056.
37. Megwalu UC, Ma Y. Racial disparities in oropharyngeal cancer survival. *Oral Oncol.* 2017;65:33−37. https://doi.org/10.1016/j.oraloncology.2016.12.015.
38. Lenze NR, Farquhar DR, Mazul AL, Masood MM, Zevallos JP. Racial disparities and human papillomavirus status in oropharyngeal cancer: a systematic review and meta-analysis. *Head Neck.* 2019;41(1):256−261. https://doi.org/10.1002/hed.25414.
39. Stein E, Lenze NR, Yarbrough WG, Hayes DN, Mazul A, Sheth S. Systematic review and meta-analysis of racial survival disparities among oropharyngeal cancer cases by HPV status. *Head Neck.* 2020;42(10):2985−3001. https://doi.org/10.1002/hed.26328.
40. Shin JY, Truong MT. Racial disparities in laryngeal cancer treatment and outcome: a population-based analysis of 24,069 patients. *Laryngoscope.* 2015;125(7):1667−1674. https://doi.org/10.1002/lary.25212.
41. Chen S, Dee EC, Muralidhar V, Nguyen PL, Amin MR, Givi B. Disparities in mortality from larynx cancer: implications for reducing racial differences. *Laryngoscope.* 2021;131(4):E1147−E1155. https://doi.org/10.1002/lary.29046.
42. Misono S, Marmor S, Yueh B, Virnig BA. Treatment and survival in 10,429 patients with localized laryngeal cancer: a population-based analysis. *Cancer.* 2014;120(12):1810−1817. https://doi.org/10.1002/cncr.28608.
43. Hou WH, Daly ME, Lee NY, Farwell DG, Luu Q, Chen AM. Racial disparities in the use of voice preservation therapy for locally advanced laryngeal cancer. *Arch Otolaryngol Head Neck Surg.* 2012;138(7):644−649. https://doi.org/10.1001/archoto.2012.1021.
44. Iwata AJ, Williams AM, Taylor AR, Chang SS. Socioeconomic disparities and comorbidities, not race, affect salivary gland malignancy survival outcomes. *Laryngoscope.* 2017;127(11):2545−2550. https://doi.org/10.1002/lary.26633.
45. Russell JL, Chen NW, Ortiz SJ, Schrank TP, Kuo YF, Resto VA. Racial and ethnic disparities in salivary gland cancer survival. *JAMA Otolaryngol Head Neck Surg.* 2014;140(6):504−512. https://doi.org/10.1001/jamaoto.2014.406.
46. Patel VJ, Chen NW, Resto VA. Racial and ethnic disparities in nasopharyngeal cancer survival in the United States. *Otolaryngol Head Neck Surg.* 2017;156(1):122−131. https://doi.org/10.1177/0194599816672625.
47. Chang ET, Ye W, Zeng YX, Adami HO. The evolving epidemiology of nasopharyngeal carcinoma. *Cancer Epidemiol Biomarkers Prev.* 2021;30(6):1035−1047. https://doi.org/10.1158/1055-9965.EPI-20-1702.
48. Wang Y, Zhang Y, Ma S. Racial differences in nasopharyngeal carcinoma in the United States. *Cancer Epidemiol.* 2013;37(6). https://doi.org/10.1016/j.canep.2013.08.008.
49. Zhou L, Shen N, Li G, Ding J, Liu D, Huang X. The racial disparity of nasopharyngeal carcinoma based on the database analysis. *Am J Otolaryngol.* 2019;40(6):102288. https://doi.org/10.1016/j.amjoto.2019.102288.
50. Bossi P, Chan AT, Licitra L, et al. Nasopharyngeal carcinoma: ESMO-EURACAN clinical practice guidelines for diagnosis, treatment and follow-up†. *Ann Oncol.* 2021;32(4):452−465. https://doi.org/10.1016/j.annonc.2020.12.007.
51. Challapalli SD, Simpson MC, Adjei Boakye E, et al. Survival differences in nasopharyngeal carcinoma among racial and ethnic minority groups in the United States: a retrospective cohort study. *Clin Otolaryngol.* 2019;44(1):14−20. https://doi.org/10.1111/coa.13225.

52. Wang Q, Xie H, Li Y, et al. Racial and ethnic disparities in nasopharyngeal cancer with an emphasis among Asian Americans. *Int J Cancer.* 2022;151(8):1291−1303. https://doi.org/10.1002/ijc.34154.

53. Choi SH, Terrell JE, Fowler KE, et al. Socioeconomic and other demographic disparities predicting survival among head and neck cancer patients. *PLoS One.* 2016;11(3): e0149886. https://doi.org/10.1371/journal.pone.0149886.

54. Russo DP, Tham T, Bardash Y, Kraus D. The effect of race in head and neck cancer: a meta-analysis controlling for socioeconomic status. *Am J Otolaryngol.* 2020;41(6): 102624. https://doi.org/10.1016/j.amjoto.2020.102624.

55. Graboyes EM, Ellis MA, Li H, et al. Racial and ethnic disparities in travel for head and neck cancer treatment and the impact of travel distance on survival. *Cancer.* 2018; 124(15):3181−3191. https://doi.org/10.1002/cncr.31571.

56. Clarke JA, Despotis AM, Ramirez RJ, Zevallos JP, Mazul AL. Head and neck cancer survival disparities by race and rural-urban context. *Cancer Epidemiol Biomarkers Prev.* 2020;29(10):1955−1961. https://doi.org/10.1158/1055-9965.EPI-20-0376.

57. Dwojak SM, Finkelstein DM, Emerick KS, Lee JH, Petereit DG, Deschler DG. Poor survival for American Indians with head and neck squamous cell carcinoma. *Otolaryngol Head Neck Surg.* 2014;151(2):265−271. https://doi.org/10.1177/0194599814533083.

58. Megwalu UC, Ma Y. Racial/ethnic disparities in use of high-quality hospitals among oral cancer patients in California. *Laryngoscope.* 2022;132(4):793−800. https://doi.org/10.1002/lary.29830.

59. National Health Statistics Reports. February 11, 2022:169:15.

60. Shukla N, Ma Y, Megwalu UC. The role of insurance status as a mediator of racial disparities in oropharyngeal cancer outcomes. *Head Neck.* 2021;43(10):3116−3124. https://doi.org/10.1002/hed.26807.

61. Cannon RB, Shepherd HM, McCrary H, et al. Association of the patient protection and Affordable Care Act with insurance coverage for head and neck cancer in the SEER database. *JAMA Otolaryngol Head Neck Surg.* 2018;144(11):1052−1057. https://doi.org/10.1001/jamaoto.2018.1792.

62. Agarwal P, Agrawal RR, Jones EA, Devaiah AK. Social determinants of health and oral cavity cancer treatment and survival: a competing risk analysis. *Laryngoscope.* 2020; 130(9):2160−2165. https://doi.org/10.1002/lary.28321.

63. Panth N, Barnes J, Sethi RKV, Varvares MA, Osazuwa-Peters N. Socioeconomic and demographic variation in insurance coverage among patients with head and neck cancer after the Affordable Care Act. *JAMA Otolaryngol Head Neck Surg.* 2019;145(12): 1144−1149. https://doi.org/10.1001/jamaoto.2019.2724.

64. Babu A, Wassef DW, Sangal NR, Goldrich D, Baredes S, Park RCW. The Affordable Care Act: implications for underserved populations with head & neck cancer. *Am J Otolaryngol.* 2020;41(4):102464. https://doi.org/10.1016/j.amjoto.2020.102464.

65. Murphy CT, Galloway TJ, Handorf EA, et al. Survival impact of increasing time to treatment initiation for patients with head and neck cancer in the United States. *J Clin Oncol.* 2016;34(2):169−178. https://doi.org/10.1200/JCO.2015.61.5906.

66. Liao DZ, Schlecht NF, Rosenblatt G, et al. Association of delayed time to treatment initiation with overall survival and recurrence among patients with head and neck squamous cell carcinoma in an underserved urban population. *JAMA Otolaryngol Head Neck Surg.* 2019;145(11):1001−1009. https://doi.org/10.1001/jamaoto.2019.2414.

67. Naghavi AO, Echevarria MI, Strom TJ, et al. Treatment delays, race, and outcomes in head and neck cancer. *Cancer Epidemiol.* 2016;45:18−25. https://doi.org/10.1016/j.canep.2016.09.005.

68. Goel AN, Frangos MI, Raghavan G, et al. The impact of treatment package time on survival in surgically managed head and neck cancer in the United States. *Oral Oncol.* 2019;88:39−48. https://doi.org/10.1016/j.oraloncology.2018.11.021.

69. Guttmann DM, Kobie J, Grover S, et al. National disparities in treatment package time for resected locally advanced head and neck cancer and impact on overall survival. *Head Neck.* 2018;40(6):1147−1155. https://doi.org/10.1002/hed.25091.

70. Yarn C, Wakefield DV, Spencer S, Martin MY, Pisu M, Schwartz DL. Insurance status and head and neck radiotherapy interruption disparities in the Mid-Southern United States. *Head Neck.* 2020;42(8):2013−2020. https://doi.org/10.1002/hed.26128.

71. Nocon CC, Ajmani GS, Bhayani MK. A contemporary analysis of racial disparities in recommended and received treatment for head and neck cancer. *Cancer.* 2020;126(2):381−389. https://doi.org/10.1002/cncr.32342.

72. Parhar HS, Anderson DW, Janjua AS, Durham JS, Prisman E. Patient choice of nonsurgical treatment contributes to disparities in head and neck squamous cell carcinoma. *Otolaryngol Head Neck Surg.* 2018;158(6):1057−1064. https://doi.org/10.1177/0194599818755353.

73. Gaubatz ME, Bukatko AR, Simpson MC, et al. Racial and socioeconomic disparities associated with 90-day mortality among patients with head and neck cancer in the United States. *Oral Oncol.* 2019;89:95−101. https://doi.org/10.1016/j.oraloncology.2018.12.023.

74. Crippen MM, Elias ML, Weisberger JS, et al. Refusal of cancer-directed surgery in head and neck squamous cell carcinoma patients. *Laryngoscope.* 2019;129(6):1368−1373. https://doi.org/10.1002/lary.27116.

75. Petereit DG, Molloy K, Reiner ML, et al. Establishing a patient navigator program to reduce cancer disparities in the American Indian Communities of Western South Dakota: initial observations and results. *Cancer Control.* 2008;15(3):254−259. https://doi.org/10.1177/107327480801500309.

76. Manning M, Yongue C, Garikipati A, et al. Overall survival from a prospective multi-institutional trial to resolve black-white disparities in the treatment of early stage breast and lung cancer. *Int J Radiat Oncol Biol Phys.* 2021;111(3):S28. https://doi.org/10.1016/j.ijrobp.2021.07.091.

Disparities in the diagnosis and treatment of obstructive sleep apnea

15

Stacey L. Ishman[1,2,3], Javier J.M. Howard[4]

[1]Division of Pulmonary and Sleep Medicine, Cincinnati Children's Hospital Medical Center, Cincinnati, OH, United States; [2]Division of HealthVine, Cincinnati Children's Hospital Medical Center, Cincinnati, OH, United States; [3]Department of Otolaryngology—Head and Neck Surgery, College of Medicine, University of Cincinnati, Cincinnati, OH, United States; [4]Department of Otolaryngology—Head and Neck Surgery, School of Medicine, Stanford University, Stanford, CA, United States

Introduction

Sleep is a fundamental physiologic process undertaken by all known living organisms;[1] however, sleep disordered breathing (SDB) is one of the most prevalent chronic diseases plaguing modern human society. This group of disorders, including obstructive sleep apnea (OSA), is estimated to afflict between 9% and 38% of the world's population, with projections suggesting that the burden will continue to grow.[2]

Epidemiologic studies demonstrate that the global burden of SDB is not equally distributed across populations. A growing body of evidence reports that minoritized, marginalized, and otherwise disadvantaged populations are disproportionately impacted by SDB. The sequelae of SDB and OSA do not occur in isolation, as these disease processes are associated with cardiovascular,[3] metabolic,[4] and neurocognitive diseases, as well as increased overall healthcare utilization, workplace and motor vehicle accidents, and all-cause mortality.[5]

Since most of what is known about the epidemiology, pathophysiology, diagnosis, and treatment of OSA comes from research performed in overwhelmingly White, non-Hispanic male populations, it is difficult to extrapolate these data to apply to women and racial and ethnic minority groups. Additionally, awareness about OSA is low, and it is likely that familiarity in minority and socioeconomically disadvantaged communities, where healthcare literacy is reduced, is even lower than in the general community.[6–8] In this chapter, we seek to summarize the existing literature on this subject, as well as to highlight areas that would benefit from future research, and interventions which may improve health equity.

Epidemiology/prevalence

The prevalence of OSA is increasing in both males and females, and there is evidence that this phenomenon is closely related to the worsening obesity epidemic.[9,10] Most of the current evidence (based on biological sex) demonstrates that OSA is more common in males, and that males typically have a more severe phenotype than premenopausal females of the same age. Current estimates report a 2:1 to 3:1 male predominance for OSA in premenopausal age groups; however, prevalence is closer to 1:1 for postmenopausal age groups.[11-13] Overall, the prevalence and severity of OSA increase with age in both sexes, with females demonstrating a later onset of disease. Central obesity and hormone status appear to moderate the prevalence of OSA in females and may explain some of this disparity.[14,15]

With regard to the pediatric population, a 2008 systematic review found SDB to be more common in males compared to females, and this difference may be mediated by age due to the hormonal differences of puberty.[16] However, the vast majority of the studies use caregiver report of SBD symptoms to estimate prevalence, which is inherently imprecise and subject to bias.

There are limited data regarding the prevalence of OSA as it relates to ethnicity and race, and these results are mixed. Much of the current literature focuses on differences between White and Black populations in the United States (US), with less data focused on Latinx and Asian populations. There are little or no data on other racial and ethnic groups like indigenous populations.

The first notable examination of the relationship between ethnicity and OSA in adults was published by Villanueva in 2005.[17] They noted many challenges in comparing and interpreting existing data and estimates of prevalence and severity. These challenges included how estimates were made (i.e., self-reported questionnaires, home sleep tests, and polysomnography [PSG]) and the guidelines or criteria used to score those data (i.e., PSG scoring criteria which vary from organization to organization and have changed significantly over time). They concluded that the overall prevalence of OSA was likely similar across European, Asian, and Indian populations, ranging from 1.3% to 7.5% in males and 2% to 3.2% in females.[17]

A recent review by Hnin et al. (2018) utilized an apnea hypopnea index (AHI) or respiratory disturbance index (RDI) cutoff of ≥15 to report adult prevalence estimates by ethnicity using International Classification of Sleep Disorders (ICSD-3) criteria. They found that the prevalence and severity of OSA in these interethnic studies ranged widely. In White individuals, estimates ranged from 1.5% to 57%, Asian individuals from 14% to 39.4%, Black individuals from 16.7% to 47%, and Latinx individuals from 15.9% to 45.5%.[18]

Early data in the literature, primarily from the 1990s, demonstrated that Black populations have higher prevalence and severity of OSA across the lifespan. Black children were estimated to have upward of four to six times the OSA prevalence, along with higher severity, than their White peers.[19-21] Stepanski et al. found that Black children experienced significantly greater hypoxemia with obstructive events relative to their White and Latinx peers, suggesting that they may be at higher risk of cardiovascular consequences of SDB.[22] This is especially disconcerting given that studies in diverse samples have found the association between OSA and cardiovascular disease to be stronger in Black individuals.[23]

Similar to that in children, studies in the 1990s found that both young and elderly adult Black populations were at higher risk for OSA than their White peers.[24,25] Interestingly, more recent cohort studies, from 2010 to current day, including the Osteoporotic Fractures in Men (MrOS) Sleep Study, Multi-Ethnic Study of Atherosclerosis (MESA), study of Women's Health (SWAN), and Sleep Heart Health study have reported no significant difference in the prevalence or severity of OSA in Black American adults compared to White American adults.[26–29] Furthermore, while the MESA study did not show higher rates of PSG diagnosed SDB in Black adults relative to White adults, Black adults were found to have significantly higher rates of obstructive sleep apnea syndrome (OSAS; defined as SDB + Epworth Sleepiness Scale (ESS) > 10), short sleep duration, poor sleep quality, and daytime sleepiness relative to White adults.[26] Results from this study highlight an alarming, broader disparity in objective and subjective sleep quality and quantity in Black adults.

In addition, studies from the 1990s demonstrated that Latinx adults had 3× the prevalence of moderate or greater OSA than non-Hispanic White adults.[30] However, the majority of studies published since 2010, including MESA 1, Sleep Heart Health study, and MrOS Sleep Study reported no significant difference in prevalence between White and Latinx populations.[27,29,31] The MESA 2 study (2015), however, did report a higher prevalence of severe OSA (AHI ≥30) in Latinx compared to White Americans after adjusting for age, gender, and study site.[26]

There are limited data comparing the prevalence of OSA between Asian and White children; however, the prevalence of symptomatic OSA appears to be similar between these populations.[32–34]

Most current evidence suggests that adult Asian populations have higher prevalence and severity of OSA relative to White populations.[35,36] Data from the MESA study published in 2015 found Chinese adults had higher odds of objectively measured SDB and were 37% more likely to have severe SDB relative to White adults. Despite this, the same study found that Chinese adults had the lowest prevalence of doctor-diagnosed OSA.[26] This suggests there may be barriers to care that need to be explored more in Chinese American adult populations.

A study comparing OSA prevalence in the Japanese population as estimated by the Circulatory Risk in Communities Study (CIRCS) versus White American populations (MESA) noted significantly lower OSA prevalence and severity in the Japanese population. These differences suggest that when comparing adult Asian and White populations, BMI and sex appear to be important factors accounting for differences in prevalence between these groups.[26,37] A 2008 comparative study of adult Japanese versus White males in Brazil found that for the same OSA severity, Japanese descendants have lower BMI.[37]

To date, there are no studies reporting OSA prevalence data based on patient sexual orientation or gender identity. However, there is evidence that sexual minorities haver higher rates of all types of sleep disorders, likely associated with the increased mental, emotional, and physical stress associated with discrimination and stigmatization. A large retrospective cross-sectional study published in 2022 using a large US-based administrative claims database reported a higher burden of all sleep disorders (and mood disorders) in transgender or gender-nonconforming youth, including triple the odds of OSA compared to their cisgender peers. Interestingly, while gender-affirming therapy (GAT) has been associated with decreased odds of other sleep disorders (insomnia) in transgender youth on GAT relative to their transgender peers without GAT, no difference was seen in odds of OSA.[38] This may reflect improved mental health among transgender youth on GAT, subsequently improving sleep; however, GAT may interact with OSA physiology differently, as discussed later in this chapter.

Clinical presentation

The clinical presentation of patients with OSA has been shown to vary based on patient age, sex, and race and ethnicity. This is likely moderated by cultural, lifestyle, and ecological factors on both patients and providers, in addition to patients' comorbid disease status and access to care. Patients in certain groups may perceive certain behaviors and feelings associated with OSA to be normal (e.g., snoring runs in the family) or not of high salience.

With regard to the clinical presentation of OSA in pediatric patients based on sex, this has been sparsely examined and is inherently more complex than in adults, as caregiver perception and biases are at play. Social perceptions of what is normal and acceptable behavior in children (i.e., snoring and hyperactivity) vary based on sex, and this is further modulated by the context of culture and environment.

The data are inconsistent, but the prevalence of SDB symptoms (including snoring) may be higher among male children. A 2008 systematic review found 15 studies reporting a higher prevalence of SDB symptoms in males, while 19 studies found no difference by sex and only one study (Swedish cohort of children aged 5—7) reported a higher prevalence of snoring in females.[16,39] A challenge in interpreting data on prevalence in children is the heterogeneity of age in these studies, given the role that hormones may play in the pathogenesis of disease. It has been proposed that sex differences in SDB are more likely to emerge with the onset of puberty, and the evidence thus far suggest this hypothesis may be correct. For example, of the 15 studies in the 2008 systematic review that found higher prevalence of SDB symptoms among males, more than half of them included children older than age 13. In contrast, of the 19 studies that failed to demonstrate higher SDB symptoms among males, only 3 included children 13 and older (of note all 19 of these studies showed no difference between the sexes). All studies including males aged 17 or older found a significant sex-based difference in prevalence.[16]

Much of the early OSA literature and subsequent assumptions and stereotypes of how adult OSA patients present clinically were developed based on middle-aged

White males, and their clinical presentation is considered the "traditional" presentation. This is important to consider as males tend to present as "sleepier" than females, whereas females tend to have symptoms described as "more vague" than males[40]; these include symptoms of insomnia, fatigue, or depression, as well as a higher likelihood of presenting with conditions with similar symptom profiles like depression and hypothyroidism.[40–42]

Shepertycky and colleagues found that adult females are less likely to present with witnessed apneas and consume less caffeine per day than adult males.[41] All of these factors may contribute to misdiagnosis or delayed diagnosis of OSA in females. Interestingly, these factors, along with physiologic factors relating to estrogen, may contribute to the fact that females tend to be diagnosed with OSA at older ages, greater BMI, and larger waist-to-hip ratio than males.[12,42,43] Neck fat may also be more predictive of upper airway patency and subsequent OSA risk in females than in males.[44] Interestingly, after PSG, females tend to have a lower AHI at time of diagnosis when compared to males.[42]

In addition to biological sex, it is important to consider the ways that gender identity and gender expression may modulate the clinical presentation of OSA. However, there is no literature to date dedicated to examining or delineating differences in the clinical presentation of SDB or OSA in nonbinary or gender-nonconforming individuals.

Sexual orientation may also impact that ways which patients with OSA present (or do not present). Given that bed partner report and complaints (firsthand or otherwise) are frequently key important factors in the diagnosis and monitoring of OSA, individuals who may feel reluctance to have their bed partner accompany them to medical appointments may contribute to delayed or missed diagnosis. While there is a paucity of literature on the subject, the NEXT Generation Health Study, which is a national longitudinal cohort study of US adolescents found that sexual minority (nonheterosexual identifying) females reported significantly more self-reported daytime sleepiness and snoring than their heterosexual peers. Further analysis found these symptoms to be associated with overweight status and increased depressive symptoms, suggesting possible overall worse mental and physical health among sexual minority females.[45] No other sexual orientation sleep health disparities were identified.

The clinical presentation of patients with OSA is impacted by racial and ethnic and cultural factors (including shared beliefs and norms), as well as comorbid disease. Factors like lack of connectedness to the healthcare system may also delay or decrease the odds of diagnosis of OSA.

In children, Black race alone has been found to be an independent risk factor for OSA.[16] A 2017 study of preschoolers (64% White, 36% Black, 59% male) found that Black preschoolers were more likely to live in a single parent household (53% vs. 9%) and were more likely to share a bed with a caregiver (51% vs. 20%) than their White peers. These are interesting findings, as more frequent exposure to the child while sleeping (sharing a bed) may modulate the quality of caregiver reported sleep concerns. This study found that White children were more likely to present with insomnia symptoms, while Black children were more likely to present with SBD symptoms.[46] Rubens et al. (2016) similarly found Black children's caregivers were more likely to present with SDB concerns than White children.[47]

Black adults tend to underreport all sleep problems, contributing to their under-diagnosis.[48] For OSA specifically, Black adults typically have a higher BMI and severity at time of diagnosis. Although some studies have shown no severity differ-ence (based on AHI) in OSA at the time of diagnosis,[49] Black Americans are typi-cally five years younger at their time of diagnosis than their White counterparts.[49,50] While Thornton et al. reported these same findings, they found no difference in OSA severity between Black and White individuals when controlling for BMI and median household income.[50] They also found that for both sexes, Black adults were younger, had higher BMI, higher severity of OSA based on AHI, and were sleepier (based on ESS) than their White counterparts.[50]

Clinical presentation of SDB in preadolescent Latinx children has been high-lighted in the population-based Tuscon Children's Assessment of Sleep Apnea Study (TuCASA). In their sample of nearly 1500 children, Latinx parents reported that their children experienced significantly greater rates of snoring, excessive daytime sleepiness, witnessed apneas, and learning difficulties than White parents.[51]

With regard to Latinx adults, there are scant data on the differences in clinical presentation of OSA, but a study by Subramanian et al. found that Latinx females with OSA were more likely to complain of psychogenic insomnia, while White fe-males with OSA were more likely to complain of sleep maintenance insomnia.[42]

Similarly, there are not much data in Asian populations on clinical presentation; however, there does not appear to be a clear difference in the prevalence of habitual snoring or parent-reported witnessed apneas between Asian and White pediatric populations.[16] In Asian adults, there is evidence suggesting a tendency to underre-port OSA symptoms.[36]

Diagnosis

The detection and diagnosis of OSA is a problem broadly, across all populations, but this is likely even more challenging in minority populations.[52] There are a myriad of barriers to entering the healthcare system for patients with OSA, as discussed more extensively in a later section on awareness and knowledge. Even for patients who successfully navigate the system and are referred for PSG, it can take months to un-dergo testing, possibly even longer in underserved communities.[52] Home sleep testing (HST) may help alleviate some of these disparities, with evidence in urban Black adult populations that HST may be feasible,[53] but the study did not examine subsequent adherence to treatment or other outcomes, thus it is hard to extrapolate at this time whether HST can reduce disparities in this population.

Disparities in diagnosis have been elucidated across the lifespan. A study of chil-dren presenting with SDB in Canada (where there is universal health care) revealed that longer driving times are associated with lower odds of PSG before adenotonsillectomy (AT), even when adjusting for socioeconomic status (SES) and comorbidities. Interestingly, younger age and female sex were also associated with lower odds of PSG prior to AT.[54]

Retrospective analysis of an urban US cohort of children with SDB, referred from primary care to either subspecialty appointment or PSG, found that 50% were lost to follow up after referral on two-year follow up. Interestingly, more children (76%) were lost to follow up when referred for PSG when compared to referral to a subspecialty clinic (32%). Black patients were found to be over twice as likely to be lost to follow up relative to their White peers.[55] Other studies have demonstrated that children with public insurance experienced significantly longer intervals from initial evaluation to PSG than their peers with private insurance. They also found that half of all patients referred for PSG (regardless of SES) were lost to follow up, indicating that PSG may deter and or delay care for all children with SDB, especially those with public insurance or low SES.[56]

OSA is an underdiagnosed condition in both the US and around the world, with the Wisconsin cohort estimating that approximately only 7% of adult females and 18% of adult males with moderate-to-severe OSA had been formally diagnosed.[57] When it comes to mild OSA, it is estimated that only 2% of females and 10% of males with mild OSA have a clinical diagnosis. Studies have shown that factors associated with increased chances of clinical OSA diagnosis and treatment are male sex and elevated BMI.[58] The underlying reasons for the underdiagnosis of OSA in females have been sparsely researched to date; however, differences in clinical presentation may play a key role in many patients.

When it comes to race and ethnicity, rates of diagnosis in communities of color in the US may lag behind White populations; however, there are limited objective data in Asian, Black, and other populations. The Hispanic Community Health Study found that only 1.3% of patients had a prior diagnosis of OSA, despite finding an OSA prevalence of 25.8% in the general US population.[59] This suggests a staggeringly low level of diagnosis in the US Latinx community. In addition, there is little or no information regarding diagnosis based on sexual orientation, gender identity, or gender expression.

Treatment

First-line treatment for OSA in children is AT. However, despite the literature indicating that children in racial and ethnic minority groups in the US have a greater prevalence and severity of SDB than White children, some groups may be less likely to receive treatment. A systematic review of the literature by Boss et al. (2011) found that non-White children and those with private insurance were more likely to undergo AT.[21]

In addition, parents of Black children may be less willing to consider AT for SDB than their White peers; however, the factors associated with this have not yet been elucidated.[60] This disparity may be explained by evidence which suggests that some of these children are lost in the path to treatment. Yan et al. found that the odds of following up with an otolaryngologist after referral for SDB were 83% lower in Black children and 73% lower in Latinx children relative to their White peers.[61]

Using insurance status as a proxy for SES, children with lower SES also seem to be less likely to receive treatment. Children with public insurance had significantly lower odds than privately insured children of following up with an otolaryngologist for SDB[21] and were less likely to undergo AT for OSA.[61] Additionally, children with higher SES are reported to have lower rates of postoperative complications.[62]

There are several other studies in the US demonstrating that White children and those with private insurance are more likely than their Black and Latinx peers to undergo AT for OSA. Additionally, White children also tend to wait a shorter time until surgery.[63] No comparative data on the treatment of Asian versus White children were found.

Interestingly, a 2018 retrospective study out of Texas of over 30,000 pediatric patients (41% female, 51% White, 24% Black, 23% Latinx, 3.0% Asian) found that Black children are more likely to have respiratory complications following inpatient AT. The study used a logistical regression to control for age, gender, obesity, OSA, asthma, sickle cell anemia, and insurance status, and Black children continued to have higher rates of respiratory complications (OR 1.5, 95% CI: 1.3−1.8), respiratory interventions (OR: 1.5, 95% CI: 1.3−1.7), and all respiratory events (OR: 1.5, 95% CI: 1.4−1.6) relative to the overall population mean. White children had lower risk of respiratory events and interventions, while Latinx and Asian children did not show significant differences relative to the mean. No significant difference was noted based on gender.[64]

A large cross-sectional multicenter database review of nearly 80,000 cases of pediatric tonsillectomy in California, Iowa, Florida, and New York in 2010−11 (59% White, 23% Latinx, 10% Black, and 8% other) found that Black and Latinx children had significantly increased risk of revisit after AT and increased likelihood of acute pain at the revisit relative to White children. These authors did not find an association between race and rate of postoperative hemorrhage.[62] In this study, female sex was associated with decreased risk of posttonsillectomy hemorrhage.

With regard to geography, pediatric patients living in rural areas tend to experience longer wait times and longer driving distance to undergo AT.[65]

While the factors that lead to varied rates and patterns of treatment of OSA across populations are myriad, there has been some research to date to help elucidate these issues. The gold standard for OSA treatment remains continuous positive airway pressure (CPAP) therapy. However, getting patients diagnosed with OSA and prescribed CPAP can be wrought with a variety of challenges. Once prescribed, CPAP adherence rates (defined as use of at least 4 h per night for at least 70% of nights) are overall quite dismal, but they do tend to follow different patterns based on the patient's age, race, and SES.

In adults, White male patients who live in higher SES neighborhoods are more likely to receive treatment for OSA. Additionally, this same archetype of patient is most likely to be compliant with CPAP therapy. A single 2004 study by Scharf et al. found no significant difference in the mean number of self-reported hours of CPAP use per week between Black and White patients.[49] However, the vast majority of studies do support the notion that Latinx and Black adults have lower rates of CPAP adherence than White adults.[66–68] Published CPAP adherence data in Asian populations are scarce, with no comparative studies to non-Asian minority groups. There is also a wide variety of reported CPAP acceptance and adherence rates in different parts of Asia.[69]

In a study done by Joo et al. in 2007 with over 75% Black individuals, females were 2.5 times more likely to be noncomplaint with CPAP therapy than males when adjusting for race, marital status, and age.[68] While few studies exist comparing CPAP compliance between adult males and females, two European studies support these findings.[70,71] One Canadian study (81% male) reported higher compliance rates in females,[72] while two other European studies found no difference between sexes.[73,74]

Decreased CPAP compliance has also been observed in individuals living in lower SES zip codes.[66,75,76] Platt et al. examined veterans with OSA and found that compliance rates of individuals in neighborhoods with high SES were twice that of those who lived in low SES neighborhoods. Other studies have shown that patients with low SES have attitudes that are less receptive to CPAP and are less compliant overall.[76]

Oral appliance therapy (OAT) can be an effective nonsurgical treatment option for some OSA patients with milder disease;[77] however, no data on differences in compliance based on race, sex, sexual orientation, gender identity, or other demographic factors could be found at the time this was written.

When it comes to surgical management of OSA, the racial disparities in treatment are even more alarming. A 2022 study by Khan et al. reported on the ADHERE registry of patients who had undergone implantation of upper airway stimulation devices for the treatment of OSA in Europe and the US. Of the nearly 2755 patients in the database, only 125 identified as non-White (<5%).[78] A study by Cohen et al. performed multivariate analysis of over half a million patients with OSA from a large private insurance database and found that Black race, increased age, atrial fibrillation, obesity, and congestive heart failure were independently associated with a decreased rate of surgery for OSA. Interestingly, Asian race, hypertension, arrhythmias other than atrial fibrillation, pulmonary disease, and liver disease were independently associated with an increased risk of surgery for OSA.[79]

Although non-White adult patients are less likely to undergo surgical treatment of their OSA, the available data indicate that their adherence rates and outcomes following surgery are at least as high as their White peers. Khan et al. found no significant difference in adherence, subjective (change in ESS) efficacy, or objective (posttreatment AHI) efficacy between White and non-White individuals undergoing hypoglossal nerve stimulation (HGNS) after propensity matching and secondary analysis.[78]

Ruthberg et al. analyzed the National Inpatient Sample (NIS) database records from 2007 to 2014 for adult patients with the diagnosis of OSA who underwent either soft tissue or skeletal surgery for OSA and found that patients who underwent any type of surgery for OSA (soft tissue or skeletal) were more likely to be younger, male, of the highest income bracket, utilize private insurance, and of Latinx or Asian race.[80] Interestingly, a study by Garg et al. of over 6000 patients aged 14 and older in the NIS from 2005 to 2012 found conflicting results. Specifically, when looking at patients who had undergone jaw surgery in this cohort, females were more likely than males to receive jaw surgery (OR $= 1.68$, $P = .0007$), and racial minority individuals [Black (OR $= 0.19$, $P < .0001$), Latinx (OR $= 0.42$, $P = .0009$), Asian (OR $= 0.41$, $P = .0009$), and other non-Caucasian (OR $= 0.19$, $P = .0008$)] were less likely to undergo jaw surgery than Caucasian individuals. However, patients in lower income brackets and those with Medicare were significantly less likely to undergo jaw surgery,[81] consistent with the reports from Ruthberg et al.

A systematic review of studies published between 2016 and 2020 investigating sleep outcomes following nonnasal surgery for OSA in adults found within those studies reporting sex demographics, that only 16% of patients were female. For studies reporting data on race and ethnicity (with the exception of two studies with 100% Chinese patients) patient demographics were 87.9% White, 7.5% Asian, 0.7% Black, and 3.9% other.[82]

Mechanisms

Disparities in the diagnosis and treatment of OSA across the sexes have been demonstrated, like other disease processes. However, the biological and pathophysiological mechanisms by which males and females differ in the development of and severity of OSA have only been postulated with a small amount of evidence. The available literature is primarily retrospective and observational; thus, it is hard to deduce strong mechanistic hypotheses. Differences in the prevalence and severity of OSA in males and females are believed to be at least in part due to the protective effects of estrogen.[11,83,84] Animal and in vitro studies have demonstrated that estrogen receptors are upregulated in the genioglossus muscle, which may have a protective effect on the fatigue ability of the genioglossus tissue when exposed to intermittent hypoxia.[85]

Human studies supporting this hypothesis include a study from the late 1980s which found that females with a history of hysterectomy had a significant reduction in AHI after 1 week of conjugated hormone replacement therapy. Thus they found that the addition of exogenous estrogen may contribute to the reversal of the deleterious impact of the abrupt decrease in endogenous estrogen production associated with hysterectomy.[84] Other studies have demonstrated only slight reductions in REM sleep-related AHI with hormone replacement therapy.[86] There is also cohort-level data supporting that estrogen can be protective against OSA in premenopausal females when compared to their male peers and controlling for both age and

BMI.[11,83] Additionally, there is a significant uptick in the prevalence and severity of OSA in females who are postmenopausal when compared to premenopausal females matched for comorbidities.

There are theories that testosterone may play a role in the pathogenesis of OSA in males; however, the currently available evidence is minimal,[87,88] especially when compared to the data on the protective effect of estrogen. A 2012 study in obese males with severe OSA suggested that exogenous testosterone may mildly increase OSA severity.[89] A 2020 review of the literature on OSA and testosterone therapy concluded that short-term, high-dose testosterone may mildly worsen OSA, and that this effect is likely time limited. The mechanism of action remains unknown, but the authors postulate it is most likely related to altered hypoxic and hypercapnic ventilatory response with testosterone therapy.[88]

When it comes to mechanisms as to why there is a difference in the prevalence and severity of OSA across different racial and ethnic groups, the data are not much more compelling than that for biological sex. Some of the proposed mechanisms include differences in genetic, environmental, sociocultural, and craniofacial factors. Historically, the increased prevalence and severity of OSA in the Black population were thought to be due to increased rates of obesity. However, this has been debunked by a body of literature suggesting that the relationship between BMI and OSA is similar between Black and White adults.[25] Interestingly, Chinese individuals with OSA tend to have a more severe OSA phenotype at lower BMI than their White counterparts, suggesting that skeletal restriction may be important for OSA risk in this population.[90,91]

Craniofacial factors have been examined in OSA patients, with a handful of studies comparing these factors based on race. Patients with OSA tend to have similar craniofacial findings across all racial and ethnic groups; however, the patterns and impact of these findings may differ. Between Black and White adults, brachycephaly (wider laterally than AP) is associated with increased AHI in White adults but not in Black adults.[92] In a study of White adults, skeletal craniofacial restriction and soft tissue enlargement of tongue and soft palate were associated with OSA, while soft tissue enlargement of the tongue was the only significant factor in Black adult patients.[25]

There is almost no work published on nonbiological factors on SDB, such as environmental factors, despite the significant impact that environment has on health.[93] Data from the NHANES survey assessed OSA symptoms using questionnaire data and found a correlation between having pets in the home or living in a home with musty or mildew smell and higher risk of self-reported OSA symptoms.[94]

Knowledge/awareness

One of the major barriers to getting patients of all backgrounds engaged with the care continuum for OSA diagnosis and management is health literacy.[95] Patients with limited health literacy often have greater difficulty locating providers, communicating with them once they've found a provider, and accurately completing health forms and surveys. These patients may not be effectively identified by current screening and diagnosis methods, even if they are connected with the appropriate providers. It has been shown that greater than 55% of new patients in a British clinic (race not reported) had difficulty completing the ESS.[96] Another study showed that 44% of patients (39% Black, 59% White) with known low health literacy skills seen in a Louisiana clinic required reading assistance to interpret National Sleep Foundation (NSF) and American Academy of Sleep Medicine (AASM) brochures.[97]

Proxies of health literacy including SES and education level have been noted to directly correlate with OSA knowledge in caregivers of patients with Down syndrome (DS). In a 2022 study on patients with DS, the majority (84%) of which had a prior diagnosis of OSA, only about one in six had undergone repeat PSG to monitor disease progression. Children with caregivers who had at least a college education were nearly five times as likely to have two more sleep studies. While patients with DS often have a phenotype of OSA that is favorable for HGNS, only about one in six caregivers of patients with DS are aware of new and emerging therapy options for OSA, such as HGNS.[98] In that same cohort of caregivers, 40% were not aware of American Academy of Pediatrics (AAP) guidelines encouraging baseline PSG in children with DS by age 4 (or sooner if OSA symptoms). This is not surprising given that there is evidence that adherence to these guidelines is low.[99,100] However, children with parents who had at least a college education were nearly six times as like to be aware of the AAP guidelines.

A June 2021 study that assessed nearly 250 random parents (87% White, 79% female, 69% with college degree) presenting with their children to a pediatric otolaryngology clinic found that the average parent recognized less than half of the presenting symptoms of pediatric OSA.[101] Another study by Honaker et al. (2022) of predominately Black (60%) and female (93%) caregivers found similar degrees of knowledge on OSA, with mean scores of 56% correct.[102]

A national cross-sectional study in 2007 of a population-based sample of nearly 600 parents found that only about one-sixth of parents considered themselves to be "knowledgeable" about pediatric OSA, less than one-fifth of parents knew that it could be treated with AT, and a similar number (one-fifth) understood the sequelae of untreated OSA. Nearly 40% of parents thought that AT was an "outdated" procedure.[103] Even more alarming than lack of caregiver knowledge on OSA, the numbers are not any better among pediatricians; a study of over 600 pediatricians found a mean score of correct responses about SDB of less than 50%, with only 5% answering all questions correctly.[104]

Knowledge and awareness of OSA are further modulated by other racial and cultural factors that contribute to ongoing disparities in care. Black patients have lower rates of self-referral for OSA[49] and also have lower screening rates for medical conditions than reported for White patients, even when controlling for other factors like insurance status.[105] These low screening rates and subsequent health disparities may exist as a result of patient's knowledge, beliefs, and attitudes surrounding the disease, its implications, and its treatment.[106] This has been demonstrated in the literature for a variety of other health conditions, including hypertension,[106] HIV treatment adherence,[107,108] colorectal cancer screening,[109] and utilization of mental health services.[110] In a prior study, only about one quarter of Black patients at risk for OSA adhered to undergoing a recommended sleep evaluation.[95] Although racial and ethnic disparities for OSA and its related morbidity and mortality have been examined in the literature (primarily in Black populations compared to Whites), there is scant literature focused on understanding and addressing differences in prevalence by race and ethnicity, and almost none focused on developing targeted screening and treatment interventions.[111] It is not clear whether the disparities in screening and treatment are due to a lack of public versus healthcare provider awareness, or both.[112]

A 2010 article documented a growing interest in the use of telehealth to enhance outreach to minority communities,[113] and data from 2008 onward show that internet use in minority communities has grown substantially over the last several years.[114] These efforts have shown promise, with US minority groups reporting that online information has affected their health habits[115] and computer-based health screening has shown higher rates of acceptance in these communities relative to traditional screening methods.[116]

Gaps and future directions

While overall there is a relative paucity of literature describing disparities in the prevalence, awareness, diagnosis, and treatment of OSA, there are certain areas that are more neglected than others (Fig. 15.1). With regard to sex, the mechanisms by which sex hormones impact the severity of OSA warrants greater attention, in both the context of endogenous hormones as well as exogenous hormones of varying dosages and durations. Concerted efforts are needed to elucidate differences in the symptoms and clinical presentation of OSA across the lifespan in females, especially in pre- and postmenopausal groups, possibly with the development of newly tailored screening tools or approaches.

The impact of sexual orientation has been completely overlooked in the literature for OSA and remains neglected in sleep literature more broadly. Examining attitudes and perceptions of healthcare providers, as well as of patients that are sexual minorities, is crucial to ensure that screening tools and clinical interactions are not missing key information from bed partners due to poor wording or cultural stigma. It is important that screening tools and providers use open-ended wording rather than assuming the gender of the patient's bed partner.

Another relevant issue involves universal and consistent reporting of sex, race, and ethnicity, and other demographic data including country of origin, gender identity, and sexual orientation in all OSA related studies. A 2022 systematic review on the representation of race and sex in studies reporting outcomes on nonnasal sleep surgeries found that only 8.8% of studies reported data on race or ethnicity, while 93% of studies reported data on sex.[82] Designing and implementing efficacious

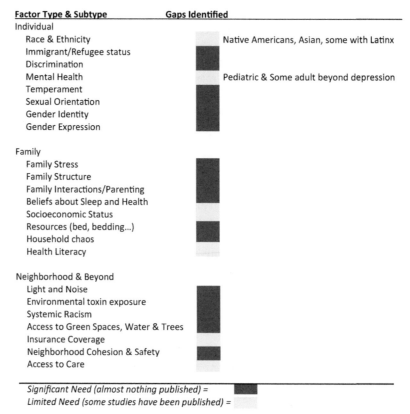

Factor Type & Subtype	Gaps Identified	
Individual		
Race & Ethnicity		Native Americans, Asian, some with Latinx
Immigrant/Refugee status		
Discrimination		
Mental Health		Pediatric & Some adult beyond depression
Temperament		
Sexual Orientation		
Gender Identity		
Gender Expression		
Family		
Family Stress		
Family Structure		
Family Interactions/Parenting		
Beliefs about Sleep and Health		
Socioeconomic Status		
Resources (bed, bedding...)		
Household chaos		
Health Literacy		
Neighborhood & Beyond		
Light and Noise		
Environmental toxin exposure		
Systemic Racism		
Access to Green Spaces, Water & Trees		
Insurance Coverage		
Neighborhood Cohesion & Safety		
Access to Care		

Significant Need (almost nothing published) =
Limited Need (some studies have been published) =

FIGURE 15.1

Gaps in health disparity research for adults and children based on socioecological factors contributing to sleep disparities assessing individual, family, and neighborhood and beyond (including broad sociocultural factors).

interventions to alleviate health disparities in the OSA disease burden across populations hinges on quality, thoughtful, clinically relevant research to bring these disparities to light. Our progress toward achieving health equity in OSA is stunted each time a study fails to collect and report demographic data.

Some groups seem to be completely overlooked in the literature on OSA, including indigenous communities, like Native Americans. This may be just a microcosm of a much larger societal issue of Native Americans being the most underrepresented group in science fields.[117] This further asserts the notion that representation matters immensely, both in clinical medicine, and academic medicine, at all levels, and in all fields. The nuanced perspectives of the individuals from the communities where these health disparities manifest may be the most adept at uncovering the solutions to achieve health equity.

References

1. Siegel JM. Do all animals sleep? *Trends Neurosci.* 2008;31(4):208–213. https://doi.org/10.1016/j.tins.2008.02.001.

2. Senaratna CV, Perret JL, Lodge CJ, et al. Prevalence of obstructive sleep apnea in the general population: a systematic review. *Sleep Med Rev.* 2017;34:70–81. https://doi.org/10.1016/j.smrv.2016.07.002.

3. Cowie MR, Linz D, Redline S, Somers VK, Simonds AK. Sleep disordered breathing and cardiovascular disease: JACC state-of-the-art review. *J Am Coll Cardiol.* 2021;78(6):608–624. https://doi.org/10.1016/j.jacc.2021.05.048.

4. Drager LF, Togeiro SM, Polotsky VY, Lorenzi-Filho G. Obstructive sleep apnea: a cardiometabolic risk in obesity and the metabolic syndrome. *J Am Coll Cardiol.* 2013;62(7):569–576. https://doi.org/10.1016/j.jacc.2013.05.045.

5. Trzepizur W, Blanchard M, Ganem T, et al. Sleep apnea-specific hypoxic burden, symptom subtypes, and risk of cardiovascular events and all-cause mortality. *Am J Respir Crit Care Med.* 2022;205(1):108–117. https://doi.org/10.1164/rccm.202105-1274OC.

6. Sia CH, Hong Y, Tan LWL, van Dam RM, Lee CH, Tan A. Awareness and knowledge of obstructive sleep apnea among the general population. *Sleep Med.* 2017;36:10–17. https://doi.org/10.1016/j.sleep.2017.03.030.

7. Mantilla R, Tafur A, Soria J, et al. Awareness of obstructive sleep apnea in a Latin American community. In: *A66. Epidemiology and Diagnosis of Sleep-Disordered Breathing.* American Thoracic Society; 2009:A2147. https://doi.org/10.1164/ajrccm-conference.2009.179.1_MeetingAbstracts.A2147.

8. Alshehri AM, Alshehri MS, Alamri OM, et al. Knowledge, awareness, and attitudes toward obstructive sleep apnea among the population of the Asir region of Saudi Arabia in 2019. *Cureus.* 2020;12(3):e7254. https://doi.org/10.7759/cureus.7254.

9. Schwartz AR, Patil SP, Laffan AM, Polotsky V, Schneider H, Smith PL. Obesity and obstructive sleep apnea: pathogenic mechanisms and therapeutic approaches. *Proc Am Thorac Soc.* 2008;5(2):185–192. https://doi.org/10.1513/pats.200708-137MG.

10. Peppard PE, Young T, Barnet JH, Palta M, Hagen EW, Hla KM. Increased prevalence of sleep-disordered breathing in adults. *Am J Epidemiol.* 2013;177(9):1006–1014. https://doi.org/10.1093/aje/kws342.

11. Bixler EO, Vgontzas AN, Lin HM, et al. Prevalence of sleep-disordered breathing in women: effects of gender. *Am J Respir Crit Care Med.* 2001;163(3 Pt 1):608–613. https://doi.org/10.1164/ajrccm.163.3.9911064.

12. Redline S, Kump K, Tishler PV, Browner I, Ferrette V. Gender differences in sleep disordered breathing in a community-based sample. *Am J Respir Crit Care Med.* 1994;149(3 Pt 1):722–726. https://doi.org/10.1164/ajrccm.149.3.8118642.

13. Young T, Shahar E, Nieto FJ, et al. Predictors of sleep-disordered breathing in community-dwelling adults: the sleep heart health study. *Arch Intern Med.* 2002;162(8):893–900. https://doi.org/10.1001/archinte.162.8.893.

14. Huang T, Lin BM, Redline S, Curhan GC, Hu FB, Tworoger SS. Type of menopause, age at menopause, and risk of developing obstructive sleep apnea in postmenopausal women. *Am J Epidemiol.* 2018;187(7):1370–1379. https://doi.org/10.1093/aje/kwy011.

15. Heinzer R, Vat S, Marques-Vidal P, et al. Prevalence of sleep-disordered breathing in the general population: the HypnoLaus study. *Lancet Respir Med.* 2015;3(4):310–318. https://doi.org/10.1016/S2213-2600(15)00043-0.

16. Lumeng JC, Chervin RD. Epidemiology of pediatric obstructive sleep apnea. *Proc Am Thorac Soc*. 2008;5(2):242−252. https://doi.org/10.1513/pats.200708-135MG.

17. Villaneuva ATC, Buchanan PR, Yee BJ, Grunstein RR. Ethnicity and obstructive sleep apnoea. *Sleep Med Rev*. 2005;9(6):419−436. https://doi.org/10.1016/j.smrv.2005.04.005.

18. Hnin K, Mukherjee S, Antic NA, et al. The impact of ethnicity on the prevalence and severity of obstructive sleep apnea. *Sleep Med Rev*. 2018;41:78−86. https://doi.org/10.1016/j.smrv.2018.01.003.

19. Redline S, Tishler PV, Schluchter M, Aylor J, Clark K, Graham G. Risk factors for sleep-disordered breathing in children. Associations with obesity, race, and respiratory problems. *Am J Respir Crit Care Med*. 1999;159(5 Pt 1):1527−1532. https://doi.org/10.1164/ajrccm.159.5.9809079.

20. Marcus CL, Moore RH, Rosen CL, et al. A randomized trial of adenotonsillectomy for childhood sleep apnea. *N Engl J Med*. 2013;368(25):2366−2376. https://doi.org/10.1056/NEJMoa1215881.

21. Boss EF, Smith DF, Ishman SL. Racial/ethnic and socioeconomic disparities in the diagnosis and treatment of sleep-disordered breathing in children. *Int J Pediatr Otorhinolaryngol*. 2011;75(3):299−307. https://doi.org/10.1016/j.ijporl.2010.11.006.

22. Stepanski E, Zayyad A, Nigro C, Lopata M, Basner R. Sleep-disordered breathing in a predominantly African-American pediatric population. *J Sleep Res*. 1999;8(1):65−70. https://doi.org/10.1046/j.1365-2869.1999.00136.x.

23. Geovanini GR, Wang R, Weng J, et al. Association between obstructive sleep apnea and cardiovascular risk factors: variation by age, sex, and race. The multi-ethnic study of Atherosclerosis. *Ann Am Thorac Soc*. 2018;15(8):970−977. https://doi.org/10.1513/AnnalsATS.201802-121OC.

24. Ancoli-Israel S, Klauber MR, Stepnowsky C, Estline E, Chinn A, Fell R. Sleep-disordered breathing in African-American elderly. *Am J Respir Crit Care Med*. 1995;152(6 Pt 1):1946−1949. https://doi.org/10.1164/ajrccm.152.6.8520760.

25. Redline S, Tishler PV, Hans MG, Tosteson TD, Strohl KP, Spry K. Racial differences in sleep-disordered breathing in African-Americans and Caucasians. *Am J Respir Crit Care Med*. 1997;155(1):186−192. https://doi.org/10.1164/ajrccm.155.1.9001310.

26. Chen X, Wang R, Zee P, et al. Racial/ethnic differences in sleep disturbances: the multi-ethnic study of Atherosclerosis (MESA). *Sleep*. 2015;38(6):877−888. https://doi.org/10.5665/sleep.4732.

27. Song Y, Ancoli-Israel S, Lewis CE, Redline S, Harrison SL, Stone KL. The association of race/ethnicity with objectively measured sleep characteristics in older men. *Behav Sleep Med*. 2011;10(1):54−69. https://doi.org/10.1080/15402002.2012.636276.

28. Hall MH, Matthews KA, Kravitz HM, et al. Race and financial strain are independent correlates of sleep in midlife women: the SWAN sleep study. *Sleep*. 2009;32(1):73−82.

29. Baldwin CM, Ervin AM, Mays MZ, et al. Sleep disturbances, quality of life, and ethnicity: the sleep heart health study. *J Clin Sleep Med*. 2010;6(2):176−183.

30. Kripke DF, Ancoli-Israel S, Klauber MR, Wingard DL, Mason WJ, Mullaney DJ. Prevalence of sleep-disordered breathing in ages 40-64 years: a population-based survey. *Sleep*. 1997;20(1):65−76. https://doi.org/10.1093/sleep/20.1.65.

31. Yamagishi K, Ohira T, Nakano H, et al. Cross-cultural comparison of the sleep-disordered breathing prevalence among Americans and Japanese. *Eur Respir J*. 2010;36(2):379−384. https://doi.org/10.1183/09031936.00118609.

32. Ip MS, Lam B, Lauder IJ, et al. A community study of sleep-disordered breathing in middle-aged Chinese men in Hong Kong. *Chest*. 2001;119(1):62−69. https://doi.org/10.1378/chest.119.1.62.

33. Ip MSM, Lam B, Tang LCH, Lauder IJ, Ip TY, Lam WK. A community study of sleep-disordered breathing in middle-aged Chinese women in Hong Kong: prevalence and gender differences. *Chest*. 2004;125(1):127−134. https://doi.org/10.1378/chest.125.1.127.

34. Young T, Palta M, Dempsey J, Skatrud J, Weber S, Badr S. The occurrence of sleep-disordered breathing among middle-aged adults. *N Engl J Med*. 1993;328(17):1230−1235. https://doi.org/10.1056/NEJM199304293281704.

35. Leong WB, Arora T, Jenkinson D, et al. The prevalence and severity of obstructive sleep apnea in severe obesity: the impact of ethnicity. *J Clin Sleep Med*. 2013;9(9):853−858. https://doi.org/10.5664/jcsm.2978.

36. Ong KC, Clerk AA. Comparison of the severity of sleep-disordered breathing in Asian and Caucasian patients seen at a sleep disorders center. *Respir Med*. 1998;92(6):843−848. https://doi.org/10.1016/s0954-6111(98)90386-9.

37. Genta PR, Marcondes BF, Danzi NJ, Lorenzi-Filho G. Ethnicity as a risk factor for obstructive sleep apnea: comparison of Japanese descendants and white males in São Paulo, Brazil. *Braz J Med Biol Res*. 2008;41(8):728−733. https://doi.org/10.1590/s0100-879x2008000800015.

38. Gavidia R, Whitney DG, Hershner S, Selkie EM, Tauman R, Dunietz GL. Gender identity and transition: relationships with sleep disorders in US youth. *J Clin Sleep Med*. 2022;18(11):2553−2559. https://doi.org/10.5664/jcsm.10158.

39. Smedje H, Broman JE, Hetta J. Parents' reports of disturbed sleep in 5-7-year-old Swedish children. *Acta Paediatr Oslo Nor 1992*. 1999;88(8):858−865. https://doi.org/10.1080/08035259950168793.

40. Eliasson AH, Kashani MD, Howard RS, Vernalis MN, Modlin RE. Integrative Cardiac Health Project Registry. Fatigued on Venus, sleepy on Mars-gender and racial differences in symptoms of sleep apnea. *Sleep Breath Schlaf Atm*. 2015;19(1):99−107. https://doi.org/10.1007/s11325-014-0968-ys.

41. Shepertycky MR, Banno K, Kryger MH. Differences between men and women in the clinical presentation of patients diagnosed with obstructive sleep apnea syndrome. *Sleep*. 2005;28(3):309−314.

42. Subramanian S, Guntupalli B, Murugan T, et al. Gender and ethnic differences in prevalence of self-reported insomnia among patients with obstructive sleep apnea. *Sleep Breath Schlaf Atm*. 2011;15(4):711−715. https://doi.org/10.1007/s11325-010-0426-4.

43. Subramanian S, Jayaraman G, Majid H, Aguilar R, Surani S. Influence of gender and anthropometric measures on severity of obstructive sleep apnea. *Sleep Breath Schlaf Atm*. 2012;16(4):1091−1095. https://doi.org/10.1007/s11325-011-0607-9.

44. Simpson L, Mukherjee S, Cooper MN, et al. Sex differences in the association of regional fat distribution with the severity of obstructive sleep apnea. *Sleep*. 2010;33(4):467−474. https://doi.org/10.1093/sleep/33.4.467.

45. Luk JW, Sita KR, Lewin D, Simons-Morton BG, Haynie DL. Sexual orientation and sleep behaviors in a national sample of adolescents followed into young adulthood. *J Clin Sleep Med*. 2019;15(11):1635−1643. https://doi.org/10.5664/jcsm.8030.

46. Williamson AA, Rubens SL, Patrick KE, Moore M, Mindell JA. Differences in sleep patterns and problems by race in a clinical sample of black and white preschoolers. *J Clin Sleep Med*. 2017;13(11):1281−1288. https://doi.org/10.5664/jcsm.6798.

47. Rubens SL, Patrick KE, Williamson AA, Moore M, Mindell JA. Individual and socio-demographic factors related to presenting problem and diagnostic impressions at a pediatric sleep clinic. *Sleep Med.* 2016;25:67–72. https://doi.org/10.1016/j.sleep.2016.06.017.

48. Jean-Louis G, Magai CM, Cohen CI, et al. Ethnic differences in self-reported sleep problems in older adults. *Sleep.* 2001;24(8):926–933. https://doi.org/10.1093/sleep/24.8.926.

49. Scharf SM, Seiden L, DeMore J, Carter-Pokras O. Racial differences in clinical presentation of patients with sleep-disordered breathing. *Sleep Breath Schlaf Atm.* 2004;8(4):173–183. https://doi.org/10.1007/s11325-004-0173-5.

50. Thornton JD, Dudley KA, Saeed GJ, et al. Differences in symptoms and severity of obstructive sleep apnea between black and white patients. *Ann Am Thorac Soc.* 2022;19(2):272–278. https://doi.org/10.1513/AnnalsATS.202012-1483OC.

51. Goodwin JL, Kaemingk KL, Fregosi RF, et al. Parasomnias and sleep disordered breathing in Caucasian and Hispanic children – the Tucson children's assessment of sleep apnea study. *BMC Med.* 2004;2:14. https://doi.org/10.1186/1741-7015-2-14.

52. Medicine I of, Policy B on HS, Research C on SM. *Sleep Disorders and Sleep Deprivation: An Unmet Public Health Problem.* National Academies Press; 2006.

53. Garg N, Rolle AJ, Lee TA, Prasad B. Home-based diagnosis of obstructive sleep apnea in an urban population. *J Clin Sleep Med.* 2014;10(8):879–885. https://doi.org/10.5664/jcsm.3960.

54. Radhakrishnan D, Knight B, Gozdyra P, et al. Geographic disparities in performance of pediatric polysomnography to diagnose obstructive sleep apnea in a universal access health care system. *Int J Pediatr Otorhinolaryngol.* 2021;147:110803. https://doi.org/10.1016/j.ijporl.2021.110803.

55. Harris VC, Links AR, Kim JM, Walsh J, Tunkel DE, Boss EF. Follow up and time to treatment in an urban cohort of children with sleep-disordered breathing. *Otolaryngol–Head Neck Surg Off J Am Acad Otolaryngol-Head Neck Surg.* 2018;159(2):371–378. https://doi.org/10.1177/0194599818772035.

56. Boss EF, Benke JR, Tunkel DE, Ishman SL, Bridges JFP, Kim JM. Public insurance and timing of polysomnography and surgical care for children with sleep-disordered breathing. *JAMA Otolaryngol– Head Neck Surg.* 2015;141(2):106–111. https://doi.org/10.1001/jamaoto.2014.3085.

57. Young T, Evans L, Finn L, Palta M. Estimation of the clinically diagnosed proportion of sleep apnea syndrome in middle-aged men and women. *Sleep.* 1997;20(9):705–706. https://doi.org/10.1093/sleep/20.9.705.

58. Kapur V, Strohl KP, Redline S, Iber C, O'Connor G, Nieto J. Underdiagnosis of sleep apnea syndrome in U.S. communities. *Sleep Breath Schlaf Atm.* 2002;6(2):49–54. https://doi.org/10.1007/s11325-002-0049-5.

59. Redline S, Sotres-Alvarez D, Loredo J, et al. Sleep-disordered breathing in Hispanic/Latino individuals of diverse backgrounds. The Hispanic community health study/study of Latinos. *Am J Respir Crit Care Med.* 2014;189(3):335–344. https://doi.org/10.1164/rccm.201309-1735OC.

60. Cooper JN, Koppera S, Bliss AJ, Lind MN. Characteristics associated with caregiver willingness to consider tonsillectomy for a child's obstructive sleep disordered breathing: findings from a survey of families in an urban primary care network. *Int J Pediatr Otorhinolaryngol.* 2022;158:111143. https://doi.org/10.1016/j.ijporl.2022.111143.

61. Yan F, Pearce JL, Ford ME, Nietert PJ, Pecha PP. Examining associations between neighborhood-level social vulnerability and care for children with sleep-disordered breathing. *Otolaryngol–Head Neck Surg Off J Am Acad Otolaryngol-Head Neck Surg.* 2022;166(6):1118–1126. https://doi.org/10.1177/01945998221084203.

62. Bhattacharyya N, Shapiro NL. Associations between socioeconomic status and race with complications after tonsillectomy in children. *Otolaryngol–Head Neck Surg Off J Am Acad Otolaryngol-Head Neck Surg.* 2014;151(6):1055–1060. https://doi.org/10.1177/0194599814552647.

63. Pecha PP, Chew M, Andrews AL. Racial and ethnic disparities in utilization of tonsillectomy among medicaid-insured children. *J Pediatr.* 2021;233:191–197.e2. https://doi.org/10.1016/j.jpeds.2021.01.071.

64. Kou YF, Sakai M, Shah GB, Mitchell RB, Johnson RF. Postoperative respiratory complications and racial disparities following inpatient pediatric tonsillectomy: a cross-sectional study. *Laryngoscope.* 2019;129(4):995–1000. https://doi.org/10.1002/lary.27405.

65. Yan F, Levy DA, Wen CC, et al. Rural barriers to surgical care for children with sleep-disordered breathing. *Otolaryngol–Head Neck Surg Off J Am Acad Otolaryngol-Head Neck Surg.* 2022;166(6):1127–1133. https://doi.org/10.1177/0194599821993383.

66. Billings ME, Auckley D, Benca R, et al. Race and residential socioeconomics as predictors of CPAP adherence. *Sleep.* 2011;34(12):1653–1658. https://doi.org/10.5665/sleep.1428.

67. Dunietz GL, Chervin RD, Burke JF, Braley TJ. Obstructive sleep apnea treatment disparities among older adults with neurological disorders. *Sleep Health.* 2020;6(4):534–540. https://doi.org/10.1016/j.sleh.2020.01.009.

68. Joo MJ, Herdegen JJ. Sleep apnea in an urban public hospital: assessment of severity and treatment adherence. *J Clin Sleep Med.* 2007;3(3):285–288.

69. Lee CHK, Leow LC, Song PR, Li H, Ong TH. Acceptance and adherence to continuous positive airway pressure therapy in patients with obstructive sleep apnea (OSA) in a Southeast Asian privately funded healthcare system. *Sleep Sci.* 2017;10(2):57–63. https://doi.org/10.5935/1984-0063.20170010.

70. Pelletier-Fleury N, Rakotonanahary D, Fleury B. The age and other factors in the evaluation of compliance with nasal continuous positive airway pressure for obstructive sleep apnea syndrome. A Cox's proportional hazard analysis. *Sleep Med.* 2001;2(3):225–232. https://doi.org/10.1016/s1389-9457(00)00063-0.

71. Woehrle H, Graml A, Weinreich G. Age- and gender-dependent adherence with continuous positive airway pressure therapy. *Sleep Med.* 2011;12(10):1034–1036. https://doi.org/10.1016/j.sleep.2011.05.008.

72. Sin DD, Mayers I, Man GCW, Pawluk L. Long-term compliance rates to continuous positive airway pressure in obstructive sleep apnea: a population-based study. *Chest.* 2002;121(2):430–435. https://doi.org/10.1378/chest.121.2.430.

73. Gagnadoux F, Le Vaillant M, Goupil F, et al. Influence of marital status and employment status on long-term adherence with continuous positive airway pressure in sleep apnea patients. *PLoS One.* 2011;6(8):e22503. https://doi.org/10.1371/journal.pone.0022503.

74. McArdle N, Devereux G, Heidarnejad H, Engleman HM, Mackay TW, Douglas NJ. Long-term use of CPAP therapy for sleep apnea/hypopnea syndrome. *Am J Respir Crit Care Med.* 1999;159(4 Pt 1):1108–1114. https://doi.org/10.1164/ajrccm.159.4.9807111.

75. Simon-Tuval T, Reuveni H, Greenberg-Dotan S, Oksenberg A, Tal A, Tarasiuk A. Low socioeconomic status is a risk factor for CPAP acceptance among adult OSAS patients requiring treatment. *Sleep.* 2009;32(4):545−552. https://doi.org/10.1093/sleep/32.4.545.

76. Platt AB, Field SH, Asch DA, et al. Neighborhood of residence is associated with daily adherence to CPAP therapy. *Sleep.* 2009;32(6):799−806. https://doi.org/10.1093/sleep/32.6.799.

77. Marklund M, Carlberg B, Forsgren L, Olsson T, Stenlund H, Franklin KA. Oral appliance therapy in patients with daytime sleepiness and snoring or mild to moderate sleep apnea: a randomized clinical trial. *JAMA Intern Med.* 2015;175(8):1278−1285. https://doi.org/10.1001/jamainternmed.2015.2051.

78. Khan M, Stone A, Soose RJ, et al. Does race-ethnicity affect upper airway stimulation adherence and treatment outcome of obstructive sleep apnea? *J Clin Sleep Med.* 2022. https://doi.org/10.5664/jcsm.10068.

79. Cohen SM, Howard JJM, Jin MC, Qian J, Capasso R. Racial disparities in surgical treatment of obstructive sleep apnea. *OTO Open.* 2022;6(1). https://doi.org/10.1177/2473974X221088870, 2473974X221088870.

80. Ruthberg J, Summerville L, Cai Y, Boas S, Otteson T, Kumar A. Utilization of surgical treatment for sleep apnea: a study of health disparities. *Am J Otolaryngol.* 2020;41(6):102670. https://doi.org/10.1016/j.amjoto.2020.102670.

81. Garg RK, Shan Y, Havlena JA, Afifi AM. Disparities in utilization of jaw surgery for treatment of sleep apnea: a nationwide analysis. *Plast Reconstr Surg Glob Open.* 2016;4(12):e1047. https://doi.org/10.1097/GOX.0000000000001047.

82. Debbaneh P, Ramirez K, Block-Wheeler N, Durr M. Representation of race and sex in sleep surgery studies. *Otolaryngol–Head Neck Surg Off J Am Acad Otolaryngol-Head Neck Surg.* 2022;166(6):1204−1210. https://doi.org/10.1177/01945998221088759.

83. Shahar E, Redline S, Young T, et al. Hormone replacement therapy and sleep-disordered breathing. *Am J Respir Crit Care Med.* 2003;167(9):1186−1192. https://doi.org/10.1164/rccm.200210-1238OC.

84. Pickett CK, Regensteiner JG, Woodard WD, Hagerman DD, Weil JV, Moore LG. Progestin and estrogen reduce sleep-disordered breathing in postmenopausal women. *J Appl Physiol Bethesda Md 1985.* 1989;66(4):1656−1661. https://doi.org/10.1152/jappl.1989.66.4.1656.

85. Lu Y, Liu Y, Li Y. Comparison of natural estrogens and synthetic derivative on genioglossus function and estrogen receptors expression in rats with chronic intermittent hypoxia. *J Steroid Biochem Mol Biol.* 2014;140:71−79. https://doi.org/10.1016/j.jsbmb.2013.12.006.

86. Cistulli PA, Barnes DJ, Grunstein RR, Sullivan CE. Effect of short-term hormone replacement in the treatment of obstructive sleep apnoea in postmenopausal women. *Thorax.* 1994;49(7):699−702. https://doi.org/10.1136/thx.49.7.699.

87. Hanafy HM. Testosterone therapy and obstructive sleep apnea: is there a real connection? *J Sex Med.* 2007;4(5):1241−1246. https://doi.org/10.1111/j.1743-6109.2007.00553.x.

88. Payne K, Lipshultz LI, Hotaling JM, Pastuszak AW. Obstructive sleep apnea and testosterone therapy. *Sex Med Rev.* 2021;9(2):296−303. https://doi.org/10.1016/j.sxmr.2020.04.004.

89. Hoyos CM, Killick R, Yee BJ, Grunstein RR, Liu PY. Effects of testosterone therapy on sleep and breathing in obese men with severe obstructive sleep apnoea: a randomized

placebo-controlled trial. *Clin Endocrinol.* 2012;77(4):599−607. https://doi.org/10.1111/j.1365-2265.2012.04413.x.

90. Liu Y, Lowe AA, Zeng X, Fu M, Fleetham JA. Cephalometric comparisons between Chinese and Caucasian patients with obstructive sleep apnea. *Am J Orthod Dentofac Orthop Off Publ Am Assoc Orthod Its Const Soc Am Board Orthod.* 2000;117(4):479−485. https://doi.org/10.1016/s0889-5406(00)70169-7.

91. Lee RWW, Vasudavan S, Hui DS, et al. Differences in craniofacial structures and obesity in Caucasian and Chinese patients with obstructive sleep apnea. *Sleep.* 2010;33(8):1075−1080. https://doi.org/10.1093/sleep/33.8.1075.

92. Cakirer B, Hans MG, Graham G, Aylor J, Tishler PV, Redline S. The relationship between craniofacial morphology and obstructive sleep apnea in whites and in African-Americans. *Am J Respir Crit Care Med.* 2001;163(4):947−950. https://doi.org/10.1164/ajrccm.163.4.2005136.

93. Evans GW, Kantrowitz E. Socioeconomic status and health: the potential role of environmental risk exposure. *Annu Rev Publ Health.* 2002;23:303−331. https://doi.org/10.1146/annurev.publhealth.23.112001.112349.

94. Ansarin K, Sahebi L, Sabur S. Obstructive sleep apnea syndrome: complaints and housing characteristics in a population in the United States. *Sao Paulo Med J Rev Paul Med.* 2013;131(4):220−227. https://doi.org/10.1590/1516-3180.2013.1314451.

95. Li JJ, Appleton SL, Wittert GA, et al. The relationship between functional health literacy and obstructive sleep apnea and its related risk factors and comorbidities in a population cohort of men. *Sleep.* 2014;37(3):571−578. https://doi.org/10.5665/sleep.3500.

96. Ghiassi R, Murphy K, Cummin AR, Partridge MR. Developing a pictorial epworth sleepiness scale. *Thorax.* 2011;66(2):97−100. https://doi.org/10.1136/thx.2010.136879.

97. Chesson AL, Murphy PW, Arnold CL, Davis TC. Presentation and reading level of sleep brochures: are they appropriate for sleep disorders patients? *Sleep.* 1998;21(4):406−412. https://doi.org/10.1093/sleep/21.4.406.

98. Giménez S, Tapia IE, Fortea J, et al. Caregiver knowledge of obstructive sleep apnoea in Down syndrome. *J Intellect Disabil Res JIDR.* 2023;67(1):77−88. https://doi.org/10.1111/jir.12990.

99. Hsieh A, Gilad A, Wong K, Cohen M, Levi J. Obstructive sleep apnea in children with Down syndrome: screening and effect of guidelines. *Clin Pediatr.* 2019;58(9):993−999. https://doi.org/10.1177/0009922819845333.

100. Knollman PD, Heubi CH, Meinzen-Derr J, et al. Adherence to guidelines for screening polysomnography in children with Down syndrome. *Otolaryngol–Head Neck Surg Off J Am Acad Otolaryngol-Head Neck Surg.* 2019;161(1):157−163. https://doi.org/10.1177/0194599819837243.

101. DiNardo LA, Reese AD, Raghavan M, et al. Parental knowledge of obstructive sleep apnea symptoms and tonsillectomy in children. Published online July *Ann Otol Rhinol Laryngol.* 2022;21:34894221112911. https://doi.org/10.1177/00034894221112911.

102. Honaker SM, Gopalkrishnan A, Brann M, Wiehe S, Clark AA, Chung A. "It made all the difference": a qualitative study of parental experiences with pediatric obstructive sleep apnea detection. *J Clin Sleep Med.* 2022;18(8):1921−1931. https://doi.org/10.5664/jcsm.10024.

103. Strocker AM, Shapiro NL. Parental understanding and attitudes of pediatric obstructive sleep apnea and adenotonsillectomy. *Int J Pediatr Otorhinolaryngol.* 2007;71(11):1709−1715. https://doi.org/10.1016/j.ijporl.2007.07.016.

104. Owens JA. The practice of pediatric sleep medicine: results of a community survey. *Pediatrics*. 2001;108(3):E51. https://doi.org/10.1542/peds.108.3.e51.

105. Jean-Louis G, von Gizycki H, Zizi F, Dharawat A, Lazar JM, Brown CD. Evaluation of sleep apnea in a sample of black patients. *J Clin Sleep Med*. 2008;4(5):421−425.

106. Fongwa MN, Evangelista LS, Hays RD, et al. Adherence treatment factors in hypertensive African American women. *Vasc Health Risk Manag*. 2008;4(1):157−166. https://doi.org/10.2147/vhrm.2008.04.01.157.

107. Berkley-Patton J, Goggin K, Liston R, Bradley-Ewing A, Neville S. Adapting effective narrative-based HIV-prevention interventions to increase minorities' engagement in HIV/AIDS services. *Health Commun*. 2009;24(3):199−209. https://doi.org/10.1080/10410230902804091.

108. Bogart LM, Wagner G, Galvan FH, Banks D. Conspiracy beliefs about HIV are related to antiretroviral treatment nonadherence among african american men with HIV. *J Acquir Immune Defic Syndr 1999*. 2010;53(5):648−655. https://doi.org/10.1097/QAI.0b013e3181c57dbc.

109. Menon U, Szalacha LA, Belue R, Rugen K, Martin KR, Kinney AY. Interactive, culturally sensitive education on colorectal cancer screening. *Med Care*. 2008;46(9 Suppl 1):S44−S50. https://doi.org/10.1097/MLR.0b013e31818105a0.

110. Ayalon L, Alvidrez J. The experience of Black consumers in the mental health system−identifying barriers to and facilitators of mental health treatment using the consumers' perspective. *Issues Ment Health Nurs*. 2007;28(12):1323−1340. https://doi.org/10.1080/01612840701651454.

111. Young T, Finn L. Epidemiological insights into the public health burden of sleep disordered breathing: sex differences in survival among sleep clinic patients. *Thorax*. 1998;53(Suppl 3):S16−S19. https://doi.org/10.1136/thx.53.2008.s16.

112. Chung SA, Jairam S, Hussain MR, Shapiro CM. Knowledge of sleep apnea in a sample grouping of primary care physicians. *Sleep Breath Schlaf Atm*. 2001;5(3):115−121. https://doi.org/10.1007/s11325-001-0115-4.

113. Goodall K, Ward P, Newman L. Use of information and communication technology to provide health information: what do older migrants know, and what do they need to know? *Qual Prim Care*. 2010;18(1):27−32.

114. Khan SA, Ancker JS, Li J, et al. GetHealthyHarlem.org: developing a web platform for health promotion and wellness driven by and for the Harlem community. *AMIA Annu Symp Proc AMIA Symp*. 2009;2009:317−321.

115. Computer use, internet access, and online health searching among Harlem adults - PubMed. Accessed September 28, 2022. https://pubmed-ncbi-nlm-nih-gov.laneproxy.stanford.edu/21534835/.

116. Cohall A, Dini S, Nye A, Dye B, Neu N, Hyden C. HIV testing preferences among young men of color who have sex with men. *Am J Publ Health*. 2010;100(10):1961−1966. https://doi.org/10.2105/AJPH.2008.140632.

117. Chow-Garcia N, Lee N, Svihla V, et al. Cultural identity central to Native American persistence in science. *Cult Stud Sci Educ*. 2022;17(2):557−588. https://doi.org/10.1007/s11422-021-10071-7.

Health disparities in facial plastic surgery

16

Oneida A. Arosarena[1,2], Victor O. Jegede[3]

[1]*Department of Otolaryngology, Lewis Katz School of Medicine at Temple University, Philadelphia, PA, United States;* [2]*Center for Urban Bioethics, Lewis Katz School of Medicine at Temple University, Philadelphia, PA, United States;* [3]*Lewis Katz School of Medicine at Temple University, Philadelphia, PA, United States*

Introduction

While the research on health disparities has increased exponentially since 1966,[1] research in plastic surgery health disparities, and specifically facial plastic reconstructive surgery (FPRS), is in its relative infancy as compared to other specialties. In a recent systematic review of health disparities research in plastic surgery, including articles published in the United States (US) between 1997 and 2019, Baxter et al. demonstrated that research in craniofacial and cosmetic surgical health disparities was lacking in comparison to research on breast reconstruction health disparities. Of the 147 articles that met inclusion criteria for this review, the majority obtained data from large databases, which while useful, lack information on treatment decision making, patient satisfaction and long-term outcomes.[2]

Similarly, in a review of rural otolaryngologic care disparities, Urban et al. found large gaps in the literature, most notably in FPRS. All of the FPRS articles included in their review, which comprised only 5.1% of the 79 studies that met inclusion criteria, had to do with facial trauma.[3] Like most of the literature on health disparities, most studies of FPRS health disparities describe epidemiology, patient behaviors, and practice patterns, with comparatively few studies describing interventions.[2,3]

This chapter reviews the current literature addressing health disparities in FPRS including aesthetics, craniofacial surgery, posttraumatic reconstruction, laryngectomy reconstruction, rhinoplasty, patient educational resources, and disparities in the FPRS workforce.

Redefining aesthetic ideals and anthropometric norms

It is well known that facial appearance can influence the assignment of positive or negative attributes.[4,5] While beauty is often associated with positive attributes, defining beauty is difficult.[5] Concepts such as symmetry, balance, averageness, and youthfulness have been used to characterize beauty, but even these concepts are subjective and may be culturally shaped.[5–9] A study assessing observer perceptions of patients postrhinoplasty demonstrated greatest recognition ability when there was racial congruence between the observer and the patient. This "other race effect" may indicate different cultural aesthetic priorities.[10] Similarly, a study of Miss Universe and Miss World beauty pageant winners found that the concept of ideal nasal anatomy varies between ethnicities.[9]

Historic mathematical proportions used to define facial symmetry have been based on neoclassical standards which had their basis in the High Classical Period of ancient Greece. The golden ratio (ϕ, approximately 1:1.618) is found throughout nature, and was thought by the ancient Greeks to represent perfect harmony, including facial harmony (Fig. 16.1).[5,6] Polykleitos, an ancient Greek sculptor, was thought to be the first to demonstrate how mathematical proportions of the body produced beauty in a treatise he called "The Canon."[9] This was used by European Renaissance artists to define neoclassical facial proportion canons that influenced facial plastic surgeons of the past century. However, the validity of those canons in defining beauty has been called into question.

In a study of 153 North American Caucasian young adults, Farkas et al. demonstrated a large variability in size of features in faces considered normal. The two canons found to be valid most often were horizontal proportions that were valid in only 37%–40% of the tested population, indicating that the neoclassical canons were not representative of average facial proportions in this population.[11] Similarly, the neoclassical canons were found to be invalid in a study of Greek young adults[12] and young White Brazilians.[13] Several studies have found that the neoclassical canons are even less valid in other racial and ethnic groups (Fig. 16.2).[8,14–24]

In a study comparing the validity of neoclassical canons in African American and Caucasian young adults, Farkas et al. found that 24.8% of the canons were valid in Caucasian individuals, while only 3.5% were valid in African American individuals.[14] Similarly, in an anthropometric study of African American male faces, Porter found that only 12% of the 109 subjects fit the neoclassical proportions.[15] Other studies have found significant divergence between the neoclassical canons and typical facial proportions in Nigerian,[16] Arabian,[17] Turkish,[18] and Asian[8,20–23] subjects. Within racial groups, anthropometric differences also exist between geographic locations.[21–23] Thus, the neoclassical canons should be considered rudimentary, and not representative of the complexity that comprises ethnic diversity.[9]

The need to establish anthropometric norms for various populations has been recognized in order to treat congenital or posttraumatic disfigurements successfully.[19] A comparative study of Asian and White patients with Crouzon's syndrome found that Asian Crouzon patients developed a more narrowed cranial base angle on the intracranial side of the basicranium, while White Crouzon patients developed more separated lateral pterygoids and increased angle of the sphenoid wing. Because the anterior skull base tends to be shorter in normal Asian patients than in normal White patients, the deformity in Asian Crouzon patients was not found to be as

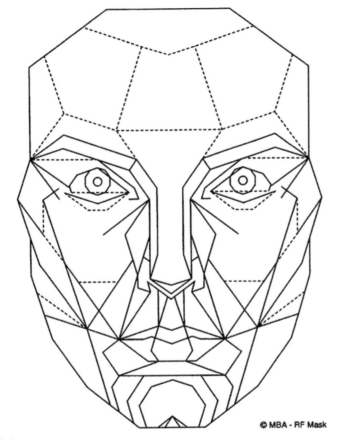

© MBA - RF Mask

FIGURE 16.1

Phi mask. The phi ratio (1:1.618) is seen repeatedly in beautiful things in nature such as the design of the snail shell and DNA. This ratio is used to create phi elements including the phi decagon. A series of phi decagons are used to construct the phi mask, a representation of the ideal relationship of facial features.

Source: Sturm-O'Brien A.K., Brissett A.E., Brissett A.E. Ethnic trends in facial plastic surgery. Facial Plast Surg. May 2010;26(2):69–74. https://doi.org/10.1055/s-0030-1253496. Phi mask used courtesy of Dr. Stephen R. Marquardt; www.beautyanalysis.com.

severe in comparison to controls matched for race, gender, and age. Therefore, the authors recommended individualization in surgical planning for patients with Crouzon syndrome.[25]

As the US becomes more diverse through immigration and interracial marriage, traditional stereotypes of beauty have become less applicable as new, uniquely beautiful facial proportions have emerged.[5] These demographic changes require facial plastic reconstructive surgeons to not only be familiar with diverse anthropometric norms, but more importantly to assess each patient's individual goals and anatomic

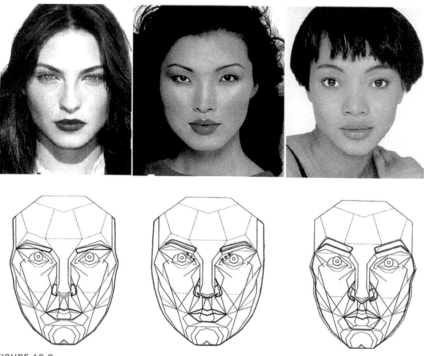

FIGURE 16.2

Ethnic variations of the phi mask. The phi mask, created from the phi ratio, represents the ideal relationship of facial features. Adjustments were made to the original mask to more accurately represent the Caucasian, Asian, and African faces.

Source: Sturm-O'Brien A.K., Brissett A.E., Brissett A.E. Ethnic trends in facial plastic surgery. Facial Plast Surg. May 2010;26(2):69–74. https://doi.org/10.1055/s-0030-1253496. Variations of phi mask used courtesy of Dr. Stephen R. Marquardt; www.beautyanalysis.com.

limitations rather than simply aspiring to achieve neoclassical proportions.[5,7,9,26] This is particularly important as more ethnic and racial minority individuals request cosmetic procedures.[6,27–29]

Care for congenital craniofacial anomalies
Cleft lip and palate

Poverty, lack of private insurance, residing in rural areas, and being non-White have long been recognized as barriers to care, particularly specialty care, for children in the US.[30–34] Orofacial clefting (OFC) is one of the most common birth defects and requires protracted care including several surgical procedures and other interventions by a multidisciplinary team of specialists (Fig. 16.3). Habilitation of

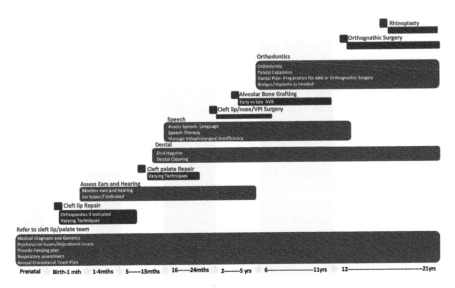

FIGURE 16.3

Longitudinal, multidisciplinary treatment required for comprehensive cleft care.

Reference Wolfswinkel EM, Howell AC, MacDonald B, Wilson JP, Howell LK. American Indian and Alaska native accessibility to comprehensive cleft lip and palate treatment. Cleft Palate Craniofac J. May 31, 2022: 10556656221104942. https://doi.org/10.1177/10556656221104942.

individuals with clefts requires significant financial and social resources.[35,36] Several studies have documented how sociodemographic factors impact the care of patients with clefts.

Delays in cleft repair. Several studies have demonstrated disparate delays in repair of OFC, which can negatively impact feeding, speech, and hearing. These problems can subsequently have long-term impacts on educational attainment and employment.[37] Increasing mean neighborhood income is positively correlated with nutritional status in patients with OFC independent of race.[37] A study using the Pediatric Health Information System, a national database of pediatric hospitals, demonstrated that age at palate repair was significantly delayed for patients who were publicly insured, of non-White race or ethnicity, and who had a diagnosis of cleft lip in addition to cleft palate.[38] In a study of Medicaid enrollees with OFC in North Carolina, children of Black mothers were 70% less likely and children of Hispanic mothers were 14% less likely to have timely cleft repair than children of White mothers.[39] Similarly, a single-institution retrospective study revealed that having Spanish as a primary language and having government insurance was associated with delay in cleft surgery.[40]

A study using the National Surgical Quality Improvement Program Pediatric (NSQIP-P) database of the American College of Surgeons confirmed that non-White patients underwent cleft repair at later ages than White patients. Asian patients were found to have the highest rates of delayed surgery due to the higher rate of international adoption of Asian children. Black patients had the highest rates of comorbidities and cardiopulmonary risk factors. The authors argued that public insurance, difficulties navigating the healthcare system, language barriers, and unmet childcare needs could be contributors to these disparities.[41]

In a retrospective study of a single institution's experience primarily serving an urban population, Zaluzec et al. found delays in cleft lip repair in patients whose parents were not native English speakers; this study excluded adopted children.[42] A study using the Health Care Cost and Utilization Project Kid's Inpatient Database (KID) also found that non-White children with cleft palate were repaired later than their White counterparts. Children from affluent families underwent repair earlier than children from poor backgrounds.[43]

Accessibility of OFC care. Cassell et al. demonstrated that North Carolina children living adjacent to small metropolitan or micropolitan areas were 77% less likely to undergo timely cleft repair than children living in large metropolitan areas.[39] Similarly, Harb et al. demonstrated that children in the Midwest underwent repair later than children in other regions, which the authors attribute to lack of easy accessibility to cleft centers.[43]

A cross-sectional study used Geographic Information Systems to overlay the locations of American Cleft Palate-Craniofacial Association-accredited centers (ACPA centers) along with census data to approximate the population distribution of American Indian/Alaska Native (AI/AN) communities. Resultant mapping showed geographic isolation between AI/AN populations and ACPA centers (Fig. 16.4), though these communities have the highest incidence of OFC. Two states with large AI/AN populations (North Dakota and Wyoming) had no ACPA centers. Only 41.7% of the ACPA centers located on AI/AN land had craniofacial fellowship-trained surgeons as compared to 78.9% of ACPA centers nationally.[44]

Complications after cleft repair. Mullen et al. demonstrated that Black and Hispanic patients were 80% more likely to be readmitted after cleft lip repair. Hispanic patients had the highest rate of requiring nutritional support after cleft palate repair.[41] Another study using the KID confirmed that non-White children had more complications and longer length of stay after cleft palate repair than White children. Increased patient age at the time of surgery, Charlson Comorbidity Index, payer, and income quartile were associated with increases in complications. The authors recommended earlier referral of minority patients for surgical repair and increased diversity among craniofacial surgeons to reduce disparities.[45]

Care following primary cleft repair. A retrospective study from the University of Michigan revealed that factors associated with missed appointments by patients with clefts included Black race, Medicaid insurance, receiving need-based financial assistance for travel, and being from an unstable social background. Having a religious affiliation resulted in keeping more appointments, perhaps pointing to the social support afforded by faith communities (Fig. 16.5). The authors recommended proactive social work resources for individuals at risk for missed appointments,

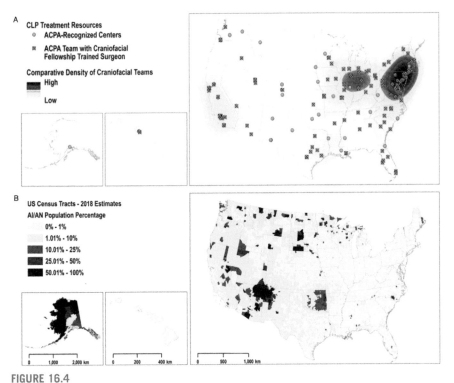

FIGURE 16.4

(A) American Cleft Palate-Craniofacial Association-recognized cleft care teams, both with and without craniofacial-trained surgeons are mapped demonstrating low to high density. (B) Those that identified as American Indians and Alaska Natives in the US census tract 2018 data were mapped by population percentage.

Reference Wolfswinkel EM, Howell AC, MacDonald B, Wilson JP, Howell LK. American Indian and Alaska native accessibility to comprehensive cleft lip and palate treatment. Cleft Palate Craniofac J. May 31, 2022: 10556656221104942. https://doi.org/10.1177/10556656221104942.

and "cleft care super days" in which patients see multiple providers in a single visit, lessening the need for parents to travel and miss work.[36]

A multiinstitutional, prospective study assessing rates of completion of secondary surgery after primary cleft repair revealed that families of children with nonprivate insurance were more likely to postpone recommended surgeries. Hispanic/Latino and Asian children had fewer recommended surgeries as compared to White children.[46] Similarly, a study of attrition rates in patients with OFC and nonsyndromic single-suture craniosynostosis found that underrepresented minorities in the cleft group were more likely to be lost to follow-up. In this study, socioeconomic status, insurance status, and distance traveled to clinic did not appear to correlate with attrition.[47]

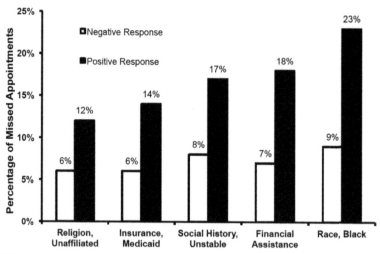

FIGURE 16.5

Significant impact of religion, insurance, social history, financial history, and race on percentage of missed appointments. The overall average rate of missed appointments was 9.6%.

Reference Lynn JV, Ranganathan K, Bageris MH, Hart-Johnson T, Buchman SR, Blackwood RA. Sociodemographic predictors of missed appointments among patients with cleft lip and palate. Cleft Palate Craniofac J. November 2018; 55(10):1440–1446. https://doi.org/10.1177/1055665618764739.

Orthodontic treatment and maxillary expansion. Currently, there is no federal mandate for orthodontic treatment of patients with congenital craniofacial anomalies, and a minority of states have such mandates.[48] Cost, frequent clinic appointments, challenging anatomy, and appliance positioning have been identified as significant barriers for cleft patients with public insurance who would benefit from nasoalveolar molding (NAM). NAM was developed to decrease cleft size and improve nasal symmetry, thus allowing for fewer reconstructive surgeries and a better aesthetic outcome.[49,50]

In a retrospective case-control study, Esmonde et al. identified female sex, bilateral clefting, travel distance, and public-payer insurance as predictors of nonadherence to NAM.[49] Another retrospective cohort study demonstrated that having private insurance was positively correlated with pursuit of NAM, while greater than 90-mile driving distance to the cleft center and Asian race were negatively associated with pursuit of NAM. The treating surgeon also affected the caregivers' decisions to pursue NAM, indicating that surgeons' biases may impact the approach used to discuss treatment options.[50]

Alveolar bone grafting (ABG) is a time-sensitive procedure completed between the ages of 8 and 12 years. ABG repairs the cleft maxillary arch, preventing tooth loss, providing a bony scaffold for dental implants, closing the vestibular and palatal oronasal fistulae, and improving nasal symmetry by providing a base for the nasal ala on the cleft side.[51] Typically, orthodontic treatment and maxillary expansion precede ABG.

Silvestre et al. demonstrated delays in ABG surgeries in African American and Hispanic children in their center. In this study, insurance status did not affect the timing of ABG.[52] Another study using the NSQIP database revealed that race and ethnicity had significant influences on timing of ABG, with African American and Hispanic patients receiving late ABG at the highest rates (29.3% and 24.4%, respectively). Asian patients had the highest rates of receiving ABG at the recommended ages (80.9%), while White patients had the highest rates of early ABG (5.4%). The authors recognized the need to identify individual, cultural, and structural barriers to timely cleft management, and the need to provide families with resources.[53]

Another retrospective study demonstrated that 67% of White and Asian patients received recommended management of the cleft alveolus (ABG or medically appropriate delay) as compared to 35% of underrepresented minority (African American, Hispanic, and Native American) patients. Reasons for delayed ABG included noncompliance (including loss to follow-up) or refusal (63%), comorbidity or medical complexity (13%), orthodontic unpreparedness (13%), and inaccurate assessment of alveolar insufficiency (13%). Reasons for lack of ABG included noncompliance or refusal (7%), comorbidity or medical complexity (2%), and orthodontic unpreparedness (2%). Families with private insurance or the ability to pay out of pocket had ABG at a significantly higher rate than families with Medicaid. The authors realized that most cases of ABG delay or absence were due to loss to follow-up, and recommended better familial educational strategies and minimization of caretaker burden to improve adherence to treatment recommendations.[51]

Badiee et al. confirmed disparities in timing of ABG in their single-institution, retrospective study. In this study, yearly income below $50,000 and non-White race were predictors of older age at ABG. Female patients and those with private insurance were more likely to undergo dental implantation. Measures recommended to improve oral habilitation for underserved children included enlisting the aid of social workers and care navigators; rescheduling missed visits in a timely fashion; using telehealth in order to minimize missed days of work and school, as well as travel costs; improving insurance coverage of orthodontic treatment; seeking philanthropic coverage of dental implants; and encouraging providers to examine their practice patterns in order to identify implicit biases.[54]

Quality of life. Children with OFC have lower Oral Health-Related Quality of Life (OHRQoL) scores than children without clefts. A multi-institutional study using the Child Oral Health Impact Profile (COHIP) compared OHRQoL between White and ethnic minority youths with clefts. The COHIP domains include oral health (specific oral health symptoms), functional wellbeing (ability to carry out tasks such as eating), emotional wellbeing (peer interactions and mood), school tasks, and self-esteem. The study found that Black, Latino, and mixed ethnicity youths with clefts had significantly lower scores than their White and Asian counterparts. Individuals without private insurance had lower scores than those with private insurance. The authors suggest that these differences may be related to restrictive healthcare coverage (e.g., coverage for scar revision, revision rhinoplasty, implants, and orthodontic care) for patients receiving public assistance. They identified the need for longitudinal investigations of patient-oriented outcomes to measure treatment effectiveness to influence health policy.[35]

Medical missions. In a transparent assessment of the impact of medical missions to low- and middle-income countries sponsored by the American Academy of Facial Plastic and Reconstructive Surgery (AAFPRS) Face to Face program, Rousso et al. identified disparities between patients treated on mission trips in comparison to those in higher income countries. Patients undergoing primary cleft lip and/or palate repair during the mission trips were significantly older than what is recommended in the literature. Care was preferentially given to younger patients with unrepaired clefts, and patients with palatal fistulas were more likely to return for follow-up visits. These data demonstrate the need for standardized postoperative visits by mission teams as well as additional resource allocation.[55]

Craniosynostosis

Craniosynostosis is defined as premature fusion of the cranial sutures, which can lead to increased intracranial pressure and neurocognitive decline. It affects 0.03%−0.06% of live births and surgical intervention is recommended within the first year of life to prevent increased intracranial pressure and associated cognitive impairment.[56] Studies using the KID determined that White patients were admitted at much earlier ages than Black and Hispanic patients. Hispanic and Black patients were more likely to have public medical assistance and to receive surgery past the recommended optimum age for surgical intervention.[56,57] Black and Hispanic patients also had longer lengths of stay.[56] One proposed consideration for the delay in care is that postoperative molding helmets used in younger children undergoing minimally invasive craniosynostosis repair are not covered by Medicaid. This limitation may necessitate that children with Medicaid undergo open cranial vault remodeling techniques. Having two or more chronic conditions was also predictive of delayed surgery.[57] Black patients were more likely to be admitted under urgent or emergent circumstances.[56] A retrospective, single-institution study of children with craniosynostosis identified a correlation with greater age at initial consultation, but not with time to surgery for African American patients compared to White patients.[58]

Orthognathic surgery

Orthognathic surgery may be performed for treatment of obstructive sleep apnea (OSA), malocclusion, or for correction of congenital anomalies including OFC and craniosynostosis. A study utilizing the KID revealed that White patients were more likely to receive orthognathic surgery for malocclusion than non-White patients. Non-White patients were more likely to be treated for OSA and congenital anomalies. Compared to White patients, Hispanic patients were more likely to have complications after having surgery for OSA and malocclusion. Hospital length of stay was increased in non-White patients. The authors attributed the increased length of stay in minority patients to increased care complexity likely related to lower use of preoperative dental and orthodontic care.[59]

Facial trauma
Pediatric

While rare in children, traumatic injuries account for significant morbidity and mortality. Among adults and children, there are differences in the craniofacial structure that are responsible for variations in the rate, severity, and location of facial fractures. Studies have shown that facial trauma distribution, causality, and management may be impacted by factors such as race, socioeconomic status, sex, and insurance status.[60,61]

In a retrospective study aimed at identifying the presence of differences in facial laceration care, Amanullah et al. found that those with private insurance were more likely to receive specialist care and procedural sedation than those with public insurance. It was also noted that patients with public insurance were routinely classified as low acuity cases while patients with private insurance carriers were regularly classified at a higher medical acuity level. According to the authors, the reason for these disparities is that parents of children covered by public insurance are less likely to seek specialty treatment for facial lacerations due to insufficient medical knowledge and possible bias on the part of healthcare providers.[62]

Disparities in pediatric facial trauma care can also be seen in the setting of long-term management. A study utilizing the KID found that children from low-income households, females, Medicaid recipients, and those treated at either metropolitan, government, or teaching hospitals were more likely to have increased lengths of stay. Medicaid patients were also found to receive higher overall hospital charges compared to those with private insurance.[63]

Another study using data from the KID found that after the passage of the Affordable Care Act, more pediatric patients who were female, in the bottom quartile of household income, on Medicaid, and identified as either African American, Hispanic, or Asian race or ethnicity began receiving inpatient management for their fractures (Fig. 16.6). The study also found that after the passage of this act, patients' race became less of a contributing factor to mortality. Authors argued that these findings directly show a reduction in racial disparities in both management and outcomes following targeted policy change.[64]

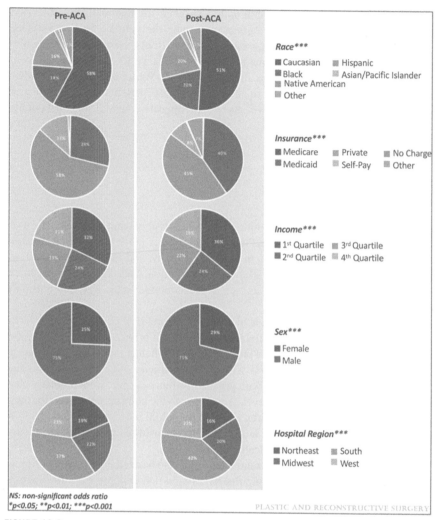

FIGURE 16.6

Patient and hospital characteristics before and after implementation of the Affordable Care Act, including bivariate analysis.

Reference Jenny HE, Yesantharao P, Redett RJ, Yang R. National trends in pediatric facial fractures: the impact of health care policy. Plast Reconstr Surg. February 1, 2021; 147(2):432–441. https://doi.org/10.1097/PRS.0000000000007537.

Adult

A significant portion of hospital admissions are due to facial injuries, with over 3 million being admitted annually. Race, insurance, gender, and geographic location all play a role in the frequency, management, and outcomes of these injuries.[65–67]

An analysis of the National Trauma Data Bank (NTDB) revealed racial disparities in facial trauma mechanisms. It was found that non-White patients had higher rates of facial injuries due to assault, while White patients were more likely to be injured via accidents or falls. In addition, factors such as being female, non-White, and uninsured were all independently associated with a decreased likelihood of early facial fracture repair. The authors argue that a portion of the disparities in care are related to pervasive racial, sex, and socio-economic intrinsic biases of the healthcare system.[68]

A similar trend can be seen in the study by Cohn et al. that also utilized patient data from the NTDB. In this analysis, it was found that urban facial trauma patients were more likely to be African American or Hispanic, have injuries involving the mandible or orbit, and to be assaulted at unknown locations by unknown attackers. The urban population was also more likely to have Medicaid insurance and less likely to have private insurance than those in the NTDB. Moreover, neighborhoods with higher maxillofacial trauma incidences were located near trauma centers, where poverty rates were high, which indicated a direct correlation between poverty and assault.[69]

It is also important to consider how insurance status affects the long-term treatment of facial trauma. A cross-sectional study comparing craniomaxillofacial (CMF) trauma coverage between Medicaid and private insurance policies found that those with private insurance were more likely to be covered for surgical, medical, and psychosocial services following traumatic facial injuries. It was noted that these disparities are due to state demographic conditions and geopolitical factors. The authors argue that physicians, medical systems, insurers, and legislators should collaborate to provide the long-term care needed after traumatic CMF injuries.[70] Fazzalari et al. found that while Medicare and non-Medicare patients received equal care in the acute setting, there were notable differences in long-term care. Medicare patients were more likely to be discharged home, while non-Medicare patients were more likely to be discharged to rehabilitation or skilled nursing facilities.[71]

Laryngectomy reconstructive outcomes

A retrospective cohort analysis of risk factors associated with development of pharyngocutaneous fistulas after total laryngectomy found that female sex and Hispanic ethnicity were significantly associated with fistula formation regardless of the reconstructive method. The study used the NSQIP database, and controlled for factors such as perioperative blood transfusion, wound classification, and associated neck dissection. Non-White patients comprising Asian, AI/AN, and Native Hawaiian/Pacific Islander races were more likely to have a regional flap closure of the laryngectomy defect instead of primary closure when compared to other racial and ethnic groups. Hispanic patients were more likely to undergo primary closure, and less likely to undergo free tissue transfer than other ethnic and racial groups. Women were more likely to undergo free tissue transfer than regional flap closure. While the study could not control for preoperative radiation therapy, the authors recommended that female laryngectomy candidates be offered vascularized closure and be screened for hypothyroidism given their increased odds of wound break down. Because Hispanics constituted only 6% of the study cohort, the authors could not draw conclusions about the increased rate of wound-related complications, and recommended future studies regarding wound healing complications in this population.[72]

Rhinoplasty outcomes

Black patients and those with lower socioeconomic status have higher odds of readmission after major surgery.[73,74] Similarly, a retrospective cohort analysis using data from the Healthcare Cost and Utilization Project revealed that Black patients, those with Medicaid or Medicare, those with conchal cartilage grafting, and those with a greater number of medical comorbidities were more likely to revisit the hospital (usually the emergency room) after undergoing septorhinoplasty. Because hospital revisit rates in this study did not correlate with the Current Procedural Terminology codes and therefore the complexity of surgery (tip rhinoplasty, osteotomies, etc.), the authors concluded that preoperative risk factors were the determinants of revisit rates.[75] Another retrospective comparative study of patients privately insured and those with Medicaid at one institution found that Medicaid patients had greater improvement in Nasal Obstruction Symptom Evaluation scores following functional rhinoplasty than privately insured patients.[76]

Patient educational resources

An increasing number of patients are accessing online health information for facial plastic surgery procedures.[27,77–79] While accessing online health information can facilitate information exchange during appointments and encourage patient participation in their care, not all online health information is accurate, comprehensible, or culturally appropriate. Well-informed consumers have been shown to have better outcomes.[27,77] Limited health literacy and English language proficiency can create significant barriers to comprehension.[27]

The 2006 National Assessment of Adult Literacy revealed that only 12% of US adults have a proficient health literacy level. The survey also revealed that older adults, ethnic and racial minorities, patients with Medicaid, patients who have not completed high school, and those for whom English is a second language are more likely to have lower health literacy.[80] Despite this, several studies demonstrate that online patient information regarding facial plastic surgery procedures is generally written at a ninth grade reading level or higher.[27,77,81,82] Suggested measures to make online medical communications more accessible include simplification of vocabulary and syntax, use of short sentences, elimination of medical jargon, use of simple definitions for potentially confusing terms, and complementary use of multimedia and visual aids, as well as providing patients with a list of specific questions to ask a provider.[27,77]

Cultural insensitivity in educational resources has also been identified as an impediment to patient engagement. A study of cosmetic surgery websites geared toward Spanish speakers found that these websites were difficult to encounter, and only 36% met or exceeded cultural sensitivity thresholds. Multiple websites were poorly translated, and no website included images aligned with the targeted demographic. Moreover, most materials emphasized procedural benefits, and either minimized or omitted risks.[27] Another study of online marketing of academic plastic surgery practices found significantly lower representation of non-White skin in comparison to census demographics. The authors suggest that lack of targeted advertising to non-White patients may subconsciously deter them from pursuing some surgical options.[83]

The facial plastic reconstructive surgery workforce

Though most medical students are now women, the proportion of women entering surgical specialties remains lower than those entering nonsurgical specialties. As of 2017, women made up only 7.8% of the AAFPRS membership. A cross-sectional survey of AAFPRS members revealed that posttraining, men were more likely to hold leadership positions though women were more likely to aspire to leadership positions. Women were more likely to feel that their gender limited their career advancement.[84]

Similarly, a cross-sectional survey of members of the American Society of Craniofacial Surgeons, the American Society of Maxillofacial Surgeons, and the International Society of Craniofacial Surgery demonstrated that more women have entered this subspecialty since 2012. US craniofacial surgeons reported more racial and sexual orientation—based discrimination than international craniofacial surgeons. Female craniofacial surgeons reported more personal discrimination encounters and reported earlier planned retirement than their male counterparts. The survey found that craniofacial surgery was less racially and ethnically diverse than plastic surgery as a whole.[85]

Another recent study contacted craniofacial fellowship programs listed in the American Society of Craniofacial Surgeons fellowship directory to identify graduates from the past 15 years and used an internet search where information was not available. Surgeon profiles and literature databases were used to obtain practice demographics and publications. This study confirmed that more women are graduating from craniofacial fellowships but continue to be a minority. There was no difference in the numbers of leadership roles between male and female craniofacial surgeons, though men had more publications than women in the field.[86]

Conclusion

While the FPRS health disparities literature is nascent, the current literature reveals disparities across the lifespan. As the population becomes more diverse, there is a need to broaden our understanding of aesthetic norms and ethnic facial proportions. There is also a need to investigate possible disparities in postablative reconstruction and cosmetic facial plastic surgery. Disparities in CMF surgery are better documented, and to a large extent are attributable to socioeconomic and geopolitical factors, which present opportunities for advocacy on the part of healthcare professionals. Factors such as physician bias, and patient beliefs, perceptions, and preferences may also play a role in perpetuating these disparities and require exploration. There is a need for educational resources that are culturally appropriate and accessible. Moreover, there is a need for increased diversity in the FPRS workforce to help eliminate disparities.

References

1. Collyer TA, Smith KE. An atlas of health inequalities and health disparities research: "How is this all getting done in silos, and why?" *Soc Sci Med.* November 2020;264: 113330. https://doi.org/10.1016/j.socscimed.2020.113330.
2. Baxter NB, Howard JC, Chung KC. A systematic review of health disparities research in plastic surgery. *Plast Reconstr Surg.* March 1, 2021;147(3):529–537. https://doi.org/10.1097/PRS.0000000000007682.
3. Urban MJ, Shimomura A, Shah S, Losenegger T, Westrick J, Jagasia AA. Rural otolaryngology care disparities: a scoping review. *Otolaryngol Head Neck Surg.* June 2022; 166(6):1219–1227. https://doi.org/10.1177/01945998211068822.
4. Nellis JC, Ishii M, Bater KL, et al. Association of rhinoplasty with perceived attractiveness, success, and overall health. *JAMA Facial Plast Surg.* March 1, 2018;20(2):97–102. https://doi.org/10.1001/jamafacial.2017.1453.
5. Hicks KE, Thomas JR. The changing face of beauty: a global assessment of facial beauty. *Otolaryngol Clin North Am.* April 2020;53(2):185–194. https://doi.org/10.1016/j.otc.2019.12.005.
6. Sturm-O'Brien AK, Brissett AE, Brissett AE. Ethnic trends in facial plastic surgery. *Facial Plast Surg.* May 2010;26(2):69–74. https://doi.org/10.1055/s-0030-1253496.
7. Bueller H. Ideal facial relationships and goals. *Facial Plast Surg.* October 2018;34(5): 458–465. https://doi.org/10.1055/s-0038-1669401.
8. Husein OF, Sepehr A, Garg R, et al. Anthropometric and aesthetic analysis of the Indian American woman's face. *J Plast Reconstr Aesthetic Surg.* November 2010;63(11): 1825–1831. https://doi.org/10.1016/j.bjps.2009.10.032.
9. Saad A, Hewett S, Nolte M, Delaunay F, Saad M, Cohen SR. Ethnic rhinoplasty in female patients: the neoclassical canons revisited. *Aesthetic Plast Surg.* April 2018;42(2): 565–576. https://doi.org/10.1007/s00266-017-1051-4.
10. Darrach H, Ishii LE, Liao D, et al. Assessment of the influence of "Other-Race Effect" on visual attention and perception of attractiveness before and after rhinoplasty. *JAMA*

Facial Plast Surg. March 1, 2019;21(2):96−102. https://doi.org/10.1001/jamafacial. 2018.1697.

11. Farkas LG, Hreczko TA, Kolar JC, Munro IR. Vertical and horizontal proportions of the face in young adult North American Caucasians: revision of neoclassical canons. *Plast Reconstr Surg*. March 1985;75(3):328−338. https://doi.org/10.1097/00006534-198503000-00005.

12. Zacharopoulos GV, Manios A, De Bree E, et al. Neoclassical facial canons in young adults. *J Craniofac Surg*. November 2012;23(6):1693−1698. https://doi.org/10.1097/SCS.0b013e31826b816b.

13. Gonzales PS, Machado CEP, Michel-Crosato E. Analysis of neoclassical facial canons for Brazilian white young adults and comparison with North American Caucasian population. *J Craniofac Surg*. July−August 2020;31(5):e432−e435. https://doi.org/10.1097/SCS.0000000000006339.

14. Farkas LG, Forrest CR, Litsas L. Revision of neoclassical facial canons in young adult Afro-Americans. *Aesthetic Plast Surg*. May−June 2000;24(3):179−184. https://doi.org/10.1007/s002660010029.

15. Porter JP. The average African American male face: an anthropometric analysis. *Arch Facial Plast Surg*. March−April 2004;6(2):78−81. https://doi.org/10.1001/archfaci. 6.2.78.

16. Olusanya AA, Aladelusi TO, Adedokun B. Anthropometric analysis of the Nigerian face: any conformity to the neoclassical canons? *J Craniofac Surg*. October 2018; 29(7):1978−1982. https://doi.org/10.1097/SCS.0000000000004831.

17. Al-Sebaei MO. The validity of three neo-classical facial canons in young adults originating from the Arabian Peninsula. *Head Face Med*. March 13, 2015;11:4. https://doi.org/10.1186/s13005-015-0064-y.

18. Borman H, Ozgur F, Gursu G. Evaluation of soft-tissue morphology of the face in 1,050 young adults. *Ann Plast Surg*. March 1999;42(3):280−288. https://doi.org/10.1097/00000637-199903000-00009.

19. Farkas LG, Katic MJ, Forrest CR, et al. International anthropometric study of facial morphology in various ethnic groups/races. *J Craniofac Surg*. July 2005;16(4): 615−646. https://doi.org/10.1097/01.scs.0000171847.58031.9e.

20. Le TT, Farkas LG, Ngim RC, Levin LS, Forrest CR. Proportionality in Asian and North American Caucasian faces using neoclassical facial canons as criteria. *Aesthetic Plast Surg*. January−February 2002;26(1):64−69. https://doi.org/10.1007/s00266-001-0033-7.

21. Choe KS, Sclafani AP, Litner JA, Yu GP, Romo 3rd T. The Korean American woman's face: anthropometric measurements and quantitative analysis of facial aesthetics. *Arch Facial Plast Surg*. Jul-Aug 2004;6(4):244−252. https://doi.org/10.1001/archfaci.6.4.244.

22. Zhao Q, Zhou R, Zhang X, et al. Morphological quantitative criteria and aesthetic evaluation of eight female Han face types. *Aesthetic Plast Surg*. April 2013;37(2):445−453. https://doi.org/10.1007/s00266-013-0081-9.

23. Wang D, Qian G, Zhang M, Farkas LG. Differences in horizontal, neoclassical facial canons in Chinese (Han) and North American Caucasian populations. *Aesthetic Plast Surg*. July−August 1997;21(4):265−269. https://doi.org/10.1007/s002669900123.

24. Fang F, Clapham PJ, Chung KC. A systematic review of interethnic variability in facial dimensions. *Plast Reconstr Surg*. February 2011;127(2):874−881. https://doi.org/10.1097/PRS.0b013e318200afdb.

25. Lu X, Forte AJ, Fan F, et al. Racial disparity between Asian and Caucasian Crouzon syndrome in skull morphology. *J Craniofac Surg*. November/December 2020;31(8):2182–2187. https://doi.org/10.1097/SCS.0000000000006741.

26. Miller LE, Kozin ED, Lee LN. Reframing our approach to facial analysis. *Otolaryngol Head Neck Surg*. May 2020;162(5):595–596. https://doi.org/10.1177/0194599820912031.

27. Johnson AR, Bravo MG, Granoff MD, Lee BT. Cultural insensitivity pervasive in Spanish online cosmetic surgery resources: a call to action. *Ann Plast Surg*. April 2019;82(4S Suppl 3):S228–S233. https://doi.org/10.1097/SAP.0000000000001841.

28. Prendergast TI, Ong'uti SK, Ortega G, et al. Differential trends in racial preferences for cosmetic surgery procedures. *Am Surg*. August 2011;77(8):1081–1085.

29. Alotaibi AS. Demographic and cultural differences in the acceptance and pursuit of cosmetic surgery: a systematic literature review. *Plast Reconstr Surg Glob Open*. March 2021;9(3):e3501. https://doi.org/10.1097/GOX.0000000000003501.

30. Wang EC, Choe MC, Meara JG, Koempel JA. Inequality of access to surgical specialty health care: why children with government-funded insurance have less access than those with private insurance in Southern California. *Pediatrics*. November 2004;114(5):e584–e590. https://doi.org/10.1542/peds.2004-0210.

31. Wood DL, Hayward RA, Corey CR, Freeman HE, Shapiro MF. Access to medical care for children and adolescents in the United States. *Pediatrics*. November 1990;86(5):666–673.

32. Boss EF, Benke JR, Tunkel DE, Ishman SL, Bridges JF, Kim JM. Public insurance and timing of polysomnography and surgical care for children with sleep-disordered breathing. *JAMA Otolaryngol Head Neck Surg*. February 2015;141(2):106–111. https://doi.org/10.1001/jamaoto.2014.3085.

33. Bisgaier J, Rhodes KV. Auditing access to specialty care for children with public insurance. *N Engl J Med*. June 16, 2011;364(24):2324–2333. https://doi.org/10.1056/NEJMsa1013285.

34. Winters R, Pou A, Friedlander P. A "medical mission" at home: the needs of rural America in terms of otolaryngology care. *J Rural Health*. Summer 2011;27(3):297–301. https://doi.org/10.1111/j.1748-0361.2010.00343.x.

35. Broder HL, Wilson-Genderson M, Sischo L. Health disparities among children with cleft. *Am J Publ Health*. May 2012;102(5):828–830. https://doi.org/10.2105/AJPH.2012.300654.

36. Lynn JV, Ranganathan K, Bageris MH, Hart-Johnson T, Buchman SR, Blackwood RA. Sociodemographic predictors of missed appointments among patients with cleft lip and palate. *Cleft Palate Craniofac J*. November 2018;55(10):1440–1446. https://doi.org/10.1177/1055665618764739.

37. Taufique ZM, Escher PJ, Gathman TJ, et al. Demographic risk factors for malnutrition in patients with cleft lip and palate. *Laryngoscope*. July 2022;132(7):1482–1486. https://doi.org/10.1002/lary.29899.

38. Abbott MM, Kokorowski PJ, Meara JG. Timeliness of surgical care in children with special health care needs: delayed palate repair for publicly insured and minority children with cleft palate. *J Pediatr Surg*. July 2011;46(7):1319–1324. https://doi.org/10.1016/j.jpedsurg.2010.10.002.

39. Cassell CH, Daniels J, Meyer RE. Timeliness of primary cleft lip/palate surgery. *Cleft Palate Craniofac J*. November 2009;46(6):588–597. https://doi.org/10.1597/08-154.1.

40. Stoneburner J, Munabi NCO, Nagengast ES, et al. Factors associated with delay in cleft surgery at a tertiary children's hospital in a major US metropolitan city. *Cleft Palate Craniofac J.* December 2021;58(12):1508–1516. https://doi.org/10.1177/1055665621989508.

41. Mullen MC, Yan F, Ford ME, Patel KG, Pecha PP. Racial and ethnic disparities in primary cleft lip and cleft palate repair. *Cleft Palate Craniofac J.* December 30, 2021. https://doi.org/10.1177/10556656211069828, 10556656211069828.

42. Zaluzec RM, Rodby KA, Bradford PS, Danielson KK, Patel PK, Rosenberg J. Delay in cleft lip and palate surgical repair: an institutional review on cleft health disparities in an urban population. *J Craniofac Surg.* November–December 2019;30(8):2328–2331. https://doi.org/10.1097/SCS.0000000000005740.

43. Harb JL, Crawford KL, Simmonds JC, Roberts C, Scott AR. Race, income, and the timeliness of cleft palate repair in the United States. *Cureus.* February 18, 2021;13(2): e13414. https://doi.org/10.7759/cureus.13414.

44. Wolfswinkel EM, Howell AC, MacDonald B, Wilson JP, Howell LK. American Indian and Alaska native accessibility to comprehensive cleft lip and palate treatment. *Cleft Palate Craniofac J.* May 31, 2022. https://doi.org/10.1177/10556656221104942, 105566 56221104942.

45. Wu RT, Peck CJ, Shultz BN, Travieso R, Steinbacher DM. Racial disparities in cleft palate repair. *Plast Reconstr Surg.* June 2019;143(6):1738–1745. https://doi.org/10.1097/PRS.0000000000005650.

46. Ruff RR, Crerand CE, Sischo L, et al. Surgical care for school-aged youth with cleft: results from a multicenter, prospective observational study. *Cleft Palate Craniofac J.* January 1, 2018. https://doi.org/10.1177/1055665618765776, 1055665618765776.

47. Cooper DC, Peterson EC, Grellner CG, et al. Cleft and craniofacial multidisciplinary team clinic: a look at attrition rates for patients with complete cleft lip and palate and nonsyndromic single-suture craniosynostosis. *Cleft Palate Craniofac J.* November 2019;56(10):1287–1294. https://doi.org/10.1177/1055665619856245.

48. Pfeifauf KD, Snyder-Warwick A, Skolnick GB, Naidoo SD, Nissen RJ, Patel KB. Primer on state statutory mandates of third-party orthodontic coverage for cleft palate and craniofacial care in the United States. *Cleft Palate Craniofac J.* March 2018;55(3): 466–469. https://doi.org/10.1177/1055665617736765.

49. Esmonde NO, Garfinkle JS, Chen Y, Lambert WE, Kuang AA. Factors associated with adherence to nasoalveolar molding (NAM) by caregivers of infants born with cleft lip and palate. *Cleft Palate Craniofac J.* February 2018;55(2):252–258. https://doi.org/10.1177/1055665617718550.

50. Kimia R, Butler PD, Guajardo I, et al. Sociodemographic factors that influence the choice to pursue nasoalveolar molding: one pediatric hospital's experience. *Cleft Palate Craniofac J.* September 2020;57(9):1069–1077. https://doi.org/10.1177/10556656 20936056.

51. Pfeifauf KD, Cooper DC, Gibson E, et al. Factors contributing to delay or absence of alveolar bone grafting. *Am J Orthod Dentofacial Orthop.* June 2022;161(6):820–828 e1. https://doi.org/10.1016/j.ajodo.2021.01.033.

52. Silvestre J, Basta MN, Fischer JP, Lowe KM, Mayro R, Jackson O. Minority and public insurance status: is there a delay to alveolar bone grafting surgery? *Cleft Palate Craniofac J.* January 2017;54(1):e1–e6. https://doi.org/10.1597/15-173.

53. Patmon D, Carlson A, Girotto J. Racial disparities in the timing of alveolar bone grafting. *Cleft Palate Craniofac J.* April 28, 2022. https://doi.org/10.1177/10556656221097813, 10556656221097813.

54. Badiee RK, Yang SC, Alcon A, Weeks AC, Rosenbluth G, Pomerantz JH. Disparities in timing of alveolar bone grafting and dental reconstruction in patients with clefts. *Cleft Palate Craniofac J.* January 19, 2022. https://doi.org/10.1177/10556656211073049, 10556656211073049.

55. Rousso JJ, Abraham MT, Rozanski C. Analyzing our international facial reconstructive mission work: a review of patients treated by American Academy of facial plastic and reconstructive surgery sanctioned trips. *J Craniofac Surg.* March/April 2019;30(2): 390–394. https://doi.org/10.1097/SCS.0000000000005060.

56. Shweikeh F, Foulad D, Nuno M, Drazin D, Adamo MA. Differences in surgical outcomes for patients with craniosynostosis in the US: impact of socioeconomic variables and race. *J Neurosurg Pediatr.* January 2016;17(1):27–33. https://doi.org/10.3171/2015.4.PEDS14342.

57. Lin Y, Pan IW, Harris DA, Luerssen TG, Lam S. The impact of insurance, race, and ethnicity on age at surgical intervention among children with nonsyndromic craniosynostosis. *J Pediatr.* May 2015;166(5):1289–1296. https://doi.org/10.1016/j.jpeds.2015.02.007.

58. Brown ZD, Bey AK, Bonfield CM, et al. Racial disparities in health care access among pediatric patients with craniosynostosis. *J Neurosurg Pediatr.* September 2016;18(3): 269–274. https://doi.org/10.3171/2016.1.PEDS15593.

59. Peck CJ, Pourtaheri N, Shultz BN, et al. Racial disparities in complications, length of stay, and costs among patients receiving orthognathic surgery in the United States. *J Oral Maxillofac Surg.* February 2021;79(2):441–449. https://doi.org/10.1016/j.joms.2020.09.023.

60. Chan KH, Gao D, Bronsert M, Chevallier KM, Perkins JN. Pediatric facial fractures: demographic determinants influencing clinical outcomes. *Laryngoscope.* February 2016; 126(2):485–490. https://doi.org/10.1002/lary.25457.

61. Owusu JA, Bellile E, Moyer JS, Sidman JD. Patterns of pediatric mandible fractures in the United States. *JAMA Facial Plast Surg.* January–February 2016;18(1):37–41. https://doi.org/10.1001/jamafacial.2015.1456.

62. Amanullah S, Linakis JG, Vivier PM, Clarke-Pearson E, Steele DW. Differences in presentation and management of pediatric facial lacerations by type of health insurance. *West J Emerg Med.* July 2015;16(4):527–534. https://doi.org/10.5811/westjem.2015.4.25009.

63. Vyas RM, Dickinson BP, Wasson KL, Roostaeian J, Bradley JP. Pediatric facial fractures: current national incidence, distribution, and health care resource use. *J Craniofac Surg.* March 2008;19(2):339–349. https://doi.org/10.1097/SCS.0b013e31814fb5e3. discussion 350.

64. Jenny HE, Yesantharao P, Redett RJ, Yang R. National trends in pediatric facial fractures: the impact of health care policy. *Plast Reconstr Surg.* February 1, 2021;147(2):432–441. https://doi.org/10.1097/PRS.0000000000007537.

65. Whipple LA, Kelly T, Aliu O, Roth MZ, Patel A. The crisis of deficiency in emergency coverage for hand and facial trauma: exploring the discrepancy between availability of elective and emergency surgical coverage. *Ann Plast Surg.* October 2017;79(4): 354–358. https://doi.org/10.1097/SAP.0000000000001155.

66. Roden KS, Tong W, Surrusco M, Shockley WW, Van Aalst JA, Hultman CS. Changing characteristics of facial fractures treated at a regional, level 1 trauma center, from 2005 to 2010: an assessment of patient demographics, referral patterns, etiology of injury,

anatomic location, and clinical outcomes. *Ann Plast Surg.* May 2012;68(5):461–466. https://doi.org/10.1097/SAP.0b013e31823b69dd.

67. Smith H, Peek-Asa C, Nesheim D, Nish A, Normandin P, Sahr S. Etiology, diagnosis, and characteristics of facial fracture at a midwestern level I trauma center. *J Trauma Nurs.* January–March 2012;19(1):57–65. https://doi.org/10.1097/JTN.0b013e31823a4c0e.

68. Wasicek PJ, Gebran SG, Ngaage LM, et al. Contemporary characterization of injury patterns, initial management, and disparities in treatment of facial fractures using the national trauma data bank. *J Craniofac Surg.* October 2019;30(7):2052–2056. https://doi.org/10.1097/SCS.0000000000005862.

69. Cohn JE, Smith KC, Licata JJ, et al. Comparing urban maxillofacial trauma patterns to the national trauma data bank(c). *Ann Otol Rhinol Laryngol.* February 2020;129(2):149–156. https://doi.org/10.1177/0003489419878457.

70. Kotha VS, de Ruiter BJ, Nicoleau M, Davidson EH. National disparities in insurance coverage of comprehensive craniomaxillofacial trauma care. *Plast Reconstr Surg Glob Open.* November 2020;8(11):e3237. https://doi.org/10.1097/GOX.0000000000003237.

71. Fazzalari A, Alfego D, Shortsleeve JT, et al. Treatment of facial fractures at a level 1 trauma center: do medicaid and non-medicaid enrollees receive the same care? *J Surg Res.* August 2020;252:183–191. https://doi.org/10.1016/j.jss.2020.03.008.

72. Smith BD, Osazuwa-Peters OL, Cannon TY, Reed WT, Puscas L, Osazuwa-Peters N. Nonsurgical risk factors associated with pharyngocutaneous fistula in patients who have undergone laryngectomy. *JAMA Otolaryngol Head Neck Surg.* November 1, 2021;147(11):966–973. https://doi.org/10.1001/jamaoto.2021.2433.

73. Tsai TC, Orav EJ, Joynt KE. Disparities in surgical 30-day readmission rates for medicare beneficiaries by race and site of care. *Ann Surg.* June 2014;259(6):1086–1090. https://doi.org/10.1097/SLA.0000000000000326.

74. Glance LG, Kellermann AL, Osler TM, Li Y, Li W, Dick AW. Impact of risk adjustment for socioeconomic status on risk-adjusted surgical readmission rates. *Ann Surg.* April 2016;263(4):698–704. https://doi.org/10.1097/SLA.0000000000001363.

75. Spataro E, Branham GH, Kallogjeri D, Piccirillo JF, Desai SC. Thirty-day hospital revisit rates and factors associated with revisits in patients undergoing septorhinoplasty. *JAMA Facial Plast Surg.* December 1, 2016;18(6):420–428. https://doi.org/10.1001/jamafacial.2016.0539.

76. Rozanski C, Gray M, Rousso JJ, Hirsch MB, Rosenberg JD. Disparities in NOSE scores and surgical approaches among patients undergoing functional rhinoplasty. *Facial Plast Surg.* February 2019;35(1):90–95. https://doi.org/10.1055/s-0038-1676051.

77. Chang IA, Wells MW, Zheng DX, et al. A multimetric readability analysis of online patient educational materials for submental fat reduction. *Aesthetic Plast Surg.* April 2022;46(2):712–718. https://doi.org/10.1007/s00266-021-02675-9.

78. Dhanda AK, Leverant E, Leshchuk K, Paskhover B. A google trends analysis of facial plastic surgery interest during the COVID-19 pandemic. *Aesthetic Plast Surg.* August 2020;44(4):1378–1380. https://doi.org/10.1007/s00266-020-01903-y.

79. Eggerstedt M, Urban MJ, Smith RM, Revenaugh PC. Interest in facial cosmetic surgery in the time of COVID-19: a google trends analysis. *Facial Plast Surg Aesthet Med.* September 2021;23(5):397–398. https://doi.org/10.1089/fpsam.2020.0605.

80. Kutner MG E, Jin Y, Paulsen C. *The Health Literacy of America's Adults: Results from the 2003 National Assessment of Adult Literacy (NCES 2006-483).* Education USDo; 2006.

81. Misra P, Agarwal N, Kasabwala K, Hansberry DR, Setzen M, Eloy JA. Readability analysis of healthcare-oriented education resources from the American Academy of Facial Plastic and Reconstructive Surgery. *Laryngoscope.* January 2013;123(1):90–96. https://doi.org/10.1002/lary.23574.

82. Ziai H, Levin M, Roskies M. Readability of internet-based resources for cosmetic facial botulinum toxin injections. *Facial Plast Surg Aesthet Med.* March–April 2021;23(2): 146–147. https://doi.org/10.1089/fpsam.2020.0564.

83. Moss WD, King BW, Memmott S, et al. An evaluation of racial disparities in online marketing of academic plastic surgery practices. *Ann Plast Surg.* April 20, 2022. https:// doi.org/10.1097/SAP.0000000000003212.

84. Lafer MP, Frants A, Zhang Y, Wang B, Lee JW. Gender differences in compensation, mentorship, and work-life balance within facial plastic surgery. *Laryngoscope.* March 2021;131(3):E787–E791. https://doi.org/10.1002/lary.29007.

85. Blum JD, Cho DY, Villavisanis DF, et al. Update: diversity and practice patterns of international craniomaxillofacial surgeons. *J Craniofac Surg.* February 3, 2022. https:// doi.org/10.1097/SCS.0000000000008486.

86. Lala BM, Salvador TM, Wang F, Shah J, Ricci JA. Gender disparities among craniofacial surgeons. *Cleft Palate Craniofac J.* March 29, 2022. https://doi.org/10.1177/ 10556656221089828, 10556656221089828.

Index

Note: 'Page numbers followed by "*f*" indicate figures, "*t*" indicates tables.'

CPI Antony Rowe
Eastbourne, UK
September 26, 2023